T0205892

Pharmaceuticals to Nutraceuticals

A Shift in Disease Prevention

Pharmaceuticals to Nutraceuticals

A Shift in Disease Prevention

Dilip Ghosh

R. B. Smarta

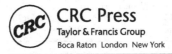

CRC Press
Taylor & Francis Group
Boca Raton London New York

CRC Press is an imprint of the
Taylor & Francis Group, an **informa** business

CRC Press
Taylor & Francis Group
6000 Broken Sound Parkway NW, Suite 300
Boca Raton, FL 33487-2742

First issued in hardback 2019

ISBN 13: 978-1-03-209752-7 (pbk)
ISBN 13: 978-1-4822-6075-5 (hbk)

This book contains information obtained from authentic and highly regarded sources. Reasonable efforts have been made to publish reliable data and information, but the author and publisher cannot assume responsibility for the validity of all materials or the consequences of their use. The authors and publishers have attempted to trace the copyright holders of all material reproduced in this publication and apologize to copyright holders if permission to publish in this form has not been obtained. If any copyright material has not been acknowledged please write and let us know so we may rectify in any future reprint.

Publisher's Note
The publisher has gone to great lengths to ensure the quality of this reprint but points out that some imperfections in the original copies may be apparent.

Library of Congress Cataloging-in-Publication Data

Names: Ghosh, Dilip K., author. | Smarta, R. B., 1944- author.
Title: Pharmaceuticals to nutraceuticals : a shift in disease prevention /
Dilip Ghosh and R. B. Smarta.
Description: Boca Raton : Taylor & Francis/CRC Press, 2017. | Includes
bibliographical references and index.
Identifiers: LCCN 2016015578 | ISBN 9781482260755 (hardback : alk. paper)
Subjects: | MESH: Dietary Supplements--standards | Functional Food--standards
| Pharmaceutical Preparations | Holistic Health
Classification: LCC RM301 | NLM QU 145.5 | DDC 615.1--dc23
LC record available at https://lccn.loc.gov/2016015578

Visit the Taylor & Francis Web site at
http://www.taylorandfrancis.com

and the CRC Press Web site at
http://www.crcpress.com

Contents

SECTION I   Introduction

SECTION II   Quality–Safety–Efficacy: Three Mantras

SECTION III   Marketing and Product Positioning

SECTION IV   Regulatory Perspective

SECTION V   Underpinning Science

SECTION VI   New Journeys through Categorization

SECTION VII   Future Trends

Authors

Dilip Ghosh, PhD, is an international speaker, facilitator, and author. He is professionally associated with Soho Flordis International (SFI) and Western Sydney University, and is an Honorary Ambassador with the Global Harmonization Initiative (GHI), all in Australia.

With more than 20 years of experience in both the pharmaceutical and food and nutrition industries, he is one of the pioneer researchers to assess the health claim opportunities of potential functional food ingredients and complementary medicines through an evaluation of the current scientific evidence–based and related claims, providing commentaries on the gaps in science, including potential requirements for research, such as human studies.

Dr. Ghosh received a PhD in biomedical science from the University of Calcutta, India, along with a BSc (Hons) and MSc in zoology/microbiology and an MPhil in environmental sciences.

Dr. Ghosh has published more than 60 papers in peer-reviewed journals and numerous articles in food and nutrition magazines and books. His recent books, *Biotechnology in Functional Foods and Nutraceuticals, Innovation of Healthy and Functional Foods*, and *Clinical Aspects of Functional Foods and Nutraceuticals,* were all published by CRC Press/Taylor & Francis in 2010, 2012, and 2014, respectively. He is the review editor of *Frontiers in Nutrigenomics* (2011–present), the *American Journal of Advanced Food Science and Technology* (2012–present), the *Journal of Obesity and Metabolic Research* (2013–present), and the *Journal of Bioethics* (2013–present). He was an associate editor and member of *Toxicology Mechanisms and Methods*, Taylor & Francis (2006–2007), and is a columnist for the *World of Nutraceuticals*. Dr. Ghosh is also in executive member and advisor of the Health Foods and Dietary Supplements Association (HADSA).

R. B. Smarta, PhD, has designed management agendas for profitable growth and relevant expansion, launching new concepts, ideas, and projects for national and global clients in pharmaceuticals, nutraceuticals, and wellness. Dr. Smarta has been in the industry for more than four decades and in consulting for a little more than three decades.

He is the founder and managing director of Interlink Marketing Consultancy Pvt. Ltd. In addition to a postgraduate degree in organic chemistry, Dr. Smarta earned an MMS in marketing from the University of Mumbai. He holds a doctorate (PhD) in management from the University of East Georgia, is a Fellow of the Royal Society of Arts and Commerce (FRSA), and is a Certified Management Consultant (CMC). He has added value and created an impact on the performance of a wide variety of clients at national and multinational corporations.

As an advocate of this nascent and essential industry of nutrition and nutraceuticals, Dr. Smarta is assisting in shaping the industry and its agenda with the help of industry leaders, members, and regulatory bodies through India's Health Foods and Dietary Supplements Association as an Honorary Secretary.

Dr. Smarta has penned eight books in the areas of pharma marketing and pharmaceutical business and nutraceuticals. Some of his titles have also been translated into German. He regularly contributes articles to several dailies and industry periodicals. He has produced video-based training packages called *Interact* for corporate trainers to enhance their skills on an ongoing basis. Dr. Smarta is a recipient of many national awards.

Contributor

Rohit Ghosh
School of Medicine
Western Sydney University
Campbeltown, Sydney, Australia

Introduction

The famous aphorism "Let food be thy medicine and medicine be thy food" (reportedly by Hippocrates) can be applied to the emerging area of research at the interface of pharmacology and nutrition. This field is currently experiencing a renewed impetus as several food components are now being employed as medicines, either directly or as prodrugs. Indeed, there are areas in which the border between "food" and "pharma" is not well defined, as the former often contains several bioactive compounds, including secondary plant molecules (polyphenols), fibers, friendly bacteria, essential fatty acids, probiotics, and other contributors. Currently, there are several drugs that are derived from natural products, including those which humans have been exposed to via diet. It is sometimes difficult to distinguish between bioactive molecules termed "drugs" and other substances that are classified as "nutrients."

Optimal health and prevention of chronic diseases can be attained (to a certain extent) by modulating the intake of macro- and micronutrients, often in pharmacological doses as in the case of supplements, nutraceuticals, and functional foods. Classic pharmacotherapy can also be accompanied by adjunct treatments with nutrition-derived remedies that are often able to decrease the doses of medicines or lessen their side effects. In summary, the border between pharma and food is becoming less distinct, and companies are marketing affordable, fast-moving nutraceutical products, with a focus on fortified foods and beverages (Street, 2015).

PARADIGM SHIFT: FROM CURE TO PREVENTION

It is generally accepted by all concerned that modern pharmaceuticals will remain out of reach of many people and "health for all" may only be realized by the use of adequately assessed nutraceutical/phytomedicinal products. Humankind has been using food bioactives or herbal medicine for healing since the beginning of civilization. In recent times, the use of herbal medicine for healthcare has increased steadily around the world, although it was neglected for decades by Western societies. However, serious concerns are being realized regarding the safety, claimed efficacy, and quality of herbal products used as herbal medicines, nutraceuticals, health foods, and cosmetics. The combination therapy of pharmaceuticals and food bioactives in disease prevention and treatment are covered in this book. A few chapters discuss the differences and similarities between foods and drugs in disease prevention and treatment. The main focus of each contribution is considered in this review. The use, including the advantages and drawbacks of combination therapy that employs drugs and foods are elaborated upon as well. A unique example is ezetimibe, which is used together with lifestyle changes (diet, weight loss, exercise) to reduce the amount of cholesterol (a fat-like substance) and other fatty substances in the blood.

CHALLENGES

The nutraceutical market is one of the most promising ones in the world. However, this market is not without its share of challenges. One of the most important fields of focus today is the need to have *evidence-based nutraceuticals*. These are also referred to as the third-generation nutraceuticals. When deriving evidence-based nutra products, it is vital that they be studied scientifically, supported on a clinical level, and contain standardized new ingredients derived from plants, foods, and so on.

The advancement of science has created three fundamental economic problems, namely, managing risk, integration, and learning. One of the most important elements of innovation is *management technology*, which is essential for a science-based business. Recombination and successful integration of the different bodies of knowledge that already exist have the potential to create breakthroughs in evidence-based nutraceutical innovation, such as traditional Chinese and Indian Ayurvedic medicines.

THE TRANSITION OF THE PHARMACEUTICAL INDUSTRY

The transition of the pharmaceutical industry from its traditional business model is ongoing. The next blockbuster molecule could be derived through the R&D intensive identification and testing in large clinical trials followed by extensive marketing (Rusu et al., 2011). It has been proposed (Anscombe et al., 2009) that the industry is challenged with three interrelated tipping points, which include what the industry sells (service models versus therapies), to whom (mass markets versus niche), and how it should organize itself (making connections versus integration).

The innovation model implies minimum changes to the current high-risk, high-margin business model, but the integration model also suggests turning pharmaceutical companies into providers of health outcomes and has been advised to move into less regulated markets such as animal and consumer health (Danner et al., 2010).

DIVERSIFICATION

Companies have started to look for alternatives to the blockbuster philosophy, which is simply, diversification. For example, Pfizer and Merck, being world leaders in consumer healthcare and animal health, are following diversification into their new business arenas. The 2009 acquisitions of Wyeth and Schering-Plough, respectively, have consolidated their market positions. Pfizer Consumer Healthcare is one of the top five over-the-counter (OTC) companies in the world. It sells two of the top ten selling OTC brands worldwide, which accounted for revenues of €2093 million after the acquisition of Wyeth (Pfizer, http://press.pfizer.com/press-release/pfizer-acquire-wyeth-creating-worlds-premier-biopharmaceutical-company, accessed on July 8, 2016). The acquisition has also allowed Pfizer to gain a foothold in the nutraceutical market, whose infant nutritionals have brought revenues of €1410 million for 2010. Pfizer Nutrition is expected to grow worldwide due to the less strictly regulated market and faces competition from other diversifiers as well as the established food industry. A clear trend here is the move into delivering not just treatments, but outcomes. An example of outcome management is the Changing Diabetes program of Novo Nordisk (http://www.novonordisk.com/about-novo-nordisk/changing-diabetes.html), which provides support such as specialized training for healthcare professionals, support for diabetes patient organizations, free blood sugar screening services, and supplying equipment for diabetes clinics.

Geographical diversification is being pursued through the numerous contributions from the world's fastest-growing, emerging markets, such as those in China, India, Brazil, Argentina, Turkey, and Romania. Despite high variations in their characteristics and stability, business in these areas offers important opportunities for growth over time. The most important strategic move is to relocate the expensive R&D activities into a lower-cost country and secure a front position in the largest emerging market through local partnerships.

In conclusion, the most innovative pharmaceutical companies are undergoing a transition from their traditional business models. The industry is attempting to control the direction of this transition by resorting to better pipeline management, mergers, and open innovation. Diversification is pursued by looking at novel scientific, business, and geographical areas.

REFERENCES

Anscombe, J., Wise, M., Cruickshank, C. et al. September 2009. Pharmaceuticals out of balance: Reaching the tipping point. A.T. Kearney, Chicago, IL. http://www.atkearney.com/index.php/Publications/pharmaceuticals-out-of-balance.html. Accessed July 8, 2016.

Danner, S., Hosseini, M., and Rimpler, M. October 2010. Fight or flight. Diversification vs. Rx focus in big pharma's quest for sustained growth. Roland Berger Strategy Consultants, Munich, Germany. http://www.rolandberger.com/expertise/industries/pharmaceuticals/2010-10-25-rbsc-pub-Fight_or_flight.html. Accessed July 8, 2016.

Rusu, A., Kuokkanen, K., and Heier, A. 2011. Current trends in the pharmaceutical industry—A case study approach. *Eur. J. Pharm. Sci.*, 44: 437–440.

Street, A. 2015. Food as pharma: Marketing nutraceuticals to India's rural poor. *Crit. Publ. Health*, 25: 361–372.

Section I

Introduction

1 Redefining Nutraceutical and Functioning Foods as Part of a Journey from Pharma to Nutra

R. B. Smarta

CONTENTS

INTRODUCTION

Achieving and maintaining a competitive advantage in any industry is neither nor has it been an easy task. The pharmaceutical and food sectors have independent as well as related challenges as both are introduced at different stages in a life cycle. The pharma sector is at a maturity stage, while the nutra and food sectors in some countries are still at the growth and infancy stages. Hence, the challenges faced by both sectors need to be examined separately and together as the population has become more sophisticated and demanding, and is expecting more product innovations; legislation also needs to cope with the environment and become more reflective and complex.

The challenges become even greater for the pharmaceutical industry that has been experiencing difficult economic conditions for the past few years and is reaching a point of falling over a patent cliff. Top management teams across the world have had to start concentrating on minimizing costs and identifying alternate revenue models. These efforts have served to only magnify the challenges.

The music and film industries have faced these challenges and they are hard nuts to crack in every sector; they are arguably even harder to crack for businesses in the food and pharmaceutical sectors. Both sectors are dependent on the health of human beings and human life is precious. Companies in these two sectors are governed by extremely rigorous standards of quality, safety, and legislation, especially in the areas of health and hygiene.

Today, the pharmaceutical industry requires total reforms from developing alternate revenue models, to driving a new focus on investments and behavior. To curb all the existing unethical practices, there is a need for better governance and transparency between the regulators and manufacturers.

CONSUMER HEALTH

Legislation and regulations are major concerns for most companies in the food and pharmaceutical sectors. The need to comply with the Food and Drug Administration (FDA), Medicines and Healthcare products Regulatory Agency (MHRA) rules, the National Food Authority (NFA) guidelines of Codex, and other food safety standards regulatory bodies and sanctioning of claims by authorities is essential. Every new product across every part of the process, from intrinsically clean environments to end-of-batch safety and quality, must be evaluated for strict compliance before implementation. This can make the process quite tough.

This is of utmost importance as the decision to buy is made by consumers. They may be influenced and, as they search for options and are in need due to health concerns, may decide to choose without a proper diagnosis. Hence, the onus of quality and safe products and providing consumers with adequate information to make informed decisions is on the industry.

EXISTENCE AND GROWTH OF THE PHARMA SECTOR

Changing market scenarios, steep increases in R&D costs, continuity in patent expirations, increasing healthcare costs, and the disease burden of every country have compelled consumers to reduce healthcare costs. In addition, the educated and health-conscious patients as consumers are moving toward wellness.

The common man today fears sickness, yet lacks the much needed awareness about the healthy habits and health benefits of any product. Thus, he is either influenced to purchase over-the-counter (OTC) products or, on the basis of his experiences, sometimes returns to the traditional medicines as they are often cost-effective and more easily available.

With the changing disease pattern and lifestyle diseases, consumers are shifting toward prevention. The utilities of both medicines and food products inclusive of nutraceutical products today coexist for the complete wellness of a patient/consumer. Usually for chronic diseases, physicians make patients aware of lifestyle changes and advise them to make the necessary changes in their lifestyle and diet.

CHALLENGES FACED BY THE PHARMACEUTICAL SECTOR

Owing to these changes in the disease pattern, consumer education and the ambition of remaining fit, drying up of new product pipelines, and expectations of the industry, patients and consumers, both sectors are going through different challenges:

1. *Patent expiries giving rise to generic medicines*: Over the last few years, many pharmaceutical companies have lost a lot of revenue simply due to one primary reason—the patent cliff, a series of expirations of blockbuster drugs. As a result of patent cliff, a multitude of small pharmaceutical companies have entered the space of mass production of generic versions of major drugs, leading to steep revenue losses for big pharmaceutical companies. The patent cliff is bound to have serious implications on the future of the pharmaceutical industry. With the market being dominated by generics, the pharmaceutical industry will face lack of funding and drive for innovation.

   A change in the development phase, particularly in market segmentation and brand development, is another challenge that pharmaceutical companies will have to face due to the patent cliff. There will be a greater need for pharmaceutical companies to create drugs that are specific and differentiable for patenting purposes and portfolio diversity.

   Apart from the pharmaceutical industry, the current healthcare industry will also experience implications in terms of facing new challenges in coverage, with physicians and hospitals providing adequate care with diminished specialty therapy.

2. *Choosing adaptable and flexible ways of corporate operations*: Having an experience of marketing medicines with higher margins for a niche group of patients with selective and particular diseases, companies will have to change to a model such that they take maximum benefit from the market evolution. Companies have to shift from serving a niche group to a bigger group of patients with not so specific but every kind of disorder or disease. They will have to operate at lower margins and perhaps at lower costs. It is quite a difficult task but Teva, Mylan, and big generic pharma companies have taken up this route, and they are making it clear to the industry that adaptability with changing environment is the choice. The challenge is to change the style of operations and orient management mind-sets to suit the new environment.

3. *Moving away from a product-centric to "patient-centric" approach as a reform*: As times change, pharmaceutical companies should develop

strategies while bearing in mind the patient-pull approach. Also, to gain higher consumption, ideally there should be a shift from R&D and product centricity toward patient centricity.

In developed nations, the emphasis needs to be on quality healthcare for the elderly as these nations have a higher mix of aged population. So, lifestyle or chronic diseases, occurring more often in the population over the age of 60, pose a grave challenge for developed nations.

4. *Need for innovations in research and development*: Higher investment and lesser output are a reality of R&D today. Hence, R&D needs to be revamped using different models to become cost-effective. A consortium is certainly a wise choice all around as it involves pairing of many companies wherein they can put their resources as a consortium and focus on a particular patient-centric goal. This also ensures that there is standardization in the processes. So, a consortium may work in the favor of the companies as these would be a group investment and the produce can be shared among them all. It is a challenge for every player in pharmaceuticals.

Emerging markets are most likely to experience a rise in chronic diseases to a larger extent in comparison to communicable diseases. In the case of developing countries, healthcare systems face a greater burden of communicable diseases. Additionally, if we take a look at the management of health around the world, in most countries this is accomplished by their respective governments, whereas in India it is not the responsibility of the central government but of the state in spite of the former having an annual health budget.

In developed countries like the United States, the United Kingdom, and Japan, a rise in the older population has stunted the growth of pharmaceuticals to as low as 2%–3%, unlike in developing nations. Also, the cost of medication is very high all over the world, with the exception of India. The common man suffers due to changing lifestyles as well as hereditary issues. These issues bring to light the need to stay healthy and fit. More and more people want to look toward alternative cures, that is, moving away from the conventional treatment and ways to prevent occurrence of diseases and disorders.

THE EMERGING ROLE OF NUTRITION ALONG WITH THE PHARMACEUTICAL SECTOR

Amino acids have added to the growth momentum in the pharma prescription market and acted as a growth driver for the past few years. Physicians have welcomed amino acids as an essential ingredient of nutrition.

After careful deliberation, the industry came to realize that amino acids could open up new business opportunities such as nutraceuticals. Thus, it would not be wrong to say that the pharmaceutical industry has adopted a shift towards nutraceuticals to grow and stay in the race to be on the top.

Total parenteral nutrition (TPN) and external nutrition (EN) have been a part of life in hospitals, but now through amino acids, it has become evident that nutrition has an essential role alongside pharma for the benefit of patients.

Taking a step ahead makes it clear that neither nutraceuticals nor pharmaceuticals are separate from each other but they coexist for the betterment of patients and medical consumers.

CHALLENGES FACED BY THE FOOD SECTORS

1. *Chances of self-medication*: The awareness about nutra products is increasing every day. With this hype, more and more people are gaining knowledge about the perceived health benefits these products offer for preventing or treating some major health disorders such as cardiovascular diseases or arthritis. This, however, may have a flipside that is often overlooked. There may be a chance that patients turn to these nutra products in lieu of taking treatment for a certain serious disorder they are experiencing. So, it would certainly be risky if a consumer starts self-medicating for the disorder experienced as he or she may be exposed to the quality issue for that particular nutra product as well, instead of turning to the much needed medical assistance.

2. *Evolving regulatory compliances*: As the field of nutra has many issues, regulations are either evolving or harmonizing all over the world. Globally, the focus is upon having pertinent regulations that are made with guidance for policy makers over high-quality scientific, technical, and regulatory nuances.

3. *Right pricing*: Since these nutrition products are made from natural plant extracts and other such ingredients, they turn out to be quite expensive as the extraction processes are extremely tedious and time-consuming. Hence, issues of pricing have become a major challenge for the nutraceutical and dietary supplement products. In order to get the right pricing, it is a general observation that such products are overpriced for a common man. In emerging or developing countries affordability becomes an important criterion for consumption. So, it is an obvious conclusion that consumers are hesitant to buy overpriced products even though they can actually be beneficial. Nutraceuticals need the right pricing to gain momentum in any market.

4. *Appropriate claims*: Various regulatory bodies in different countries around the world have created their own set of claims that nutraceutical manufacturers need to follow when making health claims on labels and market them in any country. The claims for labeling and marketing are becoming increasingly clear because of the evolving regulations.

    Manufacturers should be careful when marketing their products so they don't make claims that can be misleading and false. This is because over-claiming or wrong claims will lead to their products being vulnerable to legal action by the regulatory bodies concerned.

    Regulatory bodies now place emphasis on the importance of science-based claims that do not mislead the consumer in any way.

Stringent regulations have ensured that health claims are watertight, so manufacturers need to be cautious not to make claims over and above the existing ones for their products when marketing them. Thus, lawsuits could result if the products do not offer any of the health benefits claimed by the label.

5. *Misleading advertising and promotions*: Although it is related to health claims and their promotion to consumers, irresponsible advertising may end up misleading the consumer.

As a consumer, "taste" campaign may increase consumption, but in such products, emphasis is on the science behind the product that needs more exposure. For consumers, safety, quality, and effectiveness are the topmost concerns. There are advertising guidelines and compliances that should be enforced.

NURTURING A DOUBLE-VISION COEXISTENCE MODEL

The present model of nutraceuticals is pharma-driven. It focuses on the cure for diseases or ailments for their customers in the sick care sector. But where the needs and trends in the environment are changing, the focus of the nutraceutical model will have to shift from sick care to healthcare (i.e., preventive and promotional aspects) (Figure 1.1).

In the nutraceuticals domain, there exist peripheral opportunities for chronic lifestyle diseases and ailments prevailing in the sick care sector as well as preventive opportunities in the wellness sector. The pharma-driven model does not address the need for both prevention and promotional aspects.

With the emergence of lifestyle changes and addition of chronic lifestyle diseases and ailments such as obesity, tuberculosis, diabetes, arthritis, malaria, and cholera, diseases can be managed through preventive efforts. Although lifestyle diseases cannot be completely cured, they can be well managed through the nutra medium.

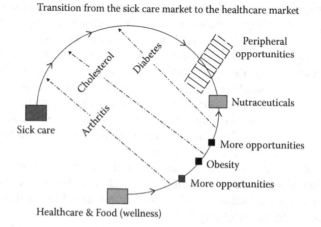

FIGURE 1.1   The conceptual nutraceutical model. (Conceptual model by Dr. R. B. Smarta.)

पथ्ये सति गदार्तस्य किमौषध निषेवणै : ।
पथ्येऽसति गदार्तस्य किमौषध निषेवणै : । । वैदयजीवन – लोलिंबराज

FIGURE 1.2

In a densely populated country like India where lifestyle diseases are catching up in the urban and rural areas, the middle-class population drives the need for conscious preventive and curative disease management rather than just the curative aspects.

There has to be a parallel opportunity between the "needs of the sick care and wellness market" and "opportunities at the peripheral for nutraceuticals." Transition from sick care to healthcare market is the need of the hour for disease management.

Physicians may not really understand nutrition as they are not formally trained. More and more physicians are realizing the need to supplement their medical treatment with a good, balanced diet and nutra products. In most healthcare facilities, focus is given not just to prescribing the right medication but also on offering the right food for quick and effective recovery of patients. This is more often done in the case of patients suffering from cardiovascular disorders. Also, in the case of diabetics, doctors recommend a strict diet along with the prescribed medication. Hospitals and big healthcare centers have dieticians and nutritionists as a part of their team that treat patients so as to create the most ideal environment for patient recovery. Lolimbraj in Vaidyajeeva stated clearly (Figure 1.2):

> In fact for those who follow the right diet where is the need for medicines and for those who do not follow the right diet what is the use of medicines?

Ancient wisdom from Ayurveda puts it wisely. It is now becoming very clear that the aftereffects of a faulty lifestyle and not following the right diet are the origin of many diseases.

MICROBIOME THEORY: THE DYSFUNCTION AND DISORDER RELATIONSHIP

About 100 trillion bacteria of several hundred species dwell in the human body. These microbes help the human body carry out their bodily functions with ease. Microbes reside in the human body or the host, and the host gets many health benefits in lieu of the provided food and shelter.

For instance, in the case of a person experiencing irritable bowel syndrome (IBS), there is an imbalance in the microbiome count. This can simply be treated by the intake of probiotics. Probiotics fall under the nutraceutical space, indicating the rising need for such products to be included in the daily diet.

The idea is to develop good diagnostic tools and combine these with drugs and nutrition. It can be said that the largest drug in a person's repertoire is the food that he or she eats three times a day, every day of their life. Instead of inventing things, one must try to see how they can work with the components—the nutrients—that are in existing food.

THE SHIFT TO INTEGRATED (HOLISTIC) MEDICINES

Integrated medicine is a new paradigm in healthcare that focuses on the synergy and deployment of the best aspects of diverse systems of medicine, including modern medicine, homeopathy, Siddha, Unani, yoga, and naturopathy, in the best interests of patients and the community (Goyal et al., 2011).

The increasing public demand for traditional medicines has led to considerable interest among policy makers, health administrators, and medical doctors regarding the possibilities of bringing together traditional and modern medicine. Traditional medicine looks at health, disease, and causes of diseases in a different way. The integration of traditional medicine with modern medicine may imply the incorporation of traditional medicine into the general health service system. The purpose of integrated medicine is not simply to yield a better understanding of differing practices, but primarily to promote the best care for patients by intelligently selecting the best route to health and wellness.

Surveys and other sources of evidence indicate that traditional medical practices are frequently utilized in the management of chronic diseases. Traditional medicine presents a low-cost alternative for rural and semiurban areas, where modern medicine is inaccessible.

An approach to harmonizing activities between modern and traditional medicine will promote a clearer understanding of the strengths and weaknesses of each and will encourage the provision of the best therapeutic option for patients.

ADVANTAGES OF INTEGRATED MEDICINE

- Provides the widest array of options to patients (one in three adults in the United States uses at least one complementary or alternative medical therapy [CAM])
- Provides an opportunity to combine the best of both conventional medicine and complementary alternative medicine
- Provides cost-effective treatment options
- Results in better patient outcomes, measured in terms of symptom relief, functional status, and patient satisfaction
- Focuses on holistic health and well-being

Technology is seen as one of the three important drivers of increasing healthcare accessibility. Selection and adoption of appropriate technology often make a critical difference in the success of healthcare reform and reengineering, and it has the capability to revolutionize the way healthcare is delivered.

Therefore, it would not be wrong to conclude that using traditional medicines and modern medicines together can be a great therapeutic option for patients. These two different schools of medicine can work in harmony so as to complement each other's strengths and weaknesses, thus providing the best of health to the individual undergoing treatment.

Of course, the amount and complexity of legislation is one thing—its rate of change is another. Simply staying abreast can be a major task in itself.

TREATMENT OF MEDICAL PROBLEMS WITH NUTRITION-BASED PRODUCTS

We will looking at three kinds of diseases. The first is metabolic syndrome (disorders that increase the risk of diabetes and heart problems). The second is gastrointestinal health (the problems that occur in the intestinal tract). The third area is a more challenging one. We believe that there is more and more evidence that good nutrition could help manage cognitive decline. After extensive research, a product like Fruitflow was launched that contains tomato extract. It can be added to yogurts, beverages, and other food products. It is the only functional food ingredient that addresses platelet aggregation by keeping them smooth, thereby avoiding their aggregation in the blood vessels.

Another notable example of nutrition for improved health is ubiquinol. It is a safe, cost-effective ingredient and the key to male infertility. Ubiquinol or coenzyme Q10 has now been used in a wide range of nutraceuticals either alone or in combination with other substances to create *all-round* fertility products.

THE CONVERGENCE OF PHARMA AND NUTRA

We believe that there is a convergence between food and pharma. Chronic diseases need more than just the traditional pharmaceutical approach. Our food and nutrition expertise can help create a new industry where nutrition plays a bigger role in helping people who live with difficult chronic medical conditions.

With the aging population, getting people healthy at the later stage of life is difficult and expensive. Healthcare is going to be in real trouble if we do not start to look at it in a different way.

This in turn will compel the policy makers, health administrators, and medical doctors to look at these alternatives. The way traditional medicines perceive health and disease and their causes is very different. Treating a patient using both modern medicines and traditional medicines goes on to imply that the general health service system can include traditional medicines.

The immense turmoil in the pharmaceutical industry has pushed them to look toward greener pastures. The nutraceutical and functional food and beverage markets are currently experiencing tremendous growth potential, which is a big attraction for pharma companies.

There was a 44% rise in the retail sales value of fortified/functional foods between 2005–2010 across 32 markets where Euromonitor International conducted its detailed health and wellness research. For functional bottled water, the global value went up by 70% in 2006–2011. On the other hand, the sales value for vitamins and dietary supplements rose by almost 50%. It has been estimated that the global nutraceutical market is likely to reach $250 billion by 2015 according to a report by Global Industry Analysts.

With great advances in biotechnology, there is great interest in using food for medical purposes. Using natural herbs and foods for treating ailments is a very old tradition in many cultures. Interest is now expanding toward food with medicinal properties (enriched foods). Probiotics, prebiotics, functional foods, clinical foods, and nutraceuticals are promoted as "good for you foods" either as a part of the daily diet or for a particular disorder treatment such as improving digestion and bone density.

THE WAY FORWARD

A CASE FOR EVIDENCE-BASED PRODUCTS

Prelicense Activities

Pharmaceutical organizations need to understand the causes of diseases and to develop compounds that can be tested in the lab for their effectiveness in treating a disease. Once these targets are identified by the research and development team, they are usually passed to a team responsible for turning these targets into medicines that can be submitted for clinical trials. After the complex clinical trial process is completed, the medicines can be submitted for regulatory approval and, if granted, sold to healthcare providers. End to end, this process of discovering and developing a new molecular entity (NME) takes an average of 13.5 years and (capitalized) costs of $1.8 billion.

The number of targets that hit the market as medicines is a small percentage that is diminishing fast. During target identification, scientists work to understand the cause of disease by looking at pathways, for example, how the disease begins and spreads.

They investigate gene expression, protein mechanisms, and many other highly complex aspects of the causes of disease.

Advances in genomics, proteomics, and protein modeling are transforming the discovery process. At the same time, the sheer volume and structure of the data are challenging leaders in the field to develop shared ontologies to express the meaning of the data.

It is in this area of intensive scientific research that collaboration and transformative partnerships between pharmaceutical companies themselves can take place. A common ontology allows a shared understanding of the semantics of the original data. The cloud offers to host large volumes of complex data in collaborative platform and at relatively low cost. This is an area where Logica and our partner ecosystem have a definite key role to play.

At the end of the discovery process, the objective is to turn target compounds into medicines. This is the expensive part of the discovery process, and the more a target falls out of the process, the greater is the loss incurred by the company. It is therefore vital that those medicines entering the later stage of clinical trials, with live patients, are targeted at a narrow, highly specific cohort.

Evidence Creation Activities

Evidence-based approaches are also being adopted by nutraceuticals for regulatory compliance, which can be ideally seen through the following examples. Fruitflow is the first natural, scientifically substantiated ingredient that contributes to healthy blood flow in the body. In 10 human trials, the consumption of Fruitflow has been proven to maintain healthy platelet aggregation and improve blood flow.

Ubiquinol/Coenzyme Q10 is an essential electron carrier in the body's mitochondrial respiratory chain. Male infertility is a worldwide health issue. For the first time, clinical usefulness of ubiquinol for the treatment of idiopathic male infertility has been documented. Ubiquinol improves semen quality and is also safe, cost-effective, and a discrete treatment for reduced sperm motility.

TNO's patented *in vitro* gastrointestinal models (TIM 1 and TIM 2) are unique gastrointestinal models that are flexible and accurate and that produce highly reproductive results. Nutritional and functional properties of foods and ingredients can be assessed under simulated physiological digestion conditions. The systems are very well validated and offer broad versatility in experimental strategies and goals.

For over 15 years, TIM models have been used successfully and the study results have been described in over 30 scientific peer-reviewed publications. The models are FDA-approved. TIM experiments are free from ethical constraints and are conducted without harming animals or humans. Thus, the nutra industry is working on a clinical evidence–based approach that is sure to work to its advantage.

A CASE FOR THE CARE OF CONSUMERS

Cycle of care can be defined as the method that carefully analyzes the present state of the healthcare process and it can be designed for any particular medical condition. It also enables us to judge how one can bring about cost-effectiveness and enhance clinical outcomes, accessibility, and quality of care for the masses.

There are different phases in the care cycle that have a close link with the stage of the disorder/disease. The phases of a care cycle are as follows: prevention, screening, diagnosis, treatment, management, and surveillance.

The final phase of a care cycle is surveillance wherein a consumer/patient has to see their doctor for checkups at foretold intervals of time. This is an extremely vital phase as it would keep the doctor informed about any possibilities of a recurrence of the disease. A perfect example of this would be a cancer patient as there can be regular follow-ups postcure.

So, it would be apt to say that a cycle of care ideally takes care of an individual's health condition. In this process, the patient's condition transforms from being sick/ill to being fit and fine.

The various phases of cycle of care are a part of healthcare such that the two concepts are not very different from each other. Healthcare can be simply defined as the prevention, treatment, and management of an illness, while at the same time ensuring complete wellness through preservation of mental and physical well-being. This can be done with ease through the cooperation of medical and allied healthcare professionals. In a number of emerging and developing economies, healthcare systems are facing major risks because of excessive demands and costs, low quality of care, and restricted access that is not properly coordinated.

There is a relation between the cycle of care and the health outcomes. This is because the quality of care, cost of treatment, and access are the major attributes in determining whether the actual health outcomes are in sync with the optimum achievable outcome for the same. There are three different levels of healthcare, namely, primary, secondary, and tertiary healthcare.

In 1978, the WHO defined primary healthcare as essential healthcare, based on practical, scientifically sound, and socially acceptable method and technology; universal accessibility to all in the community through their full participation; affordable cost; and geared toward self-reliance and self-determination.

When medical specialists offer a service and they are not the first ones to be contacted by a patient, then it is known as secondary patient care. More often, a patient is referred to secondary care by their primary care provider (usually their GP) and is delivered in clinics or hospitals.

Tertiary care is a highly specialized consultative method of treatment in which a patient is referred from the primary or secondary healthcare professional or even inpatients in hospitals. Often, tertiary care is given by personnel and in facilities for the further medical investigations and treatment. For instance, tertiary care services are often needed when treating cancer patients, cardiac surgery patients, advanced neonatology services, and the like.

A CASE FOR BRANDING

People fundamentally enjoy having the power to choose between comparable options. In the absence of brands with a strong image, the consumer will naturally prefer to buy the cheapest product. Brands must fulfill the promises made to the market, or consumers will no longer support them with future purchases. Competitive position—innovation in product marketing—provides a competitive edge to a brand.

While developing customer-focused products that address specific needs of different customer demographics and then focusing on credibility building, lowering the price of products can help brands to be different.

Increasing awareness of a product among physicians and consumers through advertising and education in context of increasing consumer sophistication leads to more opportunities for shelf space in mainstream retailers.

There have been very few nutraceutical or functional food brands. One example that clearly stands out is Yakult (Harman, 2003). It was suggested that in the case of functional food and beverages, almost all consumer segments would be expected to make trade-offs between functional benefit, price, and carrier attributes given the complex and multifaceted nature of consumer food choice.

CONCLUSION

Instead of there being a convergence, there is a need for both pharmaceutical and nutraceutical sectors to coexist. In a cycle of care, both the sectors are absolutely important for the betterment of society. Pharmaceuticals and nutraceuticals can work hand in hand to ensure complete wellness in the treatment cycle of healthcare as they could be used at different stages. Evidence is the heart of the product and care design through R&D clinical trials, *in vitro* studies, or human studies. Cost of R&D can be readjusted when both work together and, unlike pharma, nutraceuticals can create big healthy brands for better health.

Nutraceuticals can work at the preemptive as well as the healing stages, while surgery and specialized work will always be needed for treating a patient's ailment.

Thus, healthy living must be encouraged where importance is given to responsible nutrition as there is a swift move from preventive methods of treatment to a curative one. The advancements in technology and increasing innovation in nutraceuticals have given rise to more and more high-quality nutra products. Now, it is possible to even cure diseases with these nutra products. This is especially useful in the case of chronic diseases. The treatment of a chronic disease through the use of pharmaceutical products can be further hastened if it is supported by nutraceutical products.

It is important to remember that in Eastern knowledge systems, a patient is treated for an ailment or disorder using a proper diet. Diet or the food eaten was considered as the remedial medicine. So, it can be observed that medication and diet are interwoven and both pharma and nutra can be used in a synergistic way for curing a patient.

Therefore, nutraceutical space will experience a tremendous amount of growth, but that would not imply that the nutra space will overshadow the pharma space in any way. This is because for swift and wholesome treatment, both sectors have to coexist in the future.

For this coexistence between the two sectors, it is vital to improve the level of education on the nutraceutical products available on the market. This education has to begin with the doctors as they need to understand how nutraceutical products can not only aid but even cure diseases and disorders. Thus, the syllabus for doctors has to be amended. Consumer awareness certainly varies for different demographics and those who have access to the Internet and such mediums are aware of the health benefits nutra products offer. But for those who do not have access to advanced mediums of communication, health awareness campaigns are a good option. There has to be awareness on all levels, apart from the ones mentioned previously, like pharmacists and regulators.

REFERENCES

Aarikka-Stenroos, L. and Sandberg, B. 2011. From new-product development to commercialization through networks. *J. Bus. Res.*, 65(2): 198–206.

Behner, P., Edmunds, R., Ehrhardt, M. et al. 2013. *2013 Life Sciences (Pharmaceuticals) Industry Perspective*. Booz & Company.

Bogue, J. 2009. Cross-category innovativeness as a source of new product ideas: Consumers' perception of over-the-counter pharmacological beverages. *Food Qual. Prefer.*, 20(5): 363–371.

Boogaard, P.J. October 2012. Facing cross-industry challenges in the food and pharma industries. Scientificcomputing.com. http://www.industriallabautomation.com/Facing.php.

Capaldo, A. and Peruzzelli, A. 2011. In search of alliance-level relational capabilities: Balancing innovation value creation and appropriability in R&D alliances. *Scand. J. Manag.*, 27(3): 273–286.

Department of Pharmaceuticals. 2012. National pharmaceutical pricing policy. http://apps.who.int/medicinedocs/en/m/abstract/Js20106en/. Accessed July 20, 2016.

Ernst & Young. 2010. Progressions Pharma 3.0. In 2010, EY acquired Terco, the Brazilian member firm of Grant Thornton.

Gebhart, F. December 2012. Retail pharmacists find opportunity in the growing medical food market. *Drug Topics*. http://drugtopics.modernmedicine.com/drug-topics/news/modernmedicine/modern-medicine-feature-articles/retail-pharmacists-find-opportunity. Accessed July 20, 2016.

Gopakumar, K.M. and Santhosh, M.R. 2012. An unhealthy future for the Indian pharmaceutical industry? *Third World Resurgence*, 259(March): 9–14. http://www.twnside.org.sg/title2/resurgence/2012/pdf/259.pdf.

Goyal, P., Midha, T. et.al. 2011. Utilization of Indian Systems of Medicine and Homeopathy(ISM&H): A cross-sectional study among school students of Kanpur city. *Indian J. Prev. Soc. Med.*, 42(3): 326–328.

Grant Thornton and FICCI. 2012. Nutraconsensus: Emerging insights on nutraceuticals— Players and policy makers.

Harman, C. 2003. *The Global Report on Nutraceuticals*. ABOUT Publishing Group, London, UK.

Integrative Medicine and Complete Wellness Nutrition as Medicine. The Firshein Center for Comprehensive Medicine, New York. www.firsheincenter.com/nutrition-as-medicine.html.

Interlink Knowledge Cell. 2011. White paper on regulatory perspective of nutraceuticals in India. http://interlinkconsultancy.com/white_paper/index.html. Accessed July 20, 2016.

Jaswal, I. and Kandal, N. 2013. Indian pharmaceutical industry: Boon or bane. Social Science Research Network. Working Paper Series. http://papers.ssrn.com/sol3/papers.cfm?abstract_id=2200406.

Karim, N.K. June 2012. Challenges and opportunities for pharma industry. *Pharmabiz*. http://pharmabiz.com/ArticleDetails.aspx?aid=69654&sid=9. Accessed July 20, 2016.

Lockwood, G.B. 2007. The hype surrounding nutraceutical supplements: Do consumers get what they deserve. *Nutrition,* 23(10): 771–772. http://www.nutrociencia.com.br/upload_files/artigos_download/suplementos.pdf.

PricewaterhouseCoopers. 2012. Food as pharma. http://www.pwc.com/en_GX/gx/retail-consumer/pdf/rc-worlds-newsletter-foods-final.pdf. Accessed July 20, 2016.

Rao, M. and Mant, D. May 2012. Strengthening primary healthcare in India: White paper on opportunities for partnership. *BMJ*, 344. http://www.bmj.com/content/344/bmj.e3151.

Smarta, R.B. 2012. Market: Focused innovation in food and nutrition. In *Innovations in Healthy & Functional Foods* (eds.) Dilip Ghosh, Shantanu Das, Debasis Bagchi, and R.B. Smarta, pp. 511–512, Chapter 30. CRC Press, Boca Raton, FL.

Verbeek, X.A.A.M. and Lord, W.P. 2007. The care cycle: An overview. Biomedical Informatics Department, Philips Medical Systems. http://incenter.medical.philips.com/doclib/enc/fetch/2000/4504/577242/577256/588821/5050628/5313460/5318705/8_Care_Cycle.pdf%3fnodeid%3d5318718%26vernum%3d1.

2 Holistic Health through Nutrition, Diet, and Nutraceuticals for Prevention and Treatment

R. B. Smarta

CONTENTS

INTRODUCTION

Health and cheerfulness naturally beget each other.

—Joseph Addison

Health is a state of complete harmony of the body, mind and spirit. When one is free from physical disabilities and mental distractions, the gates of the soul open.

—B.K.S. Iyengar

Health is the level of functional or metabolic efficiency of a living organism (Huber and Knottnerus, 2011). In the case of human beings, good health is a general condition when a person's mind and body is free from any illness, injury, or pain. In 1946, the World Health Organization (WHO) defined health, in its broader sense, as a state of complete physical, mental, and social well-being and not merely the absence of disease or infirmity.

THE CONCEPT OF HOLISTIC HEALTH

Holistic health is principally an approach toward a healthy life. While it is obvious that preventing illness is crucial, the concept of holistic health goes beyond this and emphasizes attaining higher levels of wellness. The ancient approach toward health takes into consideration the whole person and how they interact with their environment, rather than concentrating on the illness, specific conditions, or parts of the body. The concept of holistic health stresses the connection of mind, body, and spirit. The objective of this approach is to achieve maximum well-being, wherein the entire body is functioning at its very best. In the holistic health approach, individuals are required to accept and take responsibility for their own level of health and well-being.

The concept of holistic health in medical practice involves all aspects related to a person's health, including psychological, physical, and social well-being. These aspects take into account the individual as a whole, thus the term "holistic health".

By incorporating the approaches of holistic health, people can enjoy the resulting vitality and well-being by combining positive lifestyle changes as per the holistic health approach, and, also due to the positive effects, people are motivated to further continue this process throughout their lives.

RELEVANCE IN TODAY'S WORLD

The concept of holistic medicines has been used for treating and preventing illnesses/health conditions. This concept is practiced in many countries such as the United States, Sweden, and India. Holistic medicine practitioners use different forms of medicine (allopathic, alternative, homeopathy) and therapies for treatment, prevention, or management of illness; some practitioners use alternative medicine exclusively.

According to the American Holistic Medical Association, it is essential to take into consideration the spiritual element when assessing a person's overall well-being. Holistic health is based on the law of nature that a whole is made up of interdependent parts (The Rosen Publishing Group, 1999, American Holistic Health Association). The earth is made up of several elements such as air, water, land, plants, and animals. All these elements are important for sustenance of life and if they are separated, any effect or interaction with one is also felt by the other systems. In the same way, an individual is considered as a whole that is made up of interdependent parts/elements, such as *physical, mental, emotional,* and *spiritual.* If any one of the elements is not working at its best, it affects all the other elements/parts of the individual. Furthermore, this whole person, including all of the parts, is constantly interacting with everything in the surrounding environment. For example, when an individual is anxious, his or her nervousness may result in a physical reaction such as a headache or a stomachache. When people suppress anger over a long period of time, they often develop a serious illness such as migraine headaches, emphysema, or even arthritis.

According to American Holistic Health Association's, Suzan Walter's principles of holistic health state that health is more than just not being sick. Holistic health is an ongoing process. As a lifestyle, it includes a personal commitment. No matter what their current health status is, people can improve their level of well-being. Even when there are temporary setbacks, movement should always be headed toward wellness.

The most obvious choices people make each day are what they "consume" both physically and mentally. The cells in a person's body are constantly being replaced. New cells are built from what is available. Harmful substances or the lack of building blocks needed in the body can result in imperfect cells that are unable to do what is required to keep the person healthy. Similarly, on the nonphysical level, a person's mental attitudes are "built" from what they see and hear.

The majority of the illnesses and premature deaths can be traced to lifestyle choices. The impact of excesses of sugar, caffeine and negative attitudes goes unheeded. Combined with deficiencies in exercise, nutritious foods, and self-esteem, these gradually accumulate harmful effects. Over time, they diminish the quality of the "environment" within that human being and can set the stage for illness to take hold. The quality of life, now and in the future, is actually being determined by a multitude of seemingly unimportant choices made every day (Nancy, 1999) (Figure 2.1).

The biopsychosocial–spiritual model is a holistic approach rather than a medical approach toward promoting health and treatment of illness and pain. In this approach, spirituality and religion are important beyond the treatment of an individual with a specific, diagnosed medical condition. There are two key components to this model that encompass a way to address spirituality and religion in physical health and mental health.

1. Holistic health includes the support and promotion of overall health and well-being of individuals, families, and communities. Holistic health is deeply associated with spirituality and religion. They support and enhance physical and mental health and well-being. For example, many traditions address caring for the body, avoiding behaviors that degrades the body and spirit, or supporting healthy diet choices. Holistic health approaches can offer opportunities to promote spiritual well-being as well.

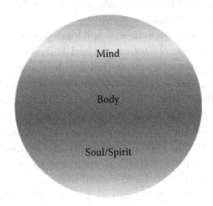

FIGURE 2.1   The biopsychosocial–spiritual model for holistic health. (Adapted from Maloof 1996.)

2. Holistic health recognizes the fact that for certain people and their families, the experience of illness and pain may relate to spiritual concerns and that those concerns may manifest as physical or emotional symptoms.

Holistic health approaches not only address curing or treating a specific physical ailment but also ensuring that support and comfort are provided to the individual and his or her family and community. Thus, holistic care can address the care and support of families who have a child or other member who is seriously or chronically ill or has a disability. It can address the pain of the bereaved. Part of that support can include spiritual and religious resources.

When seeking quality care, references to holistic health are often made.

At an individual level, the complexity of this holistic view can be seen in the diagram shown earlier. Any "disease" in one of these three parts may be manifested in another area, so physical and psychological symptoms or pain may be indicators of "spiritual distress."

METHODS USED IN THE HOLISTIC HEALTH APPROACH

Some of the most popular methods of this approach include the following:

Meditation/prayer: Meditation is one of the effective alternative therapies. Meditation has positive effects on physical illnesses. By incorporating meditation into your daily routine, you can use your energies to be free of diseases or illnesses. The approach of meditation considers that the root cause of many physical illnesses lies in the mind; thus it calms the mind, empowers it, and uses the mental energies that can tackle physical illnesses. Nowadays, meditation is used by most people to reduce the stress in their day-to-day lives. Apart from this, meditation has been found to be effective in treating a wide range of disorders such as anxiety, migraines, depression, insomnia, and high blood pressure. Meditation is one of the key methods in any holistic health approach.

Yoga: Yoga is a physical, mental, and spiritual practice or discipline that originated in India (*OED Online*, Oxford University Press, September 2015). Yoga is a form of exercise that involves specific postures, positions, movements, and stretches that are designed to tone the body and clear the mind. Today, apart from spiritual goals, the physical postures of yoga are used to alleviate health problems, reduce stress, and so on. Yoga is also used as a complete exercise program and physical therapy routine (Douglas and Rebecca, 2006). Yoga in its literal sense means "unison of body, mind, and spirit to attain ultimate salvation." But today, yoga is mostly practiced for physical and mental fitness.

Acupuncture: Acupuncture is a medical practice that involves the use of needles to puncture certain points on the body in order to ease pain or relieve diseases. It is one of the key components of traditional Chinese medicine (TCM). Acupuncture has been mostly used for pain relief, though it is also used for a wide range of other health conditions. Acupuncture is traditionally based on the fact that in humans the nerves operate on energy and that they are electrical; if there is a problem in the body and the energy is disrupted, then through acupuncture one can open up the block relieving the pain.

THE ROLE OF NUTRITION AND DIET (FIGURE 2.2)

In 400 BC, Hippocrates said, "Let food be your medicine and medicine be your food." Today, good nutrition is more important than ever. The nutrients obtained from food are essential for the natural processes that constantly take place inside the body. In today's fast-paced and highly demanding lifestyle, people focus more on the convenience of food they eat rather than on its nutrition. People have become used to packaged and canned foods. Nowadays, when hunger strikes, it is much easier to pop a tin or open a package or ready-made food than to actually cook or prepare a fresh meal (lack of consumption of fresh food). These convenient packaged foods may have adverse effects on our health. There have been numerous studies that link an individual's health to his or her diet; hence, nutritionists advise looking toward food and nutrition as a way not only to satisfy hunger but also for prevention of diseases and maintenance of health.

Food alone is not the key to a healthier life; along with good food, good nutrition, healthy lifestyle, and regular exercise should be made part of our lives in order to lead a healthy life.

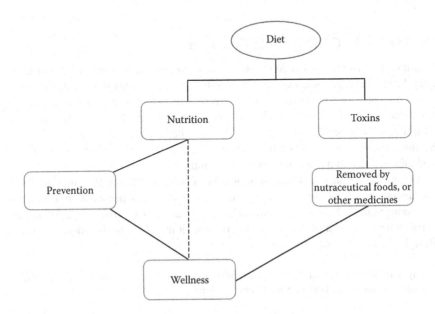

FIGURE 2.2 Role of nutrition and diet.

Some of the examples of diseases that can be prevented or managed by food are illustrated here:

Osteoporosis: In osteoporosis, a person's bones become brittle and thin due to loss of tissue, as a result of a deficiency in calcium or vitamin D or hormonal changes. This gradual thinning of bones can be slowed if enough calcium is consumed along with supplementation of vitamin D. Similarly, the intake of sufficient calcium and vitamin D can also help prevent osteoporosis.

Hyperlipidemia: Hyperlipidemia refers to high lipid levels. It includes several conditions, like high cholesterol and high triglyceride levels. Hyperlipidemia can be reduced by making certain changes in the diet, such as reducing the intake of saturated and trans fats along with increasing the intake of poly- and monounsaturated fats, plant stanols or sterols, and so on.

Diabetes: Diabetes is a group of metabolic diseases that are related to high blood sugar levels over a prolonged period. If diabetes is not treated or managed in time, then it may cause many complications. With effective changes in lifestyle such as regular diet and exercise, even the severe type of diabetes can be managed and further complications can be avoided.

The key to good nutrition is balance, variety, and moderation. Moderation refers to eating neither too much nor too little of any food or nutrient. Too much food can result in overweight or obesity; even too much of certain nutrients can have adverse effects, while eating too little can lead to numerous nutrient deficiencies and low body mass. Therefore, having a balanced diet is the key to good health.

THE ROLE OF FOOD IN LIFESTYLE DISEASES

With the increasing prevalence of lifestyle diseases, preventing diseases and managing health have become essential. Scientific research shows that oxidative stress or cell damage due to free radicals is the root cause of almost all lifestyle chronic degenerative diseases. Our body does not produce enough antioxidants that we need to eliminate the free radicals or at least manage the free radicals; hence, to balance the amount of antioxidants and free radicals, we need to intake antioxidants through food and/or through nutritional supplementation.

As long as adequate amounts of antioxidants are available for the amount of free radicals produced, no damage is caused to the body, but when more free radicals are produced than the available antioxidants, it results in oxidative stress. When this situation persists for a prolonged period of time, it may lead to the onset of various lifestyle chronic degenerative diseases.

Physical fitness is not only one of the most important keys to a healthy body, it is the basis of dynamic and creative intellectual activity.

—**John F. Kennedy**

THE ROLE OF NUTRACEUTICALS IN HEALTHCARE

Most of the nutraceuticals required today come from our food itself. Their absence or inadequacy in food causes various health conditions. A balanced diet along with certain vital nutraceuticals such as antioxidants, vitamins, and minerals helps restore and maintain good health. In the prevention of certain diseases or health conditions, "prebiotics" and "probiotics" act as important factors and have various added advantages such as helping in maintaining gut health and preventing colon cancer. Beyond nutraceuticals and ayurceuticals, the qualified herbal actives that are clinically proven for specific health conditions are the new hope for preventive healthcare.

INTEGRATIVE HEALTHCARE AND MEDICINE

The integrative healthcare or medicine approach is apt for holistic healthcare since it encompasses varied aspects of healthcare such as nutrition, diet, exercise, alternative medicine, conventional medicine, alternative therapies (acupuncture, naturopathy, Ayurvedic, and Chinese herbal medicines), yoga, and meditation. The integrative healthcare approach can be easily incorporated by all healthcare professionals and in all healthcare systems. This approach takes into consideration various aspects of human health by keeping the patient at the center and designing the approaches based on their condition; also the patient is informed, empowered, and made a partner in decision making. This approach takes care of the whole person and attends to an individual's current as well as long-term health requirements. The process of integrative healthcare encourages a person to lead a healthy life. An integrative form of healthcare and medicine can be implemented for all management, prevention, and treatment of diseases (up to some extent).

CONCLUSION

It is more important to know what person has the disease than what disease the person has.

Having a patient-centric model could be the future for the healthcare system, wherein the patient is at the center and all the care and treatment revolves around the patient rather than his or her disease. The care system can involve all three aspects, that is, prevention, management, and treatment of health and disease. This patient-centric, or total care, model may involve the integration of various forms of medicine such as conventional, alternative therapies, nutraceuticals, and nutrition–diet. In general, there has been an increase in the use of traditional medicine due to their lesser side effects and natural origin. Various therapies need to be integrated, such as acupuncture, herbal medicines, manual therapies, exercise, and spiritual therapies, to provide a complete holistic approach of therapies to the patient.

REFERENCES

A Bravewell Collaborative Report. Integrative medicine: Improving health care for patients and health care delivery for providers and payors.

Amy, P. February 2015. Definition of holistic nutrition. http://www.livestrong.com/article/167813-definition-of-holistic-nutrition/#sthash.7JfNpq46.dpuf. Accessed June 28, 2016.

Body/Mind/Spirit/: Towards a Biopsychosocial-Spiritual Model of Health. http://nccc.georgetown.edu/body_mind_spirit/framing-holistic.html. Accessed July 8, 2016.

Dhekne, A. May 2015. Integrative medicine: An approach towards holistic health. *Interlink Insight*, 14(1): 28.

Diabetes mellitus. Wikipedia. June 22, 2016, https://en.wikipedia.org/wiki/Diabetes_mellitus. Accessed June 28, 2016.

Douglas, D., Rebecca, F. 2006. *Yoga. Gale Encyclopedia of Medicine*, 3rd edn. Gale Publications, Detroit, MI. http://www.encyclopedia.com/doc/1G2-3451601767.html. Retrieved August 26, 2016.

Ernst, E., Lee, M.S., and Choi, T.-Y. 2011. Acupuncture: Does it alleviate pain and are there serious risks? A review of reviews. *Pain*, 152(4): 755–764.

Gregory, L.M. Hyperlipidemia, Vascular Web, Vascular Health, Hyperlipidemia. Society of Vascular Surgery. https://www.vascularweb.org/vascularhealth/Pages/hyperlipidemia.aspx. Accessed June 28, 2016.

Holistic health. Wikipedia. May 28, 2016, http://en.wikipedia.org/wiki/Holistic_health. Accessed June 28, 2016.

Nancy, A. 1999. *CMA: The Illustrated Encyclopedia of Body-Mind Disciplines*. Rosen Publishing Group, New York.

Walter, Suzan. AHHA self-help articles collection. Holistic Health, http://ahha.org/selfhelp-articles/holistic-health/. Accessed June 28, 2016.

3 A Paradigm Shift from Cure to Prevention and Treatment

R. B. Smarta

CONTENTS

INTRODUCTION

Modern medicines are well established as emergency cure aids for the treatment of diseases and health conditions. Modern medicines mainly aim at refreshing or appeasing, increasing the life span of the patient by relieving him or her from the disease or illness. The main focus of physicians and healthcare providers should be on prevention and cure, increasing the life span along with the quality of life (in terms of health and wellness). Other forms of medicine (alternative medicines—Ayurveda, homeopathy, nutraceuticals, etc.) and healing therapies have started to gain importance along with the conventional medicines.

The medicines or therapies should be such that they help a person lead a healthy life. In the journey of life, death is the ultimate destination for every individual, but medicines and therapies are needed and should be designed with an aim to provide good health in this journey and prevent premature death.

MODERN MEDICINE

Modern medicines focus mainly on relieving pain and symptoms and removing the agents causing the disease or illness. What we need today is the form of medicine or therapy that simultaneously tackles both cure and prevention of disease. Today, healthcare providers are neither preventing nor curing diseases with the exception of a few conditions; they simply control the further spread of disease and let our bodies fight the disease (in some cases, they provide medicines that enhances our body's ability to fight the disease). The essence of the situation or what has become the motto of healthcare providers can be captured in the following sentence: "To cure sometimes, to comfort always, to hurt the least, to harm never" (Singh and Singh, 2005).

Death and love for life are two factors that rule our lives; we continuously try and prevent the occurrence of death (which will ultimately occur anyway) and in doing so we forget to live and lead a healthy life than merely living or existing.

PREVENTION AND CURE: THE WATCHWORDS

Pharmacology is a compelling means, but it is mostly directed toward comforting and controlling. It must also be directed toward cure and prevention. We can observe that this shift from cure to prevention has already started taking place. The ultimate goal is longevity with well-being, of which freedom from disease is a very important aspect.

The primary goal of life should be health and well-being and the secondary goal should be to cure disease(s) if a patient comes to a hospital/clinic. The focus of preventive medicine is to avoid hospitalization.

LONGEVITY AND WELL-BEING

Longevity and well-being suggest the presence of (1) positive emotions and the absence of negative emotions; (2) mature character traits, including self-directedness, cooperativeness, and self-transcendence; (3) life satisfaction or quality of life; (4) character strengths and virtues, such as hope, compassion, and courage, all of which are now measurable by scales (Cloninger, 2008; Singh, 2010).

RESPONSIBLE HEALTHCARE: THE SHIFT TOWARD PREVENTION

With changing health trends and rising healthcare costs, responsible healthcare, accountable healthcare, or, in simple words, preventive healthcare is the best way to good health. People are becoming more and more aware of the importance of prevention and management of diseases as well as the management of good health. Moreover, rising healthcare costs increase the need to look at prevention rather than treatment.

FACTORS RESPONSIBLE FOR THE SHIFT
FROM CURE TO PREVENTION

During the last 2 to 3 years, the shift from cure to prevention has become more and more evident. Changing trends and lifestyle in general have propelled this shift toward health and prevention. Some of the factors responsible for the shift are detailed as follows:

- *Increase in chronic lifestyle diseases*: Several chronic lifestyle diseases like diabetes mellitus, hypertension, dyslipidemia, and overweight/obesity are the major risk factors for the development of CVD. With rapid economic development and increasing globalization over the past few decades, prevalence of these diseases has reached alarming proportions. The chronic lifestyle diseases affect all strata of society globally; that is, developed, developing, and underdeveloped countries. Most of these diseases can be prevented as well as managed to some extent. As these diseases are chronic in nature, people have become aware and are focusing on prevention of these diseases.
- *Increasing awareness among consumers*: The desire to remain or lead a healthy life has been driving consumers toward prevention. People have become more health conscious and have started understanding the varied benefits of proactive care. Along with the general population, there has been an increase in awareness among those in the corporate sector about the positive effects of healthy living and managing health. The cost of insurance premiums and employee medical claims is at an all-time high and continues to rise. Many corporate heads have started adopting workplace health programs to help their employees embrace healthier lifestyles and lower their risk of developing costly chronic diseases.
- *Increasing healthcare costs*: According to the National Sample Survey Office (NSSO) reports, consumer expenditure on healthcare has increased around the world; in rural India it has increased from 6.6% in 2004–2005 to 6.9% in 2011–2012, while the urban Indians' expenditure on medical care increased from 5.2% in 2004–2005 to 5.5% in 2011–2012. Medical expenses fall under the miscellaneous goods and services category in the NSSO report. These increasing costs force people to take precautions and proactive care to prevent diseases and remain healthy.
- *Health professionals focusing on the management of diseases rather than treatment*: With increasing consumer preference toward prevention and maintenance of health and management of diseases, healthcare/clinical professionals have started to adopt the approach of managing diseases rather than treating them.
- *Pharma companies venturing into the health and/or food supplement sector*: Many pharmaceutical companies are venturing into nutraceutical market owing to its exponential growth in the last few years. Apart from pharma companies, big FMCG companies are also entering the functional foods and functional beverage segment, thus giving a boost to the already growing nutraceutical market and further propelling the shift of healthcare to prevention.

A PARADIGM SHIFT IN THE HEALTHCARE INDUSTRY

The healthcare industry itself is also undergoing a shift from a fee-for-service to a value-based service paradigm due to the new reforms and efforts being adopted at a national level in various countries. Many healthcare experts believe that exigent healthcare costs are controllable by focusing on the preemptive component of healthcare. Following this trend, much emphasis has been placed on providing adequate preventative care, which provides immense opportunities for both healthcare and nonhealthcare organizations. In the area of preventive care, the products, therapies, and services can be segmented into three primary components: patient education systems (including wellness programs), aging in place services, and remote monitoring devices (Frost & Sullivan, 2013).

Other than this, a number of major global companies, worried over the increasing healthcare costs and loss of productivity, have teamed up with health professionals in a pioneering effort to shift the health paradigm from treating disease to promoting wellness, with incredible results. A number of prevention and health promotion programs are being conducted by big pharma and FMCG companies and various government and not-for-profit organizations, in an effort to educate people more on the importance of prevention.

To improve the health and quality of life of their workers, companies are installing gym facilities on-site or paying for off-site health club memberships and professional trainers, providing only healthy meals in company cafeterias and free nutritional instruction for workers and their families, as well as offering stress management counseling and other health promotion services.

A preventive healthcare system involves maintaining and managing health, which is where nutraceuticals, diet, and nutrition play important roles. The paradigm shift has not just been in the overall healthcare system, but it has also been experienced in the individual segments of the healthcare system such as in nutraceuticals, functional foods, dietary supplements, medical foods, and alternative medicine.

A PARADIGM SHIFT IN FOODS

The concept of food has undergone a tremendous change. Food has been mainly considered as only a means of satisfying hunger and as a basic necessity of life. But the benefits of food, apart from simply satisfying hunger, have long been unknown to humans. With the advancement of science and technology, these benefits have been reestablished as well as further studied. The awareness has increased about the ability of our food to prevent, manage, and treat (up to some extent) ailments. With this knowledge consumers, wanting to manage their health, create a demand for food products with enhanced characteristics and associated health benefits.

In one study, 93% of consumers believed certain foods have health benefits that may reduce the risk of disease or other health concerns. In addition, 85% expressed interest in learning more about the health benefits offered by functional foods (IFIC, 2002).

The various aspects of the paradigm shift in food include the following:

1. *Transition*: Patients are transitioning from passive healthcare recipients to active healthcare consumers.

2. *Let food be thy medicine*: People have now started adopting Hippocrates' thought of "let food be thy medicine."

3. *Self-care*: People have a greater sense of individual autonomy and an increased interest in wellness, self-education, and self-care.

4. *Traditional food paradigm*: Food has been viewed traditionally as a means of simply providing normal growth and development, but, today the food has been established to replace nutrients lost during processing and, in some cases, to prevent nutrient deficiencies in the population. Federal policies have generally required that other diseases be treated and managed through the use of drugs.

5. *Research has blurred the lines between food and medicine*: In these recent years, the scientific advances have blurred the line between food and medicine, as scientists identify bioactive food components that can reduce the risk of chronic disease, improve quality of life, and promote proper growth and development. The early nutrition research resulted in cures for numerous widespread deficiency-based diseases.

6. *New self-care paradigm*: A new self-care paradigm (adapted from Clydesdale, 1998) recognizes that foods can provide health benefits that can coexist with traditional medical approaches to disease treatment. This is backed by science that clearly demonstrates the additional dietary roles of foods in reducing disease risk and/or managing diseases.

Due to the advances in research and technologies, consumers have learned that food has a greater impact on health than previously known. At the same time, consumers have started to recognize the problems with the current healthcare system, perceiving that it is often expensive, time-constrained, and impersonal (Figure 3.1).

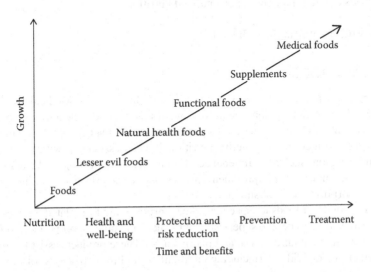

FIGURE 3.1 The changing role of food. (Adapted from Triphase Pharmaceuticals Pvt. Ltd., 2011, Presentation: Trends in Nutraceuticals.)

7. *Changing paradigm from foods to medical foods and dietary supplements*: There has been a great change in the healthcare scenario worldwide; it has changed from just food being consumed to satisfy hunger and stay alive to foods having natural functional benefits to human beings to the use of food in treatment of diseases via medical foods. The representation above shows just that.

8. *Paradigm in the role of functional foods*: Functional foods fit into a continuum that ranges from health maintenance/promotion to disease treatment. On one end of the continuum are the public health programs aimed at reducing disease risk in a large segment of the population through self-directed lifestyle changes, and on the other end of the continuum are individualized treatment programs of disease by healthcare professionals using drugs and other medical interventions. Although health professional involvement is low in self-directed treatment relative to individualized treatment, an important educational component remains. New functional foods will continue to expand the continuum, providing additional options for consumers.

   There is a role for all aspects of this paradigm in our healthcare system. Functional foods should be integral components of established public health programs to reduce the risk of specific diseases.

9. *Bio-guided processing paradigm change in food processing*: Food production and processing are evaluated in terms of yield and efficiency, but this has started to shift toward bio-guided food processing and production wherein the processing schemes will be designed keeping a focus on effective delivery of the food nutrients. This bio-guided approach to food processing will create product lines that will address individual dietary needs and facilitate more personalized nutrition.

Shift towards treatment through food.

MEDICAL FOODS

Medical food is a unique category that is regulated by the FDA. Medical food products meet distinctive nutritional requirements or metabolic deficiencies of a particular disease state. Medical foods, also regarded as foods for special medical purposes, are designed to meet the distinctive nutritional needs associated with a disease or medical condition, such as maintenance of homeostasis, adjusting to the distinctive changes in the nutritional requirements arising due to the effects of the disease process on absorption, metabolism, and excretion.

Medical foods, or foods for special medical purposes, are formulated food products intended to be used under the supervision of medical and other appropriate health professionals (e.g., dietitians, nurses, and pharmacists). These products assist the dietary management of individuals (including children) with chronic diseases, disorders, or medical conditions or during acute phases of illness, injury, or disease states.

The medical foods category is expected to play an important role in health and quality of life beyond prescription drug therapies.

THE ROLE OF NUTRACEUTICALS AND FUNCTIONAL FOODS IN DISEASE PREVENTION

Nutraceuticals have a major role to play in the maintenance/management as well as the prevention of diseases.

WELLNESS TRENDS

The shift in paradigm from cure to prevention/wellness has given rise to various new wellness trends. These trends give us clarity on which direction the world is moving in the health and wellness category. Five major trends take us from simple moderation in diet to a complex form of microbiome.

- Trend 1: *Moderation*
  More and more people are realizing that true health is about having balance. Many can benefit from a diet based on moderation, both in the types and quantities of food they consume. Besides etiquette considerations, the benefits of eating in moderation include weight loss, chronic disease management, and promotion of general health.

- Trend 2: *Genetic testing*
  DNA blueprint resultant of genetic testing can tell you how well your genes are matched to your present diet and lifestyle, as well as how you can unlock the full potential of your current and future health and wellness. Synchronizing the DNA blueprint with diet and lifestyle (also known as nutrigenomics) is the key to the exciting new realm of personalized wellness medicines.

- Trend 3: *Coconut sugar*
  Coconut sugar is a healthier option for agave sweetener, which has high fructose content and is processed. The coconut sugar is unfiltered, unbleached, and free from preservatives, thus making it a healthier option. Not only does coconut sugar have a divinely sweet taste, but it also has a low glycemic index and is rich in minerals, so it could be a good option for diabetic individuals or those predisposed to diabetes.

- Trend 4: *Naturally healthy and functional*
  Naturally healthy and functional foods are those foods/ingredients that contain components naturally beneficial to our health such as soy milk and almond milk.

- Trend 5: *Microbiomes*
  We are beginning to understand that the bacteria that live in our guts (collectively called "microbiomes") are the key to our health. Microbiomes allow us to adapt to the environment quickly, based primarily on the type of food that is available. For example, many of the traits that microbiomes can affect deal with metabolism and the ability to store and use nutrients.

Yet there is still a lot that we do not know, like exactly how do they (microorganisms) interact with other systems in our body to influence digestion and metabolism. But what we do know is that the future of food involves a personalized dietary prescription, catering to each person's unique bacterial makeup. Some of the diseases and/or disorders that may be caused by an imbalance in microbiomes are acne, antibiotic-associated diarrhea, asthma/allergies, autoimmune diseases, cancer, dental cavities, depression and anxiety, diabetes, hardening of the arteries, inflammatory bowel diseases, malnutrition, obesity, and so on.

When these trends are coupled with shifts in paradigm by consumers, anyone can observe that there is a status shift in the nutraceutical and functional food industry.

CURRENT SHIFT AREAS

In order to conclude and make all perspectives and paradigms coexist, let's consider areas in which shifts will occur and that they need to be treated differently.

A shift in the following areas will occur in nutraceuticals, dietary supplements, and functional foods:

- *Digestive health*: This megatrend is moving beyond the tipping point. Digestive health is a wellness issue and one of the biggest opportunities.
- *Convenience foods*: The ability to get healthy benefits in a conveniently sized on-the-go beverage is very appealing to consumers, particularly those with fast-paced lifestyles.
- *Benefit foods*: Functional foods and beverages that provide a benefit consumers can actually feel are important. When people can feel the benefit offered to them, they see that they are getting value for money.
- *Energy yielding and slow energy releasing*: Energy drinks are preferred more by the youngsters, but the market also attracts multitasking executives, time-pressed parents and all those who are looking for a quick supply of energy, in this hectic life.
- *Fruits and superfruits*: Superfruit refers to a fruit that combines antioxidants with high nutrient value and appealing taste. The healthy tag that has been long associated with fruits is mainly due to the innate health benefits of fruits, especially the nutrient packed superfruits.
- *Weight wellness and gluten-free*: Weight management with an increased focus on satiety, calorie-burning, gluten-free, and fat-burning ingredient properties is on the rise. People have become highly weight conscious now-a-days, giving rise to products catering to weight wellness.

CONCLUSION

The shift from cure to prevention is evident as a growing number of consumers perceive the ability to control their health by improving their present health and hedging against future diseases. Concerns related to prevention of chronic diseases and their impact on the quality of life are increasing in the world along with the concern for food safety. The increase in availability and accessibility of nutraceuticals and other wellness offerings has changed the consumer's perception about a healthy and nutritious diet. Along with consumers, governments of various nations have taken initiatives to promote health and prevent diseases.

All in all, the increasing awareness among people and initiatives from governments are expected to further propel the shift from cure to prevention.

REFERENCES

Cloninger, C.R. 2008. On well-being: Current research trends and future directions. *MSM*, 6(1): 3–9.

Clydesdale, F.M. 1998. Science, education and technology: New frontiers for health. *Crit. Rev. Food Sci. Nutr.*, 38: 397–419.

IFIC. 2002. Functional Foods Attitudinal Research. International Food Information Council, Washington, DC. http://ific.org/proactive/newsroom/release.vtml?id=20761.

Frost & Sullivan. January 23, 2013. The shift from treatment to prevention: A drive towards cutting healthcare costs. http://www.frost.com/prod/servlet/press-release.pag?docid=272751750.

Singh, A.R. 2010. Modern medicine: Towards prevention, cure, well-being and longevity. *MSM*, Jan–Dec, 8(1): 17–29.

Singh, A. and Singh, S. 2006. To cure sometimes, to comfort always, to hurt the least, to harm never. *MSM*, Jan–Dec, 4(1): 8–9.

BIBLIOGRAPHY

Pappachan, M.J. August 2011. Increasing prevalence of lifestyle diseases: High time for action. *Ind. J. Med. Res.*, 134(2): 143–145.

Rethinking the Global Health Paradigm: Making the Shift from Managing Disease to Promoting Wellness. http://www.foet.org/lectures/lecture-rethinking-health-paradigm.htm.

Richter, S. Dietary supplements—A new paradigm for manufacturers. http://www.researchgate.net/profile/Steven_Richter/publication/235655088_a_white_paper_dietary_supplements__a_new_paradigm_for_manufacturers/file/32bfe512533267c4dc.pdf. Accessed July 20, 2016.

Rising Health Care Costs Are Unsustainable. Centres for Disease Control and Prevention. http://www.cdc.gov/workplacehealthpromotion/businesscase/reasons/rising.html. Accessed July 20, 2016.

Robert, E.W., Heribert, W., Rafael, J.F., Bruce, G.J. et al. Food technology feature, bioguided processing: A paradigm change in food production. http://digitalcommons.calpoly.edu/cgi/viewcontent.cgi?article=1009&context=dsci_fac. Accessed July 20, 2016.

Safe Food and Nutritious Diet for the Consumer. Executive Summary. http://www.fao.org/worldfoodsummit/sideevents/papers/y6656e.htm. Accessed July 20, 2016.

Section 1: Health, Wellness, Fitness, and Healthy Lifestyles: An Introduction to Good Health, Wellness, Fitness, and Healthy Lifestyles Are Important for All People. www.mhhe.com/hper/physed/clw/01corb.pdf.

Sumitra, Deb Roy. March 15, 2013, 09.38 PM IST, Government incentives—FDA minister promises support with incentives for nutraceuticals industry, TNN. http://timesofindia.indiatimes.com/city/mumbai/FDA-minister-promises-support-with-incentives-for-nutraceuticals-industry/articleshow/18993461.cms. Accessed June 7, 2016.

Targeted Disease Management—Targeted Medical Pharma. http://ptlcentral.com/What-Is-a-Medical-Food.php#sthash.KpUUt70n.dpuf. Accessed June 7, 2016.

The NHS Confederation. Briefing, October 2011, Issue 224. http://www.nhsconfed.org/Publications/Documents/illness_to_wellness_241011.pdf. Accessed June 7, 2016.

4 Traditional and Modern Medicine
Filling the Gap

Dilip Ghosh

CONTENTS

INTRODUCTION

Modern medicines have been transformed hugely in the last decade due to spectacular technological advancements. Herbal medicines still remain the mainstay of medicine for most underdeveloped and developing nations. In most developed nations, increasing recognition of the value of traditional herbal healing systems is partly due to unique and affordable approach of traditional systems to the healthcare system and partly due to real and perceived limitations in conventional care. A series of plant-derived medicines have been introduced in the past but most of them never completed their journey. Traditional Chinese medicine (TCM) and Indian Ayurveda (IA), typical ethnomedicines derived from the practice of ancient Chinese and Indians, is a summary of thousands of years of clinical experiences. During its formation and development, it was greatly impacted by traditional Chinese and Indian culture and exhibited a significant cultural imprint. In contrast, modern medicine has abandoned the cultural impact and is entirely based on the experimental natural sciences. It is clear that dramatic differences have existed between traditional medicine (TM) and modern medicine in the theoretical development, the cognitive approach, and the way of thinking, and so on, which form the huge gap between them (Chen et al., 2013). This gap is affecting the potential of joint use of TM and modern medicine that can revolutionize the treatment of diseases.

A comparative analysis of the philosophy and history of science of the West and the East provides a pathway to understand transitions in social, cultural, and behavioral aspects. In the West, modern biology and modern medicine evolved through the use of reductive logic, mostly after the Renaissance. In the West, scientific and technological advances facilitated the emergence of disease-centric modern medicine, with powerful drugs, pharmaceuticals, and surgical innovations. In the East, ancient systems like Ayurveda, yoga, and TCM continued with a holistic approach to health, disease, and wellness involving body/mind/spirit. The Eastern approaches give wider recognition to the role of diet, nutrition and exercise, and lifestyle through the practices of Ayurveda, yoga, TCM, Kampo, Chi Gong, acupuncture, and natural medicines.

Internationally, TCM herbs are often criticized for not having proven effectiveness and safety, and as a result are approved as functional foods or food additives even though significant progress has been made in recent years, such as the therapeutic effect of arsenic trioxide for acute promyelocytic leukemia (APL) (Powell, 2011), and artemisinin for malaria (Klayman, 1985). The flourishing of modern biomedical technologies provides a good opportunity for TCM development (Engel and Straus, 2002). With the rise of the Chinese economy in the past 10 years, the Chinese government launched ambitious plans for the modernization and internationalization of TCM herbs (Qiu, 2007), such as the launch of the "Chinese Medicine Modernization Program" (2002–2010) and the herbalomics project (Stone, 2008), among others.

During the same time frame, there has been no significant increase in the number of FDA approved new molecular entities in the last decade that prompts us to reevaluate the drug discovery strategies (Mullard, 2012). In addition, "the failure of combinatorial chemistry and high-throughput screening (HTS) to increase new drug productivity promotes the regained enthusiasm for natural products based drug discovery as natural products provide crucial and unmatched chemical diversity to modern drug discovery programs" (Strohl, 2005). Many large international pharmaceutical companies showed great enthusiasm toward TCM and IA herbs, particularly after the approval of the Guidance for Industry Botanical Drug Products by the FDA in 2004. From drug discovery point of view, filling the gap between them is urgently needed.

PHILOSOPHICAL DIFFERENCES

Western medicine considers external factors such as viruses and bacteria as the cause of the disease, (Ackerknecht, 1982; Loudon, 1997), whereas Oriental/Asian medicine considers the nature of diseases through internal factors such as the weakening of the protective function of the body. Therefore, the prime strategy of treatment is aggressive prevention of external factors in Western medicine, and the strengthening of internal defense response in Oriental medicine. But in recent times, the Western model has met with some turbulence. In particular, the concept of "one disease— one target—one-size-fits-all" is shifting toward more personalized medicine tailored to individual patients, including the use of multiple therapeutic agents and the consideration of nutritional, psychological, and lifestyle factors when deciding the best course of treatment. This shift in strategy has been most obvious in the prevention and management of chronic diseases such as diabetes and cardiovascular disease.

The intellectual and scientific underpinnings for such a transition in medical practice are being embedded in the discipline of systems science and systems biology in the biomedical domain. Systems science aims to understand both the connectivity and interdependency of individual components within a dynamic and nonlinear system at certain organizational levels. The concepts and practices of systems biology align very closely with those of traditional Asian medicine.

Biomedicine, in contrast, is founded on the reductionist approach to health and disease, and attempts, first and foremost, to eliminate pathology. Although clinical evaluation is of paramount and critical importance, science as such is extremely impersonal, and, when treating patients, generally cuts across individual differences (genetic or other). Proneness to disease and prevention thereof are more environmental and genetic in nature than a question of "wholesome strengthening of the host." There is a strong, across-the-board underpinning of "objectivity," in diagnosis, treatment, and therapy response. Medicines are its core strength—well characterized in structure and function (usually well tested under laboratory and clinical trial conditions), with efficacy/safety trade-offs. Response is generally predictable.

THE TRANSMISSION AND TRANSFORMATION OF TRADITIONAL MEDICINAL WISDOM

Although modern medicine has evolved from herbalism and from ancient Greek traditions that share many similarities with TM, the practice of medicine was transformed by the Enlightenment and the consequent revolution in science and technology. Western-style medicine incorporated knowledge of anatomy, physiology, chemistry, and biology in the late eighteenth century, and these are considered are evidence-based methods. Although TM is starting to take on these attributes, it relies heavily on ancient records and traditional practices. In modern medicine, chronic conditions are generally treated with prolonged administration of chemical drugs, which can give rise to long-term toxicity or even resistance. Due to the different treatment regime, modernizing Asian medicines will require more than just applying modern tools and scientific techniques to ancient practices. Few active ingredients are extracted from TCM herbs by modern scientific approaches and have not been demonstrated to be clinically successful. Artemisinin and arsenic trioxide are perhaps the only two examples where the isolation of purified active molecules worked effectively (Xu, 2011). Therefore, simply extracting one active ingredient from an herb or herbal concoction and then trying to find its biological activity may not be the effective strategy in the future. The process will require a better understanding of how multiple ingredients act in synergy, and what effect they can have on multiple targets.

THE LIMITATIONS OF RANDOMIZED CONTROLLED CLINICAL TRIALS IN TRADITIONAL MEDICINE

It is widely accepted that randomized controlled trials (RCTs) are the gold standard for testing new medicines. Within an RCT, a person will be randomly allocated to a group that receives one of the treatment options or a placebo. Typically, each group should contain the same distribution of relevant demographics, such as age, sex and ethnicity, among others. The concept of the "average patient" has evolved from the rigidity of RCTs. Although such a patient does not really exist, designing a trial in this manner is not ideal for tailoring treatment to an individual. With the growing appreciation that a person's genetic variation affects his or her response to treatment, personalized trial designs must be adopted. The concept of personalized medicine has similarities with the individualized diagnostic and treatment methods of traditional Asian medicines (notwithstanding the fact that the molecular mechanisms have yet to be elucidated). Therefore, it is reasonable to assume that any clinical trial designed for personalized medicine should be adaptable for testing traditional Asian medicines. Both Western-style modern medicine and traditional Asian medicine aim to heal patients in a harmonized way and can be developed together into an integrated form of personalized medicine. Redesigning clinical trials will accelerate the blending of these two styles of healing, for the benefit of humankind (Liu, 2011).

TRADITIONAL CHINESE MEDICINES

The foundation of traditional Chinese medicine is based on 5000 years of practice and experiences. In fact, shortly after the introduction of modern medicine to China about 170 years ago, attempts have been made by some farsighted TCM experts to fill the gap. As modern (Westernized) medicine's impact increased, it led to the development of "integrative medicine" at the end of the 1950s. As a result, an academic school called converged traditional and Western medicine school was formed. However, nearly all the pioneers in the school are clinical doctors with views and perspectives mainly from TCM theories and clinical practices. Theories, therapeutic principles, technologies, and understanding of the life sciences were elaborated, and the basic structure of traditional Chinese medicine also became clearer. Most importantly, traditional Chinese medicine began to reach a common point with modern medicine.

Although the full integration of TCM with modern medicine from herb/drug, the common carrier for both, the point of view has not been performed well, it was presumed that the integration of TCM herbs with modern drugs might be a feasible and effective way to fill the gap between the two systems.

K.K. Chen is considered the first expert to use modern technologies to study Chinese herbs, but prior to that the mechanism of action of Chinese herbs was largely neglected. In his twenties, he isolated ephedrine from a Chinese herb called Mahuang and found that it had an adrenergic effect (Chen and Schmidt, 1924). This reductionist strategy is expected to find powerful and effective pure compounds from Chinese herbs by isolation, purification, and pharmacological evaluation, among others. The application of advance technologies, thus, has been considered as the critical step to success. However, no key breakthrough has been made in the modernization and internationalization of TCM herbs despite the applications of HTS (Zhu et al., 2010), high content screening (Yan and Liu, 2008), nanotechnology (Li et al., 2009), -omics (Liu and Guo, 2011; Wang et al., 2011), systems biology (van der Greef et al., 2010), and network pharmacology (Li, 2011), except the discovery of artemisinin and arsenic trioxide. Although the discovery of artemisinin is remarkable and a breakthrough, similar success stories are few and different from becoming a common drug discovery model for TCM herbs. Furthermore, such isolated pure compound-based research model has been frequently questioned and criticized due to its drift from TCM theory. Thus, new research strategies are necessary on the basis of compatibility and synergy of herbs. The combination of different herbs in clinical practice is called TCM formula that is purely based on compatibility and synergy according to the patient's condition (Tables 4.1 and 4.2). A typical formula contains at least four herbs that are addressed as the emperor, the minister, the assistant, and the envoy according to their different contributions in the formula. Generally, the emperor contributes the main therapeutic effect for the formula and the minister enhances the emperor's effect. The primary role of the assistant is to enhance the therapeutic effect of the emperor and the minister and/or eliminate or restrict their undesired side effects or potential toxicity. The envoy is considered to guide all the other herbs to reach the treatment sites and to reconcile them. Modern phytochemical studies have shown that each herb contains dozens, or even hundreds, of pure compounds (Table 4.3).

The global database indicated that, as natural products, the pure compounds isolated from TCM herbs show relatively lower pharmacological potency and selectivity. For example, the cytotoxicity of curcumin, berberine, and oridonin to many cancer line cells expressed as IC50 are approximately 5–100 M, 40–100 M, and 3–80 M, respectively (Chen et al., 2011), that are considered as low potencies. Therefore, the current single-compound-based screening strategy of TCM herbs is undoubtedly an impassable test for TCM herb–derived pure compounds.

To keep "the original taste and flavor" of TCM formula, some Chinese scholars have proposed several alternative strategies in recent years, such as the multicomponent Chinese medicine research strategy (Liang et al., 2006; Zhang and Wang, 2005) that attempts to use the active constituents or effective parts of Chinese herbs to replace the original formula. Despite some advantages by simplifying the complicated components of Chinese herbs to certain active parts and applying fingerprinting technologies to fulfill quality control, some mechanistic issues still remain to be resolved. TCM formula is an ancient empirical-based form of drug combination that requires rigorous experimental design, system evaluation, and analysis. Pure compounds combined investigations is a new trend in recent years for exploring the actions and potential mechanisms of TCM formula.

Realgar-Indigo naturalis is a formula designed by TCM practitioners in the 1980s entirely based on TCM theories and it contains realgar, *Indigo naturalis*, *Salvia miltiorrhiza*, and *Radix psudostellariae*. Multicenter clinical trials showed that this formula is very effective in acute promyelocytic leukemia (APL) patients. In this formula, realgar is considered as the principal element (the emperor), whereas *I. naturalis*, *S. miltiorrhiza*, and *R. psudostellariae* are adjuvant components to assist the effects of realgar. Tetraarsenic tetrasulfide, indirubin, and tanshinone IIA are the major active ingredients of realgar, *I. naturalis*, and *S. miltiorrhiza*, respectively. A combination of active ingredients such as tetraarsenic tetrasulfide, indirubin, and tanshinone IIA showed synergistic effect in APL models both *in vitro* and *in vivo* (Wang et al., 2008). This study is one of the good examples of the value of traditional medicine.

TABLE 4.1

A Few Ancient Herbal Formulas That Form a Consensus with Modern Medicine

Formula	Composition	Function	Traditional Application	Modern Application
Ginseng decoction	Large ginseng 20–30 g	Invigorating qi to prevent prostration	Those who have qi and blood deficiency, pale complexion, aversion to cold with fever, cold limbs, spontaneous sweating or cold sweating, and faint pulse catch this kind of disease	Hemorrhagic or cardiogenic shock
Zhenwu decoction	*Poria cocos*, Paeonia Lactiflora Pall, Ginger (sliced) each three liang, *Atractylodes macrocephala koidz* (two liang), Radix Aconiti Lateralis Preparatao (one piece, processed)	Warming yang to promote diuresis	The syndromes show as follows: Dysuria; heavy limbs with pain; hypogastralgia and diarrhea; limb swelling; white tongue coating and no eagerness to drink; deep pulse; taiyang diseases that are overused sweating method; edema due to yang insufficiency; fever; epigastric throb; dizziness; trembling body	Cardiogenic or renal edema
Yupingfeng powder	*Saposhnikovia divaricata, Radix astragali*, one liang each, *Atractylodes macrocephala koidz* (two liang) with one and a half cup of water and three pieces of ginger	Tonifying spleen and supplementing defending qi; consolidating exterior for arresting sweating	It is called a TCM immunomodulator. It treats spontaneous sweating due to deficiency of yang, susceptibility of pathogenic wind; body injury by wind, rain, cold, and dampness, and withered skin; sweating and disgusting wind; pale complexion, pale tongue, and thin–white coating, floating and deficient pulse	Rising immune functioning

Source: Adapted from Dong, J., *Evid. Based Complement. Alternat. Med.*, 2013.

TABLE 4.2
Some Common Herbs Used in Both Traditional and Modern Medicines

Herbs	Function	Traditional Application	Pharmacological Action	Modern Application
Ephedra	Antiperspiration, relieves lung congestion, antiasthmatic, diuretic	Used for respiratory infections caused by "wind," asthmatic cough and chest distress, edema caused by wind, asthma, pruritis	Ephedrine induces central nervous system excitation; improves myocardial contractility, increases cardiac output; acts on adrenoreceptor; significantly relaxes bronchial smooth muscle	Mainly used for bronchial asthma, the common cold, allergic response, nasal congestion, edema, hypotension
Datura flower	Suppresses cough and relieves dyspnea; anesthetic and odynolytic; relieves spasms and pain	Used for cough, asthma, abdominal pain; rheumatic aches, epilepsy, infantile convulsion, and anesthesia	Scopolamine and Cystospaz, two major actives that are analogous to an alpha-blocking agent; scopolamine has analgesic functions via blocking adrenergic receptors; reduces vagal inhibitory effects on the heart and stimulates the apneustic center	For gastric and duodenal ulcers and gallbladder disease, kidney disease, intestinal cramps, and can also be used for tremor palsy
Coptis	Heat dampness, fire detoxification	For hotness and humidity, vomiting, dysentery jaundice, fever, coma, upset, insomnia, hematemesis, and epistaxis due to hot blood, toothache, carbuncles	Berberine, the active component has an antimicrobial, antiarrhythmic, antihypertensive, positive inotropic effect; detoxification, anti-inflammatory, antipyretic, and antiplatelet aggregation	Commonly used to treat bacterial gastroenteritis, dysentery, and other gastrointestinal diseases
Aconite	Reviving yang for resuscitation, supplementing fire and strengthening yang, eliminating cold to stop pain	For excessive yin rejecting yang, loss of yang due to severe diaphoresis, vomiting and diarrhea, cold extremities, cold hypochondrium protrusion	The active is Myoctonine that has a cardiotonic effect, dilates blood vessels, increases blood flow, antiarrhythmic, anticold, improves tolerance to hypoxia tolerance and anti-inflammatory and analgesic effects	Clinically used to alleviate pain, especially suitable for the digestive system and cancer pain
Honeysuckle	Heat clearing and detoxicating, improves eyesight, dispels wind and heat	For anthracia and furunculosis, pharyngitis, anemopyretic cold, fever caused by warm pathogen	The main component is volatile oil. Antimicrobial, anti-inflammatory, antiendotoxin, immunostimulatory and antipyretic effects	For gastric and duodenal ulcers and gallbladder disease, kidney disease, intestinal cramps, and can also be used for tremor palsy

(Continued)

TABLE 4.2 (Continued)
Some Common Herbs Used in Both Traditional and Modern Medicines

Herbs	Function	Traditional Application	Pharmacological Action	Modern Application
Curcuma longa	Anti-inflammatory, anti-cancer	Traditionally turmeric has been used in an attempt to treat stomach and liver ailments, as well as topically to heal sores based on its supposed antimicrobial property	Curcumin is a highly pleiotropic molecule (three curcuminoids) capable of interacting with numerous molecular targets involved in inflammation	Curcumin may have potential therapeutic effects against diseases such as inflammatory bowel disease, pancreatitis, arthritis, and chronic anterior uveitis, as well as certain types of cancer
Vitis vinifera	Anti-inflammatory	Traditionally, it is utilized in the treatment of diarrhea, bleeding, hemorrhoids, varicose veins, and other circulatory and venous diseases, headache, skin disease, and vomiting	Several active components including flavonoids, polyphenols, anthocyanins, proanthocyanidins, procyanidins, and the stilbene derivative resveratrol have a broad spectrum of pharmacological effects such as antioxidative, anti-inflammatory, and antimicrobial activities, as well as having cardioprotective, hepatoprotective, and neuroprotective effects	Cardioprotective and immunemodulatory role in inflammatory conditions
Aloe vera	Anti-inflammatory	The aloe vera plant has been used for thousands of years to heal a variety of conditions, most notably burns, wounds, skin irritations, and constipation	Pharmacological activities include anti-inflammatory, antiviral and antitumor, moisturizing, anti-aging effect, antiseptic, enhances immune system, hypoglycemic, cytotoxic, antiulcer and antidiabetic effects, antibacterial effect, antioxidant, cardiovascular effect	Mostly used to speed wound healing by improving blood circulation and also for bowel diseases including ulcerative colitis, fever, itching, and inflammation

Source: Adapted from Dong, J., *Evid. Based Complement. Alternat. Med.*, 2013.

TABLE 4.3
Some Traditional Herbs Used in Modern Medicines

Formula	Composition	Function	Traditional Application	Modern Application
Artemisia apiacea	Antipyretic, antimalaria	Fever, malaria, icterus	Regulation of immune function, and anti-inflammatory, antibacterial, antimalarial role	Malaria such as encephalopathy, bilious malaria; for example, Artequick
Panax ginseng	Reinforce qi, reduce anxiety	Fatigue, chronic illness, dehydration	Improve physical, mental activity, and strengthens immunity; the pharmacological activity of ginseng has an "adaptogen"-like effect	Antitumor activity; for example, Ginsana
Scutellaria baicalensis	Heat dampness, anticoagulation, tocolysis	Cough, tocolytic, icterus	Decreases cerebral vascular resistance, improves cerebral blood circulation/flow, and antiplatelet aggregation	Paralysis after cerebrovascular disease
Bacopa monierri	The cognitive-enhancing properties of *Bacopa* are multiple and complex	Cognition, memory enhancement	Widely known herb in traditional Ayurvedic (Indian) medicine, used for various indications but most well recognized for its memory-enhancing and cognitive benefits	Supports memory, concentration, and learning retention; for example, KeenMind
Withania somnifera	Used for centuries in Ayurvedic medicine to increase longevity and vitality	Actives might help calm the brain, reduce swelling (inflammation), lower blood pressure, and alter the immune system	Ashwagandha is traditionally used as an "adaptogen" to help the body cope with daily stress, and as a general tonic	Antineoplastic agent in conjunction with radiation and chemotherapy treatment

From a pharmacology and toxicology perspective, the intelligent mixture could be easily predicted, determined, and evaluated. However, the functional identification of the rational ratio of each compound in the mixture is a big challenge because each formula contains more than one herb and nearly 100,000 formulae have been recorded in history. Fortunately, recent developments in system biology might provide technical assistance for this issue. For example, from a network perspective, methods called distance-based mutual information model (DMIM) and multicomponent synergy (NIMS) were used to identify useful relationships among herbs in numerous herbal formulae and to prioritize synergistic agent combinations in a high-throughput way (Li et al., 2011). According to the experts' opinions from both TCM and modern medicine circles, the future of TCM herbs will largely depend on their safety and efficacy.

AYURVEDA: MODERN MEDICINE INTERFACE

India is known for its traditional medicinal systems—Ayurveda, Siddha, and Unani, which are even mentioned in the ancient Vedas and other scriptures (Sharma, 1994; Valiathan, 2003). The Ayurvedic concept appeared and developed sometime between 2500 and 500 BC in India. The inner meaning of Ayurveda, "science of life," comes from the ancient Indian system of healthcare, which focuses on views of man and his illness, but its fundamentals are not based on application of pharmaceutical product from regulatory perspective. In Ayurveda, positive health means metabolically well-balanced human beings and it offers a complete system to live a long healthy life ("science of longevity") through diet and nutrition. The full philosophy of "Pathya Kalpana"—dietary regimen is that it is a magnificent remedy for few ailments and an aid to patients in cure of other diseases (Dhami, 2013). With an emphasis on self-discipline and modest living with high human values, the system strongly advocates a unique set of principles and guidelines on diet and exercise in daily healthy living.

The classical Ayurvedic system was probably driven by insight, intuition, and astute observation of human behavior and nature. "The soil is more important than the seed" concept underlies several Ayurvedic treatment strategies. A delicate balance between biophysiological forces (dosha) and constitution (prakriti) is said to determine health and disease; several other "players" such as the "mind" and "metabolic fire" (agni) also play important roles. Ayurveda's principal therapeutic aim is to harmoniously restore that balance. Cosmaceutical products also have place in bunches of buckets of Ayurveda.

Ayurveda has an extensive pharmacopoeia, predominantly herbs and minerals, whose healing properties are well summarized in modern texts (Frawley and Lad, 1994). Ayurvedic formulations, often complex with several herbal-mineral ingredients, are governed by well-described pharmacological principles of preparation, compatibility and administration (Tables 4.1 through 4.3). Ayurveda's basic perspective "no two individuals are alike" holds its promises to treat people as individual. Also, advice on diet, exercise, and lifestyle is inherently bound to its basic therapeutic approach. Rather than seeking support from laboratory or imaging investigations, Ayurvedic physicians use subtle clinical methods to diagnose and monitor therapeutic response.

India is the largest producer of medicinal plants. There are currently about 250,000 registered medical practitioners of the Ayurvedic system, as compared to about 700,000 in modern medicine. In India, around 20,000 medicinal plants have been recorded; however, traditional practitioners use only 7,000–7,500 plants for curing different diseases. The proportion of use of plants in the different Indian systems of medicine is Ayurveda 2000, Siddha 1300, Unani 1000, Homeopathy 800, Tibetan 500, Modern 200, and Folk 4500. In India, around 25,000 effective plant-based formulations are used in traditional and folk medicine. More than 1.5 million practitioners use the traditional medicinal system for healthcare in India. It is estimated that more than 7800 manufacturing units are involved in the production of natural health products and traditional plant-based formulations in India, which requires more than 2000 tons of medicinal plant raw material annually. More than 1500 herbals are sold as dietary supplements or ethnic traditional medicines (Ghosh, 2014). The renewed consumer's faith in the power of botanicals, along with the availability of a vast majority of different kinds of herbs in India, has always been a thrust behind the resurgence of this scientific art of healing under modern medicine domain.

The author is of opinion that there is mammoth potency in the field of nutraceuticals and cosmaceutical products of Ayurveda that may lead to patent grants on this account and serve masses for good health. We believe that common ground between the two systems should be explored using modern science and logic to understand Ayurveda's ancient thought and system processes. Recently, the Department of AYUSH created a new category of Ayurvedic products under the title of Ayurvedic Balya/Poshak (Ayurvedic Nutritional Products) and Ayurvedic Soundarya Prasadhak (Ayurvedic Cosmaceuticals) for licensing and exporting purposes, which may explore new opportunities for Ayurveda worldwide.

"4P HEALTHCARE"

The advent of omic technologies, which rapidly measure the entirety of the human complement of, for example, genes (genomics) or metabolites (metabonomics)—and to integrate these diverse data into a complete picture—has given rise to a new way of looking at medicine in the form of systems biology. For many traditional medicine researchers, systems biology is potentially a way to understand TM using Western scientific methodology (Peng, 2011). But it is not an easy task to translate TM experience and concepts into biochemical and biological meanings that Western scientists can understand.

Leroy Hood, president of the Institute for Systems Biology in Seattle, Washington, has first introduced what he calls "4P healthcare": predictive, personalized, preventive and participatory. This concept is the new paradigm of modern medicine within systems biology domain and focuses on the biochemical networks underlying health and disease. The aim is to treat and prevent disease by identifying and countering perturbations in the biological networks—a concept highly reminiscent of the TM philosophy. Thanks to systems biology, the gap between the two medical systems is starting to narrow. For example, the application of new phenotyping technologies simultaneously characterizes the multiple drug responses to dietary preparations, such as pu-erh tea. A human study quantitatively measured the absorption of pu-erh tea molecules, the output of gut bacteria metabolism, and the human metabolic response profile in the urine (Xie et al., 2009). The phenotyping strategy can further differentiate disease subtypes that are correlated to different TCM syndromes. This, in turn, will improve doctors' ability to personalize treatment and to predict an individual's response to a drug regimen.

CONCLUSION

There is indeed an urgent need for a paradigm shift in modern medicine toward an integrative approach for health from history, evolution, philosophy, and medicine practice perspective. No single approach can meet the changing dynamics of global health. There are various ongoing efforts in integrative healthcare occurring in different parts of the world, but the most important need is to change the mind-set from illness-, disease-, and drug-centric curatives to person-, health-, and wellness-centric approaches. The systematic promotion of health, early prediction, and prevention of ill-health should be given priority, so that the dependency on treatments and therapies can be reduced. The approaches should be personalized, where people are empowered to actively participate in maintaining their own health. The edifice of integrative health for the future must meld transdisciplinary scientific approaches to create a confluence of modern medicine and traditional systems.

Undoubtedly, modern medicine provides overwhelming symptomatic relief from diseases and disorders for patients suffering from different ailments. However, idiosyncrasy and dose-related toxicity are major obstacles, especially when long-term management is required. Under these circumstances, the potential of TM should be tested and substantiated before converting it to real-life treatment paradigms constituting an effective TM-modern medicine interface.

Although the efficacy at times is modest, safety of TM is excellent. This advantage should logically lead us to question "whether both modalities can be effectively used in conjoint treatment strategies?" Implementing this requires all-out efforts from conventional and TM physicians to see eye to eye for providing effective solutions to difficult-to-treat chronic medical disorders.

The absence of robust scientific development and controlled clinical trials has held back the integration of traditional Asian medicine with modern medicine for centuries. The tremendous safety of traditional botanicals is very reassuring and forms the foundation of the much advocated "reverse pharmacology" approach (Patwardhan et al., 2004, 2015), where clinical validation proceeds in parallel to other experimental studies. This approach significantly reduces the time and money that is required to reach the market.

REFERENCES

Ackerknecht, E.H. 1982. *A Short History of Medicine.* Johns Hopkins University Press, Baltimore, MD.

Chen, K.K. and Schmidt, C.F. 1924. The action of ephedrine, the active principle of the Chinese drug Ma Huang. *J. Pharmacol. Exp. Ther.*, 24: 339–357.

Chen, X., Pei, L., and Lu, J. 2013. Filling the gap between traditional Chinese medicine and modern medicine, are we heading to the right direction? *Complement. Ther. Med.*, 21: 272–275.

Chen, X., Pei, L., and Wang, Y. 2011. Discussion on research and development models in innovative Chinese Materia Medica. *Chin. Tradit. Herb. Drugs*, 42: 1255–1260.

Dhami, N. 2013. Trends in pharmacognosy: A modern science of natural medicines. *J. Herb. Med.*, 3: 123–131.

Dong, J. 2013. The relationship between traditional Chinese medicine and modern medicine. *Evid. Based Complement. Alternat. Med.* http://dx.doi.org/10.1155/2013/153148.

Engel, L.W. and Straus, S.E. 2002. Development of therapeutics: Opportunities within complementary and alternative medicine. *Nat. Rev. Drug Discov.*, 1: 229–237.

Frawley, D. and Lad, V. 1994. *The Yoga of Herbs*. Motilal Banarsidass Publishers Pvt Ltd., Delhi, India.

Ghosh, D. 2014. The nutraceutical potential of Ayurvedic medicine. *Nutrition Insight*, Summer Edition: 51–55.

Klayman, D.L. 1985. Qinghaosu (artemisinin): An antimalarial drug from China. *Science*, 228: 1049–1055.

Li, D.C., Zhong, X.K., Zeng, Z.P. et al. 2009. Application of targeted drug delivery system in Chinese medicine. *J. Control. Release*, 138: 103–112.

Li, S. 2011. Network target: A starting point for traditional Chinese medicine network pharmacology. *Zhongguo Zhong Yao Za Zhi*, 36: 2017–2020.

Liang, X.M., Xu, Q., Xue, X.Y., Zhang, F.F., and Xiao, Y.S. 2006. Systematic research on the multi-component Chinese medicine. *World Sci. Technol.—Modernization Tradit. Chin. Med. Mater. Med.*, 8: 16–19.

Liu, L. 2011. The clinical trial barriers. *Nature*, 480: S100.

Liu, X. and Guo, D.A. 2011. Application of proteomics in the mechanistic study of traditional Chinese medicine. *Biochem. Soc. Trans.*, 39: 1348–1352.

Loudon, I. 1997. *Western Medicine: An Illustrated History*. Oxford University Press, Oxford, UK, 1997.

Mullard, A. 2012. FDA drug approvals. *Nat. Rev. Drug Discov.*, 11: 91–94.

Patwardhan, B., Mutalik, G., and Tillu, G. 2015. *Integrative Approaches for Health*. Academic Press, Amsterdam, the Netherlands.

Patwardhan, B., Vaidya, A., and Chorghade, M. 2004. Ayurveda and natural products drug discovery. *Curr. Sci.*, 86: 789–799.

Peng, T. 2011. Where West meets East. *Nature*, 480: S84–S86.

Powell, B.L. 2011. Arsenic trioxide in acute promyelocytic leukemia: Potion not poison. *Expert Rev. Anticancer Ther.*, 11: 1317–1319.

Qiu, J. 2007. China plans to modernize traditional medicine. *Nature*, 446: 590–591.

Sharma, P.V. 1994. *Caraka Samhita* (English translation). Chaukhambia Orientalia, Delhi, India.

Stone, R. 2008. Biochemistry: Lifting the veil on traditional Chinese medicine. *Science*, 319: 709–710.

Strohl, W.R. 2005. The role of natural products in a modern drug discovery program. *Drug Discov. Today*, 5: 39–41.

Valiathan, M.S. 2003. *The Legacy of Caraka*. Orient Longman, Chennai, India.

van der Greef, J., van Wietmarschen, H., Schroen, J., Wang, M., Hankemeier, T., and Xu, G. 2010. Systems biology-based diagnostic principles as pillars of the bridge between Chinese and Western medicine. *Planta Med.*, 76: 2036–2047.

Wang, L., Zhou, G.B., Liu, P. et al. 2008. Dissection of mechanisms of Chinese medicinal formula *Realgar-Indigo naturalis* as an effective treatment for promyelocytic leukemia. *Proc. Natl. Acad. Sci. USA*, 105: 4826–4831.

Wang, X., Sun, H., Zhang, A. et al. 2011. Potential role of metabolomic approaches in the area of traditional Chinese medicine: As pillars of the bridge between Chinese and Western medicine. *J. Pharm. Biomed. Anal.*, 55: 859–868.

Xie, G., Ye, M., Wanget, Y. et al. 2009. Characterization of pu-erh tea using chemical and metabolic profiling approaches. *J. Agric. Food Chem.*, 57: 3046–3054.

Xu, Z. 2011. One step at a time. *Nature*, 480: S90–S92.

Yan, X. and Liu, C. 2008. High content screening analysis for systematic study on traditional Chinese medicine. *Chin. Tradit. Herb. Drugs*, 39: 1121–1124.

Zhang, B.L. and Wang, Y.Y. 2005. The fundamental study on critical scientific problem of prescriptions—Research and development modern Chinese medicines via the combination of standardized constituents. *Chin. J. Nat. Med.*, 3: 258–261.

Zhu, Y., Zhang, Z., Zhang, M. et al. 2010. High-throughput screening for bioactive components from traditional Chinese medicine. *Comb. Chem. High Throughput Screen.*, 13: 837–848.

Section II

Quality–Safety–Efficacy:
Three Mantras

5 Drug–Nutrient Interactions

Their Role in Clinical Outcomes

Dilip Ghosh

CONTENTS

INTRODUCTION

Drugs and nutrients share an intricate relationship in human health. Drug therapy and dietary interventions often have a complementary effect on disease prevention and therapy (Chan, 2013). In many disease states, such as hypertension, hyperlipidemia, and metabolic disorders, dietary interventions play a key role in the overall therapeutic strategy. The treatment effect is augmented by the addition of pharmacotherapy. However, in some other cases, pharmacotherapy can have a negative impact on nutrient homeostasis.

It is well established that chronic use of proton pump inhibitors to decrease gastric acid secretion may impair intestinal absorption of cobalamin, leading to anemia (McColl, 2009). Another common example is enzyme-inducing antiepileptic drugs such as carbamazepine and phenytoin that may decrease serum vitamin D concentration by increasing the metabolism of vitamin D (Lee et al., 2010). The opposite effect can also happen—changes in nutrient intake can significantly alter a patient's response to a drug. The ideal example is the relationship between vitamin K intake and the dose requirement for the anticoagulant warfarin to maintain an optimal level of anticoagulation.

The relationship between affected drugs and nutrients can be further confounded by other variables such as the route of administration, health status of the patients, end-organ function, environmental factors, and genetics (Chan, 2006). These complex interrelationships between nutrient intake and the efficacy and safety of a drug form the basis of drug–nutrient interaction research.

Diet and nutrition can have a profound effect on the therapeutic and toxic outcome of drug treatment. Conversely, drugs may induce sufficient alterations in appetite and nutritional status to produce symptoms of nutrient deficiency. In reality, clinicians frequently overlook drug–nutrient interactions as a cause of adverse drug reactions (Boullata and Hudson, 2012).

AN EVOLVING DEFINITION

A drug–nutrient interaction is defined as a physical, chemical, physiologic, or pathophysiologic relationship between a drug and a nutrient (Conner, 2005). Clinicians need more accurate predictions of the incidence and severity of drug–nutrient interactions with similar compounds, which are based on the knowledge of the mechanisms. Because we are constantly exposed to nutrients through diet, the potential for a drug–nutrient interaction is always high whenever a drug is taken by a patient. We are discussing here the drug–nutrient interaction of clinical significance that are associated with an altered physiologic response, which may lead to malnutrition, treatment failure, adverse events, or, in the most serious case, a life-threatening event, including death.

This interaction from clinical perspective raises the concern and significance that are often associated with a quantifiable alteration of the kinetic and/or dynamic profile of a drug or a nutrient. The term "kinetics" (pharmacokinetics, nutrikinetics) refers to the quantitative description of the disposition of a drug or nutrient in the human body. The kinetic profile of a target compound is usually characterized by comparing several quantifiable parameters at absorption, distribution, metabolism, and excretion levels. Physiologic half-life refers to the time it takes for the concentration (usually in the plasma) of a specific compound to reduce by one-half. This parameter is most useful as an estimate for the time it takes for a drug or nutrient to be eliminated from the body. It is also one of the parameters used to calculate the elimination rate (i.e., clearance). Bioavailability refers to the fraction of the drug or nutrient administered that becomes available to the systemic circulation in the body. By definition, intravenous administration provides 100% bioavailability.

Enteral (EN) route administration often produces lower bioavailability due to incomplete absorption or loss of the active component during the absorption phase. The rate of absorption for a particular compound can be estimated by the time taken to achieve peak plasma concentration (t_{max}). For drugs administered orally, t_{max} may provide a reasonable estimation of intestinal transit time. Finally, the area under the time-concentration curve is used to reflect the overall exposure of a drug or a nutrient by the patient during a defined period. It is affected by oral bioavailability, clearance, and, in some cases, the rate of absorption. The term "dynamics" (pharmacodynamics, nutridynamics) refers to the clinical or physiologic effects of a drug or nutrient. The mechanism of dynamic interactions often involves antagonism of the drug and nutrient at the site of action. For example, the interaction between vitamin K and warfarin can be described as a pharmacodynamic interaction as both compounds act on the clotting cascade—specifically, the enzyme vitamin K epoxide reductase (Jin et al., 2007). A precipitant agent is the drug or nutrient that causes the interaction. An interaction can be introduced by several processes: (1) the addition of a drug or nutrient, (2) the removal of a drug or nutrient from an established regimen, and (3) changing the dose of a drug or nutrient that has been administered at a stable dose for a long time. An object agent refers to the drug or the nutrient that is affected by the interaction after the introduction of the precipitant agent.

DRUG–NUTRIENT INTERACTIONS: AN OVERVIEW

Drug–nutrient interactions can be broadly classified in two categories: Direct physicochemical interaction and physiological or functional interaction. Drug–nutrient interactions can also be classified according to the site of their occurrence: within the food matrix, in the gastrointestinal tract, or during transport, metabolism, and excretion. The mechanisms and sites of drug–nutrient interactions are listed in Table 5.1.

Drug Effects on Nutritional Status

The influence of drugs on the status of a specific nutrient can also be multifactorial (Lombardi et al., 2010). Drugs can influence nutrient absorption, distribution, metabolism, and excretion. The clinical significance of changes in nutrient status as a result of drug use is based in part on the relevance of individual biomarkers. The clinical manifestations are as much patient-specific as drug-specific in relation to the change of biomarkers. Researchers are not expecting any extreme nutrient deficiency syndrome due to this interaction but lesser degree of deficit may be associated with clinical manifestations.

The concept of drug effects on nutritional status is not new. For example, the ability of carbamazepine to alter biotin status by decreasing absorption and increasing

TABLE 5.1
Mechanism and Location of Drug–Nutrient Interactions

Location	Mechanism	Clinical Effect
Food matrix	Binding and chelation	Decreases bioavailability
Gastrointestinal (GI) tract	Change in GI motility	Transit time increase reduces absorption
	Binding and chelation	Decreases bioavailability
	Change in bile acid concentration	Reduces absorption of fat soluble nutrients
	Gastric pH	Affects absorption of iron, vitamin B_{12}, and others
Circulation	Albumin concentration	Decreases transport of bound substances
	Competitive binding	Displaces albumin-bound nutrients
Target tissues	Antagonistic effect	May increase requirements for antagonized nutrients
	Enzyme activation	Reduces concentration of enzyme products
Excretion	Renal function	Lower nutrient levels and increases requirements
	Sequestration	Lower nutrient levels and increases requirements

clearance may account for some of the idiosyncratic adverse effects observed with this antiepileptic. A number of the antiepileptic medications adversely affect vitamin D metabolism and bone health (Verrotti et al., 2010). Valproic acid treatment is associated with carnitine deficiency and altered acylcarnitine subspecies that reflect impaired intermediary metabolism likely responsible for drug-induced hepatotoxicity and hyperammonemia (Werner et al., 2007). But in most of the cases, the influence on the status of a nutrient in these circumstances may or may not be adequately addressed by nutrient supplementation while the patient is taking the drug (Venhoff et al., 2002). For prophylactic nutrient supplementation for disease control, this is an area that requires more investigation to support doctor's recommendations. Conversely, there are some medication regimens that are associated with improvements in nutrient status (Drain et al., 2007). In order for clinicians to recognize, identify, prevent, or manage drug–nutrient interactions that have the potential to influence patient outcomes, a more systematic approach is necessary.

THE EFFECTS OF FOOD ON DRUG THERAPY

Oral drug administration concurrent with a diet or nutrient can alter the physico-chemical conditions within the gastrointestinal tract and may influence the rate or extent of drug absorption. A change in the extent of absorption is more clinically significant than a change in the rate of absorption because it influences bioavailability and varies with drug properties and nutrient characteristics.

Specific foods can also have a unique influence on drug disposition. Several *in vitro* and *in vivo* studies have demonstrated the possible mechanisms of these interactions. Dietary proteins as well as protein supplements have been known to increase drug metabolism (Anderson, 2010). Protein sources (e.g., soy protein isolate, casein) may have differential effects on drug disposition through induction of enzymes and transporters (Ronis et al., 2011). Several juices interact with medications by altering transporters and metabolizing enzymes to a wider degree than initially described. Grapefruit juice was the first to be identified, but others have also been shown to interact with medication based on furanocoumarin and flavonoid content (Greenblatt, 2009). Furanocoumarins appear to inhibit intestinal CYP3A isoenzymes, thereby increasing oral drug bioavailability, but can also interfere with transporters. Among the many different constituents of common berries, the anthocyanins and anthocyanidins interact with a CYP isoenzyme and transporter *in vitro* (Dreiseitel et al., 2009). The higher concentrations of isolated flavonoids and other phytochemicals found in dietary supplement products may be more cause for concern in terms of drug–nutrient interaction as well as toxicity. Their potential to interact with drug substrate of these enzymes and transporters may be greater.

PATIENT POPULATIONS AT RISK FOR ADVERSE EVENTS
ASSOCIATED WITH DRUG–NUTRIENT INTERACTIONS

There is a common belief that polypharmacy (i.e., using multiple drugs to manage different disease states) increases the risk for drug–nutrient interactions in a patient

(Salazar et al., 2007). Patients with underlying nutrient deficiencies are especially at risk of developing adverse events associated with drug–nutrient interactions. In addition, patients with multiple comorbidities or with decreased physiologic reserve are also at increased risk of experiencing adverse events. The most susceptible patients include critically ill patients—especially those who receive continuous Enteral (EN) feeding, elderly patients, and those who are obese, frail, severely malnourished, or with underlying intestinal dysfunction.

Special attention should also be paid to patients receiving EN or Parenteral (PN) support since they are at an increased risk of experiencing type I interactions. Genetics is also an important factor in determining the dose, clinical response, and threshold of interaction for a particular drug or nutrient. The significance of genetic polymorphism on drug and nutrient response is well demonstrated by the revised dosing algorithm for warfarin based on the patient's CYP2C9 and VKORC1 genotypes (Pavani et al., 2012).

Clinical Approaches toward Drug–Nutrient Interactions

For the majority of patients, most drug–nutrient interactions would not lead to an acute clinical event within days, even in the absence of an immediate intervention. This is because, with the exception of a few known drug–nutrient combinations (e.g., warfarin and vitamin K, tyramine and monoamine oxidase inhibitors), the clinical effects of most drug–nutrient interactions gradually develop over time. Interactions with a short duration rarely result in very substantial changes (e.g., >20% change from baseline) in the kinetic, dynamic, or physiologic parameters in a short period. Even if some detectable physiologic changes are present (e.g., mild changes to micronutrient status, some change in the absorption profile of a drug), most patients who are not in the high-risk categories as discussed earlier have adequate physiologic compensation to minimize the likelihood of developing adverse events. The most logical next step is to evaluate the duration of the interaction, as well as the clinical likelihood and significance of the interaction over time. Factors to be taken into account in determining the likelihood and severity of interactions include the timing and the duration of the interaction, the dose involved (if there is an established dose–response relationship between the interaction pair), whether the drug or the nutrient has a relatively narrow therapeutic window, and the time of onset and severity of the symptoms associated with supra-therapeutic/sub-therapeutic effect (Pavani et al., 2012). Drugs or nutrients that modulate the activities of metabolic enzymes or transporters, especially type IIa and IIb interactions, are more likely to cause clinically significant interactions since the change in the overall exposure of the drug–nutrient from the interaction is usually more significant than from other types of interactions. Some drug–nutrient interactions may take a long time before any symptom can be detected. For example, it will take at least a few months for patients with acid reduction therapy–associated malabsorption of iron or cobalamin to develop signs and symptoms, such as anemia, shortness of breath, and peripheral numbness (Hirschowitz et al., 2008). Similarly, vitamin D deficiency associated with the use of enzyme-inducing antiepileptic drugs takes months to years before the patient shows symptoms associated with metabolic bone disease (Menon and Harinarayan, 2010). It is therefore important to identify the surrogate markers that are specific to the clinical end point for monitoring before the patient develops disease-related symptoms. If a disease-specific surrogate marker is not available, longitudinal therapeutic monitoring of serum drug concentration or nutrient status may be necessary. The monitoring plan should be strategic, practical, end point specific, and continued as long as the risk of disease development does not exist, so that any possible signs associated with the drug–nutrient interactions can be detected at the earliest possible time.

However, if the patient belongs to the high-risk category in developing an adverse event, a relatively small change to his or her physiologic parameters may be enough to cause harm.

Although the thought process discussed earlier is still valid, early interventions may be necessary if signs and symptoms of an adverse event are suspected. The interventions may include an empirical administration of a nutrient in the event of suspected nutrient deficiency or withholding a drug in a suspected case of drug toxicity due to a drug–nutrient interaction. For example, if valproic acid–associated carnitine deficiency is highly suspected in a patient with established nutrition-associated risk factors who has been admitted to the intensive care unit with acute onset of mental status changes and hyperammonemia, it may be reasonable to start carnitine replacement therapy as soon as the blood sample has been taken for the evaluation of carnitine status. If monitoring alone is insufficient, and a change to the existing therapeutic regimen is preferred to minimize the impact of the drug–nutrient interaction, the options may include: (1) using alternative agent(s) over the interacting agent(s), (2) adjusting the dose of the object agent, (3) supplementing the object agent to replace the deficiency, (4) or using a combination of these methods. It is important to remember that drug–nutrient interaction does not always apply to the entire drug class because even a slight change in the chemical structure of a drug or nutrient may be enough to alter its binding and interaction with receptors, transporters, enzymes, and other small molecules. In many cases, an alternative drug in the same therapeutic class can be used. For example, divalent cations, dairy products, and food in general cause a type IIC interaction in the antimicrobial agents ciprofloxacin and ofloxacin. But this interaction is not observed with levofloxacin, which may be a better drug of choice for certain infections than other quinolone antibiotics in a patient receiving continuous enteral feeding (Mueller et al., 1994). Some drug–nutrient interactions, especially type I and type IIA interactions, can also be avoided by changing the route of administration. Understanding the specific mechanism of the drug–nutrient interaction can be very useful in developing an effective management strategy.

MAJOR DRUG–NUTRIENT INTERACTIONS OF CLINICAL RELEVANCE

Table 5.2 provides information on the major drug–nutrient interactions of clinical relevance (Mason, 2010). The list reflects well-known interactions of drugs that have been on the market for some time. The U.S. Food and Drug Administration (FDA) maintains an online database of recently reported interactions, as well as new drugs.

TABLE 5.2

Major Clinically Relevant Drug–Nutrient Interactions

Drug	Class	Food/Nutrient	Clinical Effect
Acarbose	Antidiabetic	Food	Delays carbohydrate breakdown and glucose absorption
Acetaminophen	Analgesic	Food	May delay extended release
Amoxicillin	Antibiotic	Food	Decreases absorption by delaying gastric emptying
Aspirin	Analgesic	Food, alcohol, curry powder	Decreases rate of absorption, gastric irritation, potential salicylate accumulation
Benzodiazepines	Anticonvulsant	Nutrient	Enhances CNS depression
Calcium carbonate	Antacid	Iron, fats	Decreases iron absorption, may cause steatorrhea
Cephalosporin	Antibiotic	Alcohol, food	Flushing, headache, nausea, vomiting, decreased rate of absorption
Chloramphenicol	Antibiotic	Iron, folic acid	Increases serum iron levels, antagonist to physiological action
Chloroquine	Antimalarial	Food	Increases bioavailability
Ciprofloxacin	Antibiotic	Caffeine, food	Decreases rate of absorption and elimination of caffeine
Codeine	Narcotic, analgesic	Alcohol, glucose	Enhances CNS effect, can cause hyperglycemia
Corticosteroid	Steroid	Calcium, phosphorus	Decreases absorption of Ca and P, and increases urinary excretion
Cyclosporine	Antirejection	Milk, fat, pineapple juice	Increases absorption
Diazepam	Anticonvulsant	Food	Increases absorption by delayed gastric emptying
Erythromycin	Antibiotic	Food	Increases absorption by delayed gastric emptying
Glipizide	Antidiabetic	Food, alcohol	Delays absorption and flushing, headache, nausea, vomiting, decreases rate of absorption
Ibuprofen	NSAID	Food (milk)	Decreases absorption
Levodopa	Anti-Parkinson	Food	Decreases absorption
Metronidazole	Antibiotic	Alcohol	Flushing, headache, nausea, vomiting, decreases rate of absorption
Nifedepine	Antihypertensive	Grapefruit juice	Increases serum level of Nifedepine
Oral contraceptives	Antiemetic	Food, vitamins, and minerals	Increases absorption, hypokalemia

(Continued)

TABLE 5.2 (*Continued*)

Major Clinically Relevant Drug–Nutrient Interactions

Drug	Class	Food/Nutrient	Clinical Effect
Salicylates	Analgesic	Iron, vitamin C	Decreases serum iron and vitamin C
Tetracycline	Antibiotic	Food, minerals, vitamins	Decreases absorption, increases urinary loss
Trimethoprim	Antibiotic	Folic acid	Decreases serum folate levels
Warfarin	Anticoagulant	Alcohol, vitamins	Inhibits warfarin metabolism and inhibits anticoagulant effects

The database can be accessed at www.fda.gov. Interested readers can also access the following databases for more information:

- http://www.drugs.com/drug_interactions.html
- http://naturaldatabase.therapeuticresearch.com/home.aspx?cs=&s=ND
- http://reference.medscape.com/drug-interactionchecker
- https://naturalmedicines.therapeuticresearch.com/

CONCLUSION

Currently, the data that guide the clinical management of most drug–nutrient interactions are mostly anecdotal experience, uncontrolled observations, and opinions. Well-controlled comparative trials with defined clinical outcomes that compare different management approaches are lacking. More importantly, carefully designed scientific research aimed at exploring and evaluating the specific mechanism of drug–nutrient interactions is extremely rare. Thus, there is a need to bridge this gap between the science and practice of drug–nutrient interactions through research.

It is hoped that the following recommendations will provide ideas for researchers and clinicians in the field to take the first few steps in achieving this goal:

- Developing a common language and concept in the understanding, evaluation, and management of drug–nutrient interactions.
- Research focusing on understanding the mechanisms of drug–nutrient interactions.
- Population- and gene-based research to compare incidence and risk factors of specific drug–nutrient interactions.
- Outcomes research that addresses the short-term and long-term clinical significance and economic impact of specific drug–nutrient interactions.

REFERENCES

Anderson, K.E. 2010. Effects of specific foods and dietary components on drug metabolism. In Boullata, J.I., Armenti, V.T., eds., *Handbook of Drug-Nutrient Interactions*, 2nd edn., pp. 243–265. Humana Press, New York.

Boullata, J.I. and Hudson, L.M. 2012. Drug–nutrient interactions: A broad view with implications for practice. *J. Acad. Nutr. Diet.*, 112: 506–516.

Chan, L.N. 2006. Drug-nutrient interactions. In Shils, M.E., Shike, M., Olson, J.A., eds., *Modern Nutrition in Health and Disease*, 10th edn., pp. 1539–1553. Lippincott Williams & Wilkins, Philadelphia, PA.

Chan, L.N. 2013. Drug–nutrient interactions. *J. Parenter. Enteral Nutr.*, 37: 450–459.

Conner, K.G. 2005. *Drug–Nutrient Interactions*, pp. 38–49. Elsevier, Amsterdam, the Netherlands.

Drain, P.K., Kupka, R., Mugusi, F. et al. 2007. Micronutrients in HIV positive persons receiving highly active antiretroviral therapy. *Am. J. Clin. Nutr.*, 85: 333–345.

Dreiseitel, A., Oosterhuis, B., Vukman, K.V. et al. 2009. Berry anthocyanins and anthocyanidins exhibit distinct affinities for the efflux transporters BCRP and MDR1. *Br. J. Pharmacol.*, 158: 1942–1950.

Greenblatt, D.J. 2009. Analysis of drug interactions involving fruit beverages and organic anion-transporting polypeptides. *J. Clin. Pharmacol.*, 49: 1403–1407.

Hirschowitz, B.I., Worthington, J., and Mohnen, J. 2008. Vitamin B_{12} deficiency in hypersecretors during long-term acid suppression with proton pump inhibitors. *Aliment. Pharmacol. Ther.*, 27: 1110–1121.

Jin, D.Y., Tie, J.K., and Stafford, D.W. 2007. The conversion of vitamin K epoxide to vitamin K quinone and vitamin K quinone to vitamin K hydroquinone uses the same active site cysteines. *Biochemistry*, 46: 7279–7283.

Lee, R.H., Lyles, K.W., and Colón-Emeric, C. 2010. A review of the effect of anticonvulsant medications on bone mineral density and fracture risk. *Am. J. Geriatr. Pharmacother.*, 8: 34–46.

Lombardi, L.R., Kreys, E., Gerry, S. et al. 2010. Nutrition in the age of polypharmacy. In Bendich, A., Deckelbaum, R.J., eds., *Preventive Nutrition*, 4th edn., pp. 79–125. Humana Press, New York.

Mason, P. 2010. Drugs and nutrition: Important drug–nutrient interactions. *Proc. Nutr. Soc.*, 69: 551–557.

McColl, K.E. 2009. Effect of proton pump inhibitors on vitamins and iron. *Am. J. Gastroenterol.*, 104 (Suppl. 2): S5–S9.

Menon, B. and Harinarayan, C.V. 2010. The effect of anti epileptic drug therapy on serum 25-hydroxyvitamin D and parameters of calcium and bone metabolism—A longitudinal study. *Seizure*, 19: 153–158.

Mueller, B.A., Brierton, D.G., Abel, S.R. et al. 1994. Effect of enteral feeding with Ensure on oral bioavailabilities of ofloxacin and ciprofloxacin. *Antimicrob. Agents Chemother.*, 38: 2101–2105.

Pavani, A., Naushad, S.M., Rupasree, Y. et al. 2012. Optimization of warfarin dose by population-specific pharmacogenomic algorithm. *Pharmacogenomics J.*, 12: 306–311.

Ronis, M.J.J., Chen, Y., Liu, X. et al. 2011. Enhanced expression and glucocorticoid-inducibility of hepatic cytochrome P450 3A involve recruitment of the pregnane-X-receptor promoter elements in rats fed soy protein isolate. *J. Nutr.*, 141: 10–16.

Salazar, J.A., Poon, I., and Nair, M. 2007. Clinical consequences of polypharmacy in elderly: Expect the unexpected, think the unthinkable. *Expert Opin. Drug Saf.*, 6: 695–704.

Venhoff, N., Setzer, B., Lebrecht, D. et al. 2002. Dietary supplements in the treatment of nucleoside reverse transcriptase inhibitor-related mitochondrial toxicity. *AIDS*, 16: 800–802.

Verrotti, A., Coppola, G., Parisi, P. et al. 2010. Bone and calcium metabolism and antiepileptic drugs. *Clin. Neurol. Neurosurg.*, 112: 1–10.

Werner, T., Treiss, I., Kohlmueller, D. et al. 2007. Effects of valproate on acylcarnitines in children with epilepsy using ESI-MS/MS. *Epilepsia*, 48: 72–76.

6 Existing and Innovative Models of Health and Disease
Elaborating on Foods versus Drugs

R. B. Smarta

CONTENTS

INTRODUCTION

A model is a theoretical way of understanding a concept. In the case of complex concepts such as health and illness, models provide various ways of approaching them. Models are used to understand the relationship between these concepts and an individual's attitude toward health and health practices.

Studying and/or the implementation of these health and disease/illness models would help healthcare professionals to provide better care by understanding their behaviors and the concepts related to health and adapting care to those of different ethnicities and cultures. Health models help us understand and act as tools for evaluating the impact of health interventions and policies at the population level.

Due to urbanization, today in any country, the population is quite diverse, so healthcare professionals are required to address and communicate to them differently. Understanding various aspects such as the pattern of a disease/illness affecting a particular sect of people, their prevention, its management by the people makes it easier for healthcare providers to better negotiate and communicate with their patients. Over the years, it has been observed that the trust between physicians and patients is dissolving.

This, along with the upsurge in technology in healthcare, has driven the medical system even further toward a "disease-based" approach to healthcare that views individuals as "cases" and underrates the sociocultural and humanistic aspects of patient care.

PREVIOUSLY ESTABLISHED MODELS

Various health and healthcare models were established as early as the 1950s. These models served the purpose of defining health, understanding the level of penetration of health-related policies and schemes among populations, understanding the nature of participation of those in healthcare programs, and so forth.

In the early 1950s, three basic types of models were established, the Health–Illness Continuum Model, the Health Belief Model, and the Revised Health Promotion Model. Each of the models was established for a different purpose.

THE HEALTH–ILLNESS CONTINUUM MODEL

This model considers health as a fluctuating dynamic state that changes as a person adapts to the changes in the internal or external environment in order to maintain a state of well-being, and illness is considered a process in which functioning of a person is diminished or impaired when compared with his/her previous condition. This model is one way to measure a person's level of health. High levels of wellness and severe illness or death are placed at the opposite ends of the healthcare continuum, hence the name health–illness continuum model, and normal health is at the center of the model (Figure 6.1).

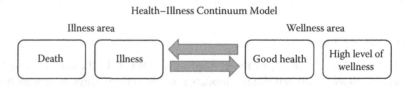

FIGURE 6.1   Health–illness continuum model. (Adapted from Milani, R.V. and Lavie, C.J., *Am. J. Med.*, 128, 337, 2015.)

THE HEALTH BELIEF MODEL

The health belief model relates to what people believe or perceive about their health and their actual condition. This model was initially developed to study the nonparticipation of people in health-screening programs and was later modified to address compliance to a therapeutic regimen. The model is built on the premise that disease prevention and curing regimens will eventually be successful and the belief that health is highly valued. Both premises need to be present in the model to be relevant in explaining healthy behavior (Martin et al., 2005).

This model is based on three aspects of a person's perception of disease:

Person's perceived susceptibility to disease: It is a person's belief that he/she will contract a disease (after exhibiting a particular type of behavior) or the complete denial of a person that he/she will contract a disease (after exhibiting a particular type of behavior).

Person's perceived seriousness of the disease: This is concerned with how much a person considers a disease seriously and weighs its further detrimental effects to take necessary action for reducing further damage.

Person's perceived benefits of the actions: This is with respect to the person's belief in the effectiveness of the measures for preventing illness. This factor is influenced by the following: (1) Faith of the person in carrying out a recommended action will prevent or modify the disease. (2) The person's perception of the cost and unpleasant effects of performing the healthy behavior.

THE REVISED HEALTH PROMOTION MODEL

The revised health promotion model is based on two components:

1. *Individual characteristics and experiences*: It can be helpful in predicting if an individual will incorporate and use health-related behaviors. If a behavior has become a habit, then it is more likely to be used again.
2. *Behavior-specific knowledge and beliefs*: These involve the belief that there will be a positive outcome from a specific health behavior, that one has the skill and competence to engage in healthy behaviors, and that one is affected by the interpersonal influences of others (especially family, peers, and healthcare providers).

Although this model has been mostly used in nursing, its components can be used to design and provide nursing interventions to promote health for individuals, families, and communities. The model describes major components and variables that influence health-promoting behaviors. The emphasis is given more to actualization of health potential and an increase in the level of well-being rather than avoidance of disease. The model has three major components of individual characteristics and experiences, behavior-specific cognition and affect, and behavioral outcome.

EXISTING AND FUTURE HEALTHCARE MODELS FOR CHRONIC DISEASES

Over the years, life expectancy has increased due to advancements in healthcare but this increase in life expectancy cannot be considered an indicator of the health status of people. In recent times due to lifestyle changes, there has been an increase in number of people getting affected by chronic diseases. According to WHO, The World Health Report 2002, chronic diseases, such as chronic diseases, such as heart disease, stroke, cancer, chronic respiratory diseases, and diabetes, have become the leading causes of mortality in the world, representing 60% of all deaths and 43% of the global burden of disease. By 2020, their contribution is expected to rise to 73% of all deaths and 60% of the global burden of disease. Moreover, 79% of the deaths attributed to these diseases occur in the developing countries. The most prominent chronic diseases are cardiovascular diseases (CVD), cancer, chronic obstructive pulmonary disease, and type 2 diabetes. Prevention of these major chronic diseases should focus on controlling the key risk factors in a well-integrated manner. Researchers suggest that existing healthcare delivery models are poorly constructed to manage chronic disease, and that reengineering of the healthcare system might offer some hope in meeting this challenge.

TRADITIONAL HEALTHCARE MODELS FOR CHRONIC DISEASES

The traditional delivery model (Figure 6.2) does not provide a holistic approach to the management of chronic diseases. The model shows less control on chronic conditions that can be treated and has a low adherence to quality indicators. There is

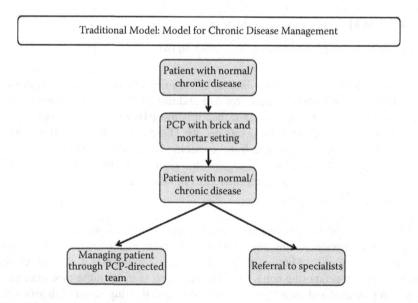

FIGURE 6.2 Traditional model for chronic disease management. (Adapted from Milani, R.V. and Lavie, C.J., *Am. J. Med.*, 128, 337, 2015.)

an emergence of various new healthcare technologies for the treatment of chronic diseases. The traditional model needs to be modified to include the new and innovative technologies in order to make it more patient-centric, having a focus on holistic patient care.

INNOVATIVE AND FUTURISTIC HEALTHCARE MODELS FOR CHRONIC DISEASES

The number of patients with chronic diseases is expected to increase in the next 4–5 years. Thus, it is essential to discover and put to use such model that overcomes the drawbacks of the traditional model for the treatment of chronic diseases. Over the years, there has been an advent in new technologies in healthcare delivery and systems. These new technologies should be incorporated in healthcare model so as to engage the patients and provide them value-based treatment/care.

The futuristic model suggested by Milani and Lavie (illustrated earlier) considers the care required for chronic disease patients in a more holistic way. This model consists of specialized Integrated Practice Units (IPUs), which organize and engage a nonphysician personnel such as pharmacists, clinicians, nurses, health educators, dietitians, and social workers around the patient's medical condition (Figure 6.3). They have also noted that social network influences have had a considerable positive impact on behaviors associated with ill habits and that social media can support successful disease management strategies that utilize the potential of social networks and these may provide a sustainable and cost-effective solution for patients with chronic diseases.

It has been observed that a physician alone is unable to cope with the necessities of superior, value- and evidenced-based care, which would yield effective changes in lifestyle and behavior of the patient. The model also involves self-monitoring, as per

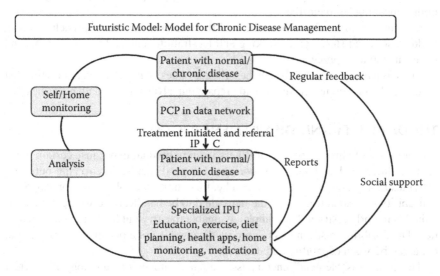

FIGURE 6.3 Futuristic disease model for chronic disease management.

the patient's own convenience, treatment, and referral-initiated Integrated Primary Care (IPC); also, during the treatment, regular feedback and reports by the IPUs and Patient Care Physician (PCP) will be provided to the patient.

According to Milani and Lavie, the model of team-based care with specialized IPUs will have the ability to deliver complete and consistent treatment as the IPUs will employ latest technologies for the better engagement of patients, in addition to providing personalized care delivery.

WHY DOES A TRADITIONAL DISEASE-BASED MODEL FAIL?

There have been many observations that a traditional disease-based model is insufficient for total patient care. In today's situations where people are aware and willing to become healthy in a holistic way rather than just treating diseases, we need a model that can address total healthcare. In the traditional model, the focus is mainly on the disease and its treatment through medications or therapies; the physicians focus on the disease and use their understanding of medicine and science to devise a plan for treatment or healthcare management. It is essential to understand the difference between a disease and illness. Disease is the pathophysiological condition, whereas illness takes into consideration many aspects related to a person, that is, physical, psychological, cultural, and social aspect. Since illness takes into consideration all aspects, physicians need to look at illness rather than just disease when planning treatment or care. For this, we need to have a patient-centric model that focuses on the patient and then the disease. People rationalize their illness experience through a complex web of personal experiences and belief systems ingrained in their cultural and social worlds. Individuals develop a personal (or adopt an existing) "explanatory model" that represents their personal conceptualization of the cause, course, and consequences of their illness. Work by medical anthropologists, sociologists, and others have paved the way for physicians to effectively "explore patient" explanatory models or the "meaning" of their illness.

Communicating and exploring beyond the standard medical approach can help build trust, avoid stereotypic thinking and frustration, and lead to an effective and honest negotiation process.

There is a requirement to change the attitude, values, and communication skills that focus on illness, not just the disease, to prepare ourselves for the challenges ahead.

THE DISABILITY AND DISABLEMENT PROCESS

The presence of chronic disease or illness in an individual may cause certain types of disabilities or disablement. *Disability* refers to difficulty in carrying out daily activities in any domain of life due to a health condition or physical problem. Such a disability may sometimes lead the individual to be handicapped wherein the individual is majorly restricted or completely unable to carry out his or her daily activities. The disability resulting from chronic diseases is not a personal characteristic, but a gap between capability and demand.

The term "disablement" encompasses all magnitudes of pathology that affect functioning. The term illustrates the effects on the functioning of an individual's body systems, day-to-day activities including physical and mental actions, as a result of chronic and acute conditions and suggests the factors that affect disablement. This disability and disablement process and models have been explained by Louis Verbrugge in the late 1980s in his various research papers.

THE BIOMEDICAL MODEL

The biomedical model is based on the concept of disease with the sequence of etiology → pathology → manifestation (Minaire, WHO, 1992). Research indicates that this biomedical model is defined not only by negative anatomical, biochemical, and physiological variables is also defined by physical, cultural, and social factors. It needs to be taken into consideration that certain variables related to disease are of prospective value for the assessment of the disablement process (Minaire, WHO, 1992). Diagnosis and lesions, symptoms, and other related indicators (physiological and economic) are useful biomedical variables that have been identified.

THE INTERNATIONAL CLASSIFICATION OF IMPAIRMENTS, DISABILITIES, AND HANDICAPS MODEL

The International Classification of Impairments, Disabilities, and Handicaps (ICIDH) were presented by WHO in 1980 (Minaire, WHO, 1992). It supported the identification of the consequences of diseases. The ICIDH model provides a common "language" that also acts as a main advantage because of the resolute shift away from the biomedical model. It also proves as an efficient teaching instrument. It is useful for prevention and planning and applicable to population surveys and samples. The ICIDH model avoids the partitioning between the medical and social consequences of the disease.

THE SITUATIONAL HANDICAP MODEL

Disablements and handicaps are a result of a diminished or complete gap between the capability and environmental demand. This model infers the integration of an individual into the environment and vis-a-vis through the concept of a situation where individual experiences are differentiated. On the other hand, it would be inappropriate and even dangerous to rely on situational experience alone for reducing the process of disablement and ignoring other factors such as the biomedical and psychological history of individual.

THE QUALITY-OF-LIFE MODEL

The quality-of-life model is based on two conceptual frameworks, namely, the ICIDH model that sees the quality of life closely related to the dimension of handicap and the concentric series of circles that determine the successive stages from disease in the center to personal functioning, psychological status, general health perception, and social or role functioning. The interrelationship between global assessment of quality of life and separate assessments of components of quality of life proves to be a difficulty in this model.

HEALTHCARE SYSTEM MODELS

The healthcare system models are mainly based on the mode and type of delivery of healthcare and funding.

THE PATIENT-CENTRIC CARE MODEL

Establishing a patient-centric model or total care model would be apt in these changing times where the patient is no longer only concerned about his/her health but more concerned about prevention and overall wellness. The patient-centric model or total care model could define the future for healthcare system.

Any existing healthcare system or model can be transformed into a patient-centric care environment or model (model for payment). The main aspect in transforming would be the shift of focus on type of care i.e. from the existing "reactive care" to "proactive care." In reactive care, the patient is diagnosed and treated as per his/her illness or symptoms presented by the patient, the overall health and wellness of the patient is secondary concern, whereas in proactive care, healthcare providers initiate a conversation with the patient and identify the health concerns rather than just focusing on the symptoms or disease. In this way, depending on the situation, an intervention that aims at the wellness of the patient is designed by the healthcare provider.

The focus today is on total healthcare. Traditional medicine can help in both the cure and prevention of diseases. Modern medicine comes into the picture for treating diseases when they progress to the acute state. Thus, total healthcare depends on working of all the above factors involved in tune with each other (Figure 6.4).

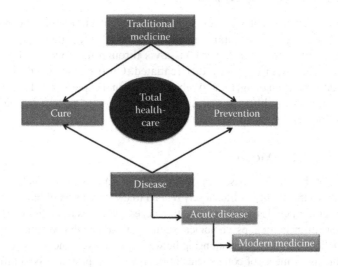

FIGURE 6.4   The total healthcare model. (From Interlink Knowledge Cell.)

MODELS FOR HEALTH MAINTENANCE AND HEALTH PROMOTION

THE HOLISTIC HEALTHCARE MODEL

Every model lacks in one or more aspects. One way to overcome or address these downfalls of individual models, is to introduce a model that takes into consideration the relationship between health and disease, wherein health goes beyond the criteria of absence of disease. We need a model or an approach that considers whole body wellness instead of treatment of a single disease.

The WHO defines health as "a state of complete physical, mental, and social well-being, and not merely the absence of disease or infirmity." This definition suggests that the mere absence of disease does not mean that a person is healthy. According to the holistic model, health is the primary concept. Healthcare professionals involved in health promotion as well as many professionals in primary healthcare have started shifting toward the holistic health model which can handle cases where the patient may seem disease-free but is actually not healthy.

The holistic health model enables individuals to enjoy their lives to the fullest by considering health as a vital state of physical, mental, social, and emotional, as well as spiritual well-being. In this model, the physician acts as a partner in the patient's care. The patient is empowered and informed and is an integral part of the decision-making process about the therapies and medications. The interventions in an integrated approach are designed to treat the illness in addition to the whole person, addressing the physical, mental, social, emotional, and spiritual factors that influence health and disease.

CONCLUSION

Just as every individual is different, every healthcare model is different and not every model can be used for every condition. Healthcare professionals cannot push through by just one therapy or one particular model. Thus, only one model cannot be used for a number of patients and for all treatments. A holistic or integrative model that would include various aspects of various different models needs to be developed so that, it can be applied to a number of treatment, management, and prevention regimens.

BIBLIOGRAPHY

Ankita, D. May 2015. Integrative medicine: An approach to holistic health, *Interlink Insight,* Mumbai, India: 14(1).

Belal Hijji, R.N. January 2012. Unit I: Concepts in health care: Health and wellness, *Legal Principles in Nursing.*

Changes in health care delivery essential to combat chronic disease: Why the disease-based model of medicine fails our patients. Elsevier, March 18, 2015.

Five steps to establishing a patient-centric care environment. March 27, 2013. http://altruistahealth.com/five-steps-to-establishing-a-patient-centric-care-environment/. Accessed December 2015.

Hofmann, B. Simplified models of the relationship between health and disease. DOI: 10.1007/s11017-005-7914-8.

Lois, M.V. and Jetie, A.M. 1994. The disablement process. *Soc. Sci. Med.*, 38(1): 1–14.

Martin, L.R., Williams, S.L., Haskard, K.B., and DiMatteo, M.R. 2005. Introduction to nursing: Models of health promotion and illness prevention. *Ther Clin. Risk Manag.* 1(3): 189–199.

Milani, R.V. and Lavie, C.J. 2015. Health care 2020: Reengineering health care delivery to combat chronic disease. *Am. J. Med.*, 128(4): 337–343.

Minaire, P. 1992. Disease, illness and health: Theoretical models of the disablement process, *Bulletin of the World Health Organization* (WHO) OMS, 70(3): 373–379.

Refat, A. Health system models—An overview. *Slideshare*, November 2012.

Small, D.C. and Small, R.M. 2011. Patients first! Engaging the hearts and minds of nurses with a patient-centered practice model, *Oregon Judicial Information Network*, 16(2).

Verbrugge, Lois M. and Jette, Alan M. 1994. The disablement process, *Social Science & Medicine*, 38(1), 1–14, http://dx.doi.org/10.1016/0277-9536(94)90294-1.

WHO, The World Health Report 2002 Risks: Promoting Healthy Life 2002.

Section III

Marketing and Product Positioning

7 Market Dynamics and Evolution in Nutraceuticals

R. B. Smarta

CONTENTS

INTRODUCTION

In any industry, it is never easy to achieve as well as maintain a competitive advantage. There are independent as well as related challenges in pharmaceutical and food sectors since both fields have been introduced at different stages of a life cycle. While the nutra and food sectors are at an early growth stage, the pharma sector has reached the maturity stage. Therefore, the challenges should be looked at from both perspectives together and individually in light of the fact that the population has now become much more demanding and sophisticated and is expecting

more innovations in products. At the same time, to cope with the changing environment, legislations should be more complex and reflective.

For the pharmaceutical industry, the challenges are even greater as the industry
has reached the stage of falling over a patent cliff. The priority of the top management teams across the organization is shifting toward reducing costs and developing alternate revenue models. But these efforts only intensified the challenges
further. Similar challenges have also been experienced in the film and music industry and they are not so very easily resolved. That is especially true for food and
pharmaceutical sectors.

Both the sectors depend on the health of human beings for their growth, and
human life is certainly precious. Stringent standards of quality, safety, and legislations, more specifically in the areas of health and hygiene, govern the companies in
both sectors. The need of the pharmaceutical industry today is total reformation, be
it creation of alternative revenue models or focusing on investments and behavior
in a novel way. Improved governance and transparency between manufacturers and
regulators are essential for putting an end to any prevalent unethical practices.

PHARMA SECTOR AND ITS GROWTH

In India, the healthcare costs need be reduced because of a number of factors such
as rising R&D costs, patent expiration, volatile market scenarios, hikes in healthcare
costs, and disease burden.

There is also a shift toward wellness among educated and health-conscious patients.
A layman does not want to become sick even if he does not possess the awareness
of healthy habits and the health benefits a product may provide. So, it is generally
observed that consumers opt for OTC products or counts on their experience, and
revert to traditional medicines, which are both readily available and cost-effective.

Consumers are now compelled to look toward prevention. For the wholesome
good health of a patient/consumer, using both medicines and food products under
nutraceuticals is done. Especially in the case of chronic diseases, doctors are creating awareness among the patients about lifestyle changes and offering advice on
changing their food habits and lifestyle.

SCIENCE-DRIVEN EVOLUTION

The dynamics and beliefs of medical consumers have changed with advancements
in science and technology. The science-driven evolution consists of evidence, education, income, and evolving thoughts.

MICROBIOME THEORY: THE DYSFUNCTION
AND DISORDER RELATIONSHIP

In the human body, there dwell about 100 trillion bacteria of many hundreds of
species. Microbiomes aid the human body in carrying out the bodily functions more
easily. These microbiomes get food and shelter in return for the health benefits the
host or the human body gets from them.

To give an example of this, the microbiome count is not in the right balance if a person is experiencing irritable bowel syndrome (IBS). This can be taken care of with the consumption of probiotics. Probiotics come under the nutraceutical sector, thus prompting the need to have these products as part of our daily diet.

Developing good diagnostic tools and combining them with drugs and nutrition is of importance here. The greatest drug in everyone's repertoire that can be followed every day of their life is the food he or she eats three times a day. It is important to see how the components—the nutrients—already existing in the food can be used before inventing anything.

Looking toward Integrated and Holistic Medicines

A new paradigm in healthcare is being brought about by integrated medicine, which emphasizes the synergy and deployment of the best aspects of the different systems of medicine, keeping in mind the best interest of the patients. These systems include modern medicine, Siddha, homeopathy, and Unani.

Naturopathy and Yoga

The rise in the demand for traditional medicines from the public has led policy makers, health administrators, and medical doctors to give serious thought to the possibility of having the traditional and modern medicine methods work together. The point of view of traditional methods toward health, disease, and the cause of the disease is different from the modern methods. The whole purpose of having integrated medicine is not just to have a good understanding of the different practices but more importantly to promote the most beneficial way to care for patients.

Traditional medical practices are being used more frequently for managing chronic diseases and this has been seen through a number of surveys and other sources of evidence. In rural and semiurban areas, traditional method of medicine is a low-cost alternative and is more easily available than modern medicine.

The New Normal World

The dynamic and fast-changing nature of the world today is best described by VUCA, a term coined by the U.S. Army War College. This term basically stands for volatility, uncertainty, complexity, and ambiguity. So, it would not be wrong to say that for companies to remain successful, timely changes should be made to their strategic plans. We are living in a world where volatility and uncertainty have become the New Normal. The Arab Spring saw a change of government in countries like Tunisia, Egypt, Libya, and Yemen. Once powerful countries in Europe are now fighting bankruptcy. We have been taking the growth in the developing part of the world for granted.

Companies that were synonymous with their product categories a few years ago are now no longer in existence for example, Kodak, the inventor of digital camera, had to wind up its operations.

What does the New Normal World mean for business? A few years ago, the Lebanese-American scholar Nicholas Taleb introduced the concept of black swans—events that are difficult to predict because they are low-probability outliers, so the past provides no reliable precedent. The natural calamities make us realize this unpredictability.

So, we now live in a VUCA world surrounded by black swans of uncertainty. This is the New Normal World!

THREE MEGATRENDS

There are three major trends that allow us to ponder what this New Normal World means. These three megatrends are as follows:

1. *Digitization*: We are increasingly living in an interconnected world and this has changed how we interact with each other and with governments and companies. Digitization is now advancing even more rapidly and fundamentally changing the way business and society works.
2. *Rise of the developing world*: The world order is changing as economic power shifts from West to East. In the last century, the developing world produced foods for the developed world to consume. But by 2020, the emerging Asia will become the world's largest consuming block, overtaking North America. This megatrend also presents both opportunities as well as risks to business.
3. *Sustainability*: The third megatrend is the changing relationship between humans and the planet we reside on. Scientific evidence has proven beyond any doubt that today we are living beyond our means.

HOW TO DEAL WITH THE CHAOS IN THE WORLD?

It has been observed that noise inside our minds creates chaos. It emerges from noise of linear ways that complicate real-world perspectives. There is a need to stop this uncertainty. There are four limits to uncertainty: the context, the determination of a player to play, the randomness of the chances, and the level of noise. Although chaos looks random, it is not. We need to change the old assumptions or context and revisit the context with respect to new situations. Chaos is a burden carried by us as a result of our perspectives to look at it; the burden comes from our inability to act, and it initially makes us indecisive and later makes us confused. So we need to change our focus from correlation of information to content of information in the context with the four limits/perspectives. There is need to work on excellence and at the same time be accountable for the decisions with determination. We need decision support in chaos.

MANAGEMENT TOOLKIT

The management toolkit will aid in dealing with the chaos. The following could be the essential components of a management toolkit:

1. Approach leadership as an experiment.
2. Boost information processing in the mind-set of action.
3. Prepare for serendipity by deliberately breaking the routine.

4. Expand the vocabulary of *yes* to overcome the glamour on *no*.
5. Take advantage of clunkers and create a culture of accepting mistakes and working on these mistakes for positivity.
6. Ensure everyone has a chance to go solo from time to time.
7. Celebrate a culture of critique and not a fault-finding mission.
8. Create minimal structure and maximum autonomy.
9. Encourage serious play. Too much control inhibits flow.
10. Cultivate provocative competence and celebrate occasions for unfamiliar terrain.
11. Perform and experiment simultaneously.

Start the process in chaos and say yes to the mess.

The Emerging Wellness Revolution

The next big thing on the horizon is the wellness revolution. This nascent industry is likely to be the next trillion-dollar industry, so much so that it would have a great impact on every aspect of people's lives. In as little as 5 years, the industry would see sales worth $1 trillion but the wellness industry is as shrouded in the dark as the automobile industry in 1908 or the personal computer industry in 1981 was. This upcoming trillion-dollar industry is on the path of growth as a result of scientific breakthroughs in biology and cellular chemistry.

The medicine business is more or less a reactive one. Even though it is large in size, people become customers only when they are affected and react to a particular condition or ailment. Here, people do not wish to be a customer. On the other hand, the wellness business is more proactive in comparison. Here, people want to become a customer by their own will so that they remain healthy, reduce the effect of aging, as well as minimize the chances of becoming a customer of the medicine business. Everyone is more than willing to be a customer of this latter approach of health.

Human beings require food every few hours for energy along with certain foods that function as building blocks and catalysts on a daily basis. Our bodies are biologically programmed in such a way that whenever there is a need of energy, we experience hunger pangs, a signal that our body requires energy (in the form of food), unfortunately, we become aware of missing building blocks or catalysts only when we become ill from nutrient deficiencies. Our bodies are also biologically programmed to seek out foods containing the highest amounts of energy: it is for this reason that we crave for foods containing sugar and fat, which have high calorific value. This has led to the success of food businesses; and in a way to the exploitation of our biological programming by entrepreneurs and commercial providers of food is the major cause of obesity and ill health in the developed world today (Dilip et al., 2011).

With regard to diet, there are three major problems worldwide today (excerpt from Dilip et al., 2011):

1. We eat too much.
2. Most people are not getting the minimum amounts of building blocks and/or catalysts that their bodies need.
3. Some sections of the population do not have food to eat.

The availability and type of food consumed, the cooking technique adopted, people's lifestyle, and dietary habits have all created challenges related to nutrition.

THE NUTRITION TRANSITION

All over the world, traditional cooking has undergone enormous changes.

The increasing pace of life, extensive use of technology, and the availability of a wide array of packaged, ready-made foods have changed basis food habits, which were mainly dependent on crops and the seasons.

As a result of this transition in lifestyle, people have become conscious about health, on the other hand though, they have made a transition in their food habits, timing, and nutrition content. This phenomenon is referred to as nutrition transition (NT). The major implications of NT can be observed in a majority of people through obesity, an imbalance in nutrition that leads to many diseases.

The writing is on the wall regarding the unhealthy shifts in food consumption and this situation needs to be checked and reversed immediately. Awareness and education need to be used extensively to counter the proliferation of NT, which has only led to degenerative and lifestyle diseases. The most susceptible people are those from the lower and middle classes in less affluent countries. Their regular intake of cheap, energy-intense, and nutrient-deficient food has led to a paradoxical situation of undernutrition (low-level intake of micronutrients and fiber) and overnutrition (high-level intake of salt, sugar, fats, etc.) This simultaneous double burden of under- and overnutrition has led to an epidemic of obesity and adult-onset diabetes. Healthcare costs to assuage the situation are steep and hence serious steps need to be taken to prevent the problem from snowballing any further.

A CHANGE IN CONSUMER PERCEPTIONS

A major section of the world's population suffers from nutritional imbalances, which indirectly affect a country's growth. Because of lifestyle changes and changing eating patterns, people today are not able to balance the recommended dietary allowance for various nutrients.

Generally, consumers consider traditional foods such as rice, wheat, bread, vegetables, and eggs to be safe. With an increase in awareness along with increased malnutrition (undernutrition as well as overnutrition), consumers have wisely started correlating nutrients to specific disease conditions. This increasing awareness has led to the emergence of a new industry or nutrient-specific products either mixed in food (functional foods) or in the form of a table/pill (supplements) to treat a particular disease.

In addition, consumers have started realizing the side effects of Western medicine and their mind-set has shifted from curative to corrective and preventive therapy. Consumers are thus developing a holistic approach to health, and food, diet, and nutrition have become the center of attraction for all stakeholders.

Consumers have also started focusing on the ingredients in food products as a solution to correct or prevent the unhealthy situation related to diet. It is predicted that by 2015, most megacities in the developing world will shift from a disease-centric to a prevention-centric medical model.

New Food Development*

With more and more people focusing on diet and the thrust on preventing and managing illnesses through intake of right food due to the Nutrition Transition, innovation and development in the food as well as nutraceutical segment has become an integral issue of the society. This represents new opportunities for both science and business.

Food, whether natural or processed, has a great impact on our body. Processed foods have been altered from their natural state for reasons related to safety and convenience. We tend to think of such modified foods as bad, but it turns out that many processed foods are not unhealthy.

So, here we are with the marketers on one side and the customers on the other. Keen on developing new markets and introducing new products, marketers are employing a multitude of services and ideas to keep pushing their products and presence in the market. With technology and globalization working full time, the competition is extreme and the law of diminishing returns is repeatedly setting in and wasting critical resources. Expensive services and inputs are being pumped in but the market, though burgeoning, is not exactly galloping.

The Role of Nutraceuticals in the Wellness Industry

Wellness is directly connected with "energy" of human beings. Human beings get energy through food, that is, their diet. Because of the changes happening due to "nutrition transition," perception of consumers about diet, and new food development, has undergone a shift and the idea about "wellness" or "being well" is getting deeply transformed.

There comes in the concept of nutrition and nutraceuticals.

The term "nutraceuticals" was originally coined in the late 1980s and has since been used to describe a wide variety of nonpharmaceutical compounds that may have an impact on health and disease states, general well-being, and performance.

It is also clear that there is a high level of consumer interest, and consequently a high demand for nutraceuticals sometimes is perceived in a more favorable light than pharmaceuticals.

Nutraceuticals are also generally easily available as over-the-counter products in supermarkets, health food shops, and pharmacies, and have not always been subject to the same level of regulatory scrutiny before they reach the marketplace. These are being seen as more "natural" and less likely to cause side effects (which is often far from true).

Over the past years, rigorous regulatory assessments for the approval of health claims, such as those carried out by the European Food Safety Authority (EFSA) in Europe and Therapeutic Goods Administration (TGA) in Australia under different levels of health claims legislation, have been implemented. These are designed to protect the consumer from misleading product communication and create a powerful research drive to substantiate nutraceutical effects according to the strictest scientific criteria.

---

* Excerpt from Dilip et al. 2011.

On August 23, 2006, the Indian Food Safety and Standards Bill (FSSB) was passed by the parliament. The food and safety laws in the country have been incorporated in the FSSAI in a way that encourages the food processing industry to develop in a scientific and systematic manner. Two important objectives of this act are

1. To propose a *single* clause relating to food
2. To ensure the *scientific development* of the food processing industry

As per the FSS Act, there are many categorizes for foods: novel foods, genetically modified foods, propriety foods, standardized foods, foods for special dietary use, and functional foods/nutraceuticals/health supplements.

Niche versus Mass Market

The functional food, beverage, and supplement (FBS) market, also known as the nutraceutical market, is defined as the aggregate sales of functional foods, beverages, and supplements fortified with bioactive ingredients, with the most notable being fiber, probiotics, protein and peptides, omega-3, phytochemicals, and vitamins and minerals. Supplements fortified with herbals are also considered part of the market. FBS market is looked upon as a market for premiumization with new value-added products promising better health through better dietary choices. For suppliers, functional FBS can provide growth opportunities as well as wider profit margins that are not available with traditional food products. Consumers are able to benefit from good health without sacrificing taste and convenience.

Drivers

The common factors driving nutraceutical market are the increase in disposable income and consciousness about one's health, particularly in Asia-Pacific regions. North America has the largest consumer base for nutraceutical products amongst all the geographies. In North America the nutraceuticals market is at mature stage and has witnessed a growth rate of more than 6% during the years 2007–2011. Developing countries like China and India possess huge potential in terms of both value and volume for nutraceutical products, as the population and disposable income are on the rise in these countries.

The major factors stimulating nutraceutical market growth in the top seven countries (the United States, Japan, the United Kingdom, Spain, Italy, Germany, and France) are as follows:

1. A growing aging population
2. A growing and affluent working population
3. Increased awareness of nutraceuticals
4. More people taking their health into their own hands
5. Top-selling ingredients in the nutritional supplement industry
6. Rising number of start-ups and supplement business owners
7. Rising focus on e-commerce among consumers

Spending on healthy and organic foods is on the rise, thus giving a boost to the overall nutraceutical market. Some of the factors restraining market growth are the lack of consumer trust about the health benefits claimed from nutraceutical products and the high prices of nutraceutical products.

SEGMENT-WISE GROWTH

According to the Freedonia Group, the top-selling group of nutraceutical ingredients in the nutritional supplement industry includes proteins, fibers, and various specialized functional additives that constitute the three major groups of nutraceutical ingredients. Proteins are projected as fastest-growing segment as manufacturers introduce innovations for protein application in foods and beverages with high-value nutrition.

Herbal and botanical extracts as well as animal- and marine-based derivatives are expected to have a steady fast growth. Global demand for these products is expected to rise 8.9% annually, through 2015.

Specialized functional additives such as omega-3 fatty acids, probiotics, vitamins, and minerals are predicted to grow at an annual increase of 6.7%, which is expected for the aforementioned group of nutraceutical ingredients, through 2015.

Innova Market Insights (2013) has identified the top five health claims for functional foods and drinks marketed to older consumers. Health optimization has become an increasing focus for an aging population, driven by rising consumer understanding of the role of a healthy diet in extending the active years. This is being reflected in promotion of the idea of healthy aging or aging well. With respect to healthy aging, the claims that are most popular are related to gut health, digestive system, immunity, energy and heart health. Such claims have a general appeal among masses. However, there are some specific, opportunities in the healthy aging segment which include brain, cognitive health, bone & joint health, eye health etc. that usually don't feature on the products. Tracked product launches using eye health claims doubled in the last 5-year period, as recorded by Innova Market Insights in 2012. A range of other ingredients claimed to be beneficial in the area of cognitive health include B vitamins, CoQ10, *Ginkgo biloba*, polyphenols, acetyl L-carnitine, and green tea, but there are few specific references to aging to date, with labeling generally simply highlighting their use and relying on consumer awareness of the benefits.

The global retail sales (in $ billion, fixed exchange rates) of health and wellness products in 2012 (Euromonitor, 2013) are as follows (Figure 7.1):

- General well-being: 397
- Weight management: 155
- Digestive health: 68
- Energy and endurance: 40
- Oral health: 18
- Cardiovascular health: 8
- Brain and memory: 0.53

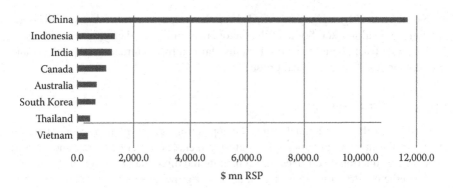

FIGURE 7.1 Health and wellness growth markets in 2011–2012. (From Hudson, E., Euromonitor, Vitafoods Europe, Geneva, Switzerland, 2013.)

Major health platforms include:

- Gut health
- Antiaging
- Weight management
- Energy and endurance
- Anxiety and depression

The Indian Market

According to estimates, the Indian nutraceutical market will grow five times its current size by the end of the current decade. Currently, the market is growing at a healthy double-digit rate and may reach Rs. 195 billion (approximately $4.2 billion) mark in the current fiscal itself. The growth of the nutraceutical market in India is largely because of the in the creased affluence and lifestyle diseases and change in consumer perception and mind-set. In addition, increase in awareness about the extra supplements among consumers and an increase in health consciousness along with rising healthcare costs are paving the way for the growth of the Indian nutraceutical market.

The market is becoming increasingly competitive with three different types of players in the market which are pharma companies, FMCG companies and pure nutraceutical manufacturers.

When nutraceuticals were introduced in India, most of the industry leaders wondered if nutritional supplements would gain acceptability in the Indian prescription-driven health and wellness industry. Contrary to their concern, nutraceuticals were well accepted, particularly by the upper-middle segment of the Indian population. However, the industry is at a nascent stage and holds ample opportunity to grow in future. There is a strong need for developing customized products, affordable pricing, and distribution strategy.

How to Leverage This Opportunity in the Market?

The question "How can companies leverage the nutraceutical market?" can be answered through these enablers (Figure 7.2).

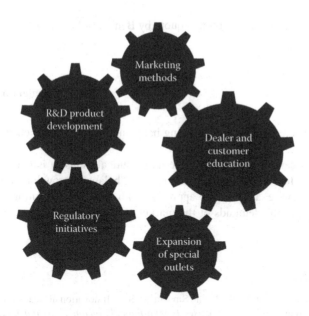

FIGURE 7.2 Nutraceutical market enablers.

R&D product development: Based on the psychodemographics of the country, new products can be developed through innovative R&D initiatives. Importance should also be given to the infrastructure requirements, quality assurance, and quality control for good-quality product development.

Regulatory initiatives: There is a need to standardize the rules and regulations for the benefit of consumers as well as stakeholders. There should be watertight laws to ensure quality compliance, adherence to scientific claims, as well as ethical marketing strategies.

Marketing methods: Companies concentrate more on making people aware of how they can improve their health through these products. So, the marketing is not simply to increase sales revenue but to also improve the health of consumers.

Customer and dealer education: This aspect can be one of the most crucial enablers of them all. The first step in this line would be dealer education. Dealers can be made aware of the health benefits every product can offer by adopting the pharma method of sales. Customers can be educated through the dealers as well as by using advertising as a medium of awareness.

Expansion of special outlets: There is a need to increase the number of wellness stores that cater these nutraceutical products to consumers. The reason being is that through these special outlets a person can get the much needed assistance for choosing the product that is right for them, whereas that may not be the case when a chemist store sells these nutra products.

These five enablers can be a way to leverage the opportunity the Indian market has to offer the nutraceutical companies.

In conclusion, let's reflect on this quote by Benjamin Franklin:

I saw few die of hunger;
Of eating, a hundred thousand

—Benjamin Franklin

Nutraceuticals are here to stay as eating habits and lifestyle have changed dramatically worldwide.

Though nascent at the moment, the nutraceutical industry is poised for a great growth ahead. Just as a balanced diet ensures a balanced growth and healthy body and mind, likewise a balanced approach with proactive planning and reactive responses, as per the demands of the market, will ensure optimal gains for players in this field.

REFERENCES

Dilip, G., Shantanu, D., Debasis, B., and Smarta, R. 2011. Innovation in Healthy and Functional Foods, Excerpt in *Market-Focused Innovation in Food and Nutrition*, Chapter 30, CRC Press, New York, 509–520 (510).

Ecosystem Convergence. 2013. Nutraceuticals: The case for inter-firewall collaboration, Mu Sigma's Point of View. Frost & Sullivan Report on Nutraceuticals, 2011.

Global Analysis of the Marine and Algae Omega-3 Ingredients Market, June 2011.

Global Business Intelligence. August 2011. Nutraceuticals Market to 2017—Food additives such as Omega-3 fatty acids, probiotics, soy and energy drinks to perform strongly.

Hudson, E. 2013. Euromonitor, Vitafoods Europe, Geneva, Switzerland.

Innovations in Healthy and Functional Foods. CRC Press.

Manwani, H. July 27, 2013. Leadership in a VUCA world. *The Hindu.*

Nutra Sector Overview (Report), 2014, Nuffoods Spectrum, MMActiv Media, Printed and Published by Jagdish Patankar on behalf of MM Activ Sci-Tech Communications, Bangalore.

Nutraceuticals product market: Global market size, segment and country analysis and forecasts (2007–2017). *Research and Markets*, March 2012.

Paul Altaffer and Grant Washington Smith. July 2011. From the Corners of the World: India: The Prowling Tiger, Nutraceuticals World. http://www.nutraceuticalsworld.com/issues/2011-07/view_columns/from-the-corners-of-the-world-india-the-prowling-t#sthash.27hpG1HC.dpuf.

Pilzer, P.Z. 2002. *The Wellness Revolution*, 2nd edn, John Wiley & Sons, Hoboken, NJ.

Report - The Indian Nutraceutical Market Valued at $1480 Million in 2011 to Grow to $2731 Million in 2016. June 2012. Frost & Sullivan. http://www.frost.com/prod/servlet/press-release.pag?docid=261666318.

Sumeet Khanna, 2011, Nutraceutical Markets on the Growth Curve: The Indian Story. Presented at 6th Nutra Summit, India. http://www.nutraceuticalsummit.in/nutra_2011/nutra_download_panel/downloads/Day1/Nutra_Markets_on_the_Growth_Curve_A_The_India_Story_B_Meta/Mr_Sumeet_Khanna.pdf.

The Freedonia Group. November 2011. World Nutraceutical Ingredients to 2015. Industry Study with Forecasts for 2015 & 2020, p. 568.

www.zyduscadila.com.

http://www.mu-sigma.com/analytics/thought_leadership/decision-sciences-nutraceuticals-the-case-for-inter-firewall-collaboration.html.

http://www.nutraceuticalsworld.com/issues/2011-07/view_columns/from-the-corners-of-the-world-india-the-prowling-t/.

http://www.nutraceuticalsummit.in/nutra_2011/nutra_download_panel/downloads/Day1/Nutra_Markets_on_the_Growth_Curve_A_The_India_Story_B_Meta/Mr_Sumeet_Khanna.pdf.

8 Business Perspective

R. B. Smarta

CONTENTS

INTRODUCTION

The nutraceutical and allied products industry is at an ever-growing phase. The dynamics of the industry are constantly changing especially in the developing markets like India, China, Mexico, and Brazil. In countries like India, nutraceuticals are already at the forefront of preventative and proactive healthcare and disease management. The global nutraceutical market accounted for $171.8 billion in 2014 and is expected to reach $295 billion by 2022. Globally, the market is estimated to be growing at a compound annual growth rate (CAGR) of 7% in the period 2014–2022. India's nutraceutical market is expected to cross $6.1 billion by 2020 from its current $2.8 billion. According to a study conducted by ASSOCHAM and RNCOS in 2014–2015, the Indian nutraceutical market was growing at CAGR of about 17% and had become one of the fastest emerging markets in the health and wellness sector. People making healthier choices are only going to further aid in the nutraceutical industry's growth.

WORLD HEALTH STATUS

Looking at today's health status of the world, it is evident that healthcare is the prime focus of every nation. The various aspects involved in healthcare are proactive care, preventive care, and diseases. The "health model" demonstrates different aspects of healthcare (Figure 8.1).

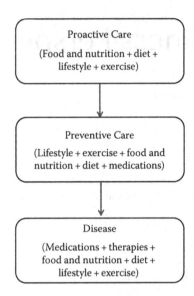

FIGURE 8.1   Health model. (From Interlink Knowledge Cell.)

Proactive care is the first aspect in this health model, which is usually taken for promotion and maintenance of good health. Proactive care is established by having a balanced diet, good food, and nutrition, making positive changes in lifestyle, increasing level of physical activities, and so on.

The second part of this model is preventive care, which involves the use of medicines. Prevention can be attained by the use of nutraceuticals, alternative medicines, or, to some extent drugs (vaccines) along with the various aspects of proactive care. The third part of this model is disease; if proactive or preventive care is not taken, one might encounter disease or illness, wherein one needs to take medicines, therapies along with good food and nutrition, balanced diet, changes in the lifestyle, and exercising. In order to remain healthy and stay fit, one needs to take proactive and/or preventive care. As more and more people are becoming aware of the importance of health, they are moving toward food, diet, and nutraceuticals.

THE GLOBAL SCENARIO OF THE NUTRACEUTICAL MARKETS

Region-wise, the United States is the leading market for nutraceuticals, with over 36% of the world's nutraceutical share. This is followed by the Asia-Pacific region with 30%, the European Union at 26%, and the rest of the world at 8%. In the Asia-Pacific region, Japan is the largest market with 14% share, followed by China with 10% share.

There has been considerable growth in the nutraceutical and functional food markets in the European Union, from approximately $1.8 billion in 1999 to $8 billion in 2006. In spite of significant growth, the market is still lagging with respect to growth observed in the counterparts of the world; that is, in 2006 the world market share represented only about 10% of total estimated world expenditures.

The United States, Japan, and South, Southeast, Far East, Middle East, and Asia-Pacific regions are the major trading partners with the European Union (Basu et al., 2007).

Together, Chinese nutraceuticals and medicinal plants are termed traditional Chinese medicines (TCMs). There are roughly 1000 small- to medium-sized enterprises located in and around China (AAFC, 2002; Patwardhan et al., 2005). Due to friendly business scenarios, these products are in huge demand and are not under strict control of branding and labeling. Strangely, TCM preparations outside China are shown to have better health and nutritional qualities than those prepared in China. However, China has a huge potential to become a global leader due to relaxed regulations, cheap labor, lower manufacturing costs, and steady demand (AAFC, 2002; Patwardhan et al., 2005). China exports its products majorly to Japan, Hong Kong, Korea, and Singapore. The Chinese herbal drugs are valued at $48 billion per annum with exports of $3.6 billion per annum (Handa, 2004).

After the United States, the second largest market for nutraceuticals is Japan. Japan has shown an annual steady average growth of 9.6% for the last 10 years. Its functional food industry was estimated to be $27.1 billion in 2006 (Functional Food Japan, Project Report, 2006). Japan's association with the use of modern functional foods dates back to the 1970s, making it a leader in the global market. As compared to the United States and the EU, the per capita consumption of nutraceuticals is considerably higher. The Japanese government has approved two types of functional foods, namely, foods with approved health claims or FOSHU (Food for Specified Health Uses) and foods that may provide health benefits (Basu et al., 2007).

THE INDIAN SCENARIO

Currently, the Indian nutraceutical market is estimated at USD 2.8 billion and is growing at a CAGR of 17% (study conducted by ASSOCHAM and RNCOS in 2014–2015). Among the emerging economies, India is one of the largest economies for nutraceuticals having high purchasing power parity. The increasing per capita income has paved way for changing lifestyles. The changing dietary habits, lack of physical activity, overconsumption of food, and increasing number of people involved in sedentary jobs all account for the changed lifestyle. This has in turn increased the incidence of lifestyle diseases. The fast-paced lifestyle has led to more consumption of processed and packaged foods that lack quality nutrients; this again contributes to the incidences of lifestyle diseases such as obesity, diabetes, and cardiovascular diseases in India. The awareness of health and fitness has increased the use of nutraceutical and allied products in India.

Traditional medicines associated with health foods in forms of recognized nutritional foods, food supplements, medicinal herbs, and crude powdered drugs derived from plant, animal, and marine sources have their roots in the Eastern cultures, particularly India and China (Banik and Basu, 2002; Dhanukar et al., 2000). The traditional Indian Ayurvedic medicines (IAMs) are common forms of functional foods and nutraceuticals in India (Patwardhan et al., 2005). India has a rich biodiversity with large varieties of medicinal herbs, spices, and tree species with no foreign competition at present. India is also a major exporter of these products to the United States, Japan, and Far East, Southeast, West, and Middle

East Asia along with parts of North Africa and the EU (Patwardhan et al., 2005). Additionally, the cost of manufacturing these products is low in India, which makes these products highly competitive in Asian and African markets. The industry in India is thus valued at $10 billion per annum with exports of $1.1 billion per annum (Singh et al., 2003).

THE NUTRACEUTICAL BUSINESS

The nutraceutical business mainly relies on the network of stakeholders and consumers. Maintaining and developing this stakeholder and consumer base is very crucial for the business.

DRIVERS OF THE NUTRACEUTICAL INDUSTRY

Some of the growth drivers of the nutraceutical industry are as follows:

- *Changing lifestyle (affordability)*: In recent years, there has been an increase in quality of life and income. This has thrown up a challenge in the form of lifestyle diseases such as obesity, diabetes, and cardiovascular diseases. Hence, nutraceuticals and foods fortified with wellness ingredients aid in providing people with more options and ease of access even in remote destinations.
- *Awareness*: Along with consumers' evolving consumption of healthy nutritional food products, the suppliers' growing efforts on building brand identity and value have created wider awareness. Retail products fortified with nutrients such as omega-3 fatty acids and vitamins are now being considered essential parts of consumables rather than niche areas.
- *Shift toward preventive therapy*: Consumers have started prioritizing prevention and wellness over treatment. The increasing understanding and perception of the relationship between diet, preventive therapies, and diseases/health conditions by consumers is creating a demand for nutra products in the market.
- *Accessibility*: Factors such as multilevel and direct marketing as practiced by companies like Amway and Herbalife have increased the accessibility of nutritional supplements to consumers.
- *Aging population*: Worldwide, the aging population is increasing and so there is an increase in age-related ailments.

In the emerging markets, the middle class is the major consumer. The desire to consume functional foods serves as a huge driver and creates a potential market for natural ingredients to be used in these foods. For health conditions that involve low risk and low involvement such as maintenance of health, gut, and weight, consumers turn to nutraceuticals rather than drugs, which are costly and may show side effects. As the cost of healthcare and medicines is increasing, consumers are looking toward nutraceuticals as an investment in health because of their preventive, rather than curative, benefits.

MARKET PERSPECTIVES

Growth is the most crucial aspect for survival in any business. Across the globe, nutraceutical industry is highly progressive and a number of companies (new stand-alone pharmaceutical and food companies) are investing in nutraceuticals. The companies wanting to make it big in the nutraceutical industry can work on these "five pillars" of nutraceutical business described next (Figure 8.2).

First, study the current regulatory guidelines and situation. Any company entering the nutraceutical business in a particular country/countries must study the regulatory aspects of that country/countries before even getting into the business. Also, if exporting to other countries, the regulatory guidelines of those countries need to be followed to ensure hassle-free export. Various regulatory-related aspects such as product approvals and registration, substantial literature for claims made on the supplement, and compliance with the existing regulatory guidelines need to be tackled so that product-related issues do not arise and the timelines do not get affected.

The second step is to develop innovative products based on scientific knowledge and new technologies, ensuring that the products are in tandem with consumer demands as well as fit in with the future. Nutraceutical companies must initially understand the needs of consumers before developing new products or developing the product strategy. Products customized per consumer needs with newer and innovative delivery formats will definitely be more accepted by consumers than other products. After innovating the products, get them approved with regulatory bodis.

Then develop marketing and branding strategy for those products keeping in mind the target audience and launching of the products. Marketing and branding is essential so as to ensure consumers' trust as well as interest. For the success of the products launched, the companies must identify growth drivers, develop brand strategy and brand perception, and assess the impact of brand strength and stature in existing environment.

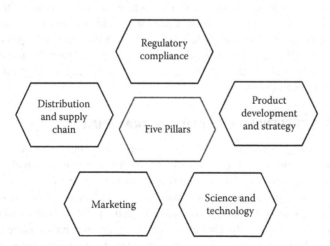

FIGURE 8.2 Five pillars of the nutraceutical business. (From Interlink Knowledge Cell.)

The last step is to select a distribution channel and ensure that the products reach the end user, that is, the consumer. The nutraceutical industry ought to establish exclusive nutraceutical distribution and supply channels as the nutraceuticals today are mostly distributed through pharmaceutical channels and others. Dedicated nutraceutical distribution channels will help make it easier for nutraceuticals to timely reach the market.

While entering the nutraceutical market or launching nutraceutical products, a company needs to take these five pillars into consideration.

MARKETING NUTRACEUTICALS EFFECTIVELY IN EMERGING MARKETS: THE INDIAN SCENARIO

During recent times the competition has greatly increased in the nutraceutical industry (internal as well as external). Moreover, there have also been a lot of foreign investors and companies entering the Indian market. The foreign competitors are expected to go after the high-end market in India; they will target the middle and subsequently the low end of the market. In this case, the main defense for Indian companies is developing stronger marketing skills, that is, strategy, innovation, differentiation, branding, and service.

Currently, in India, nutraceuticals are marketed mainly through prescription route (in association with doctors). Dietary supplements are marketed through prescription route, while other formats such as powders, functional foods, and functional beverages are mainly marketed via direct marketing (for OTC supplements) or OTC route.

While marketing any product, either nutraceuticals or pharmaceuticals, it is essential to prioritize and understand what is most important—product education, therapy education, diagnostics, or the doctor–patient matrix. The main focus of any marketer should be to indentify the potential customer, whether it is the doctor, the patient, the patient's family, or the healthcare insurance provider. Getting an answer to these questions will benefit in understanding how and to whom the marketing strategies should be targeted. In the case of nutraceuticals, we can observe that all of these are important from the marketing point of view since they are all interdependent; thus, everyone, right from the patient to the patient's family and doctors to the insurance providers, should be a focus of the marketing activities.

MAKING A DIFFERENCE THROUGH BRANDING

There are many new players worldwide in the nutraceutical industry. As mere ingredients or formulations do not drive value, some firms are simply stuck on selling generics and ingredients. Trusted brand names drive value. There are a number of products with similar vitamin and minerals, but unless we have a strong brand image, the consumer will compare the products on the price front and will go for the cheapest option. In the nutrition business, very few marketers have built really strong brand names. Thus far, there are few nutraceutical or functional food brands that can be recognized for their strong branding and their image.

Differentiating Nutraceutical Products and Ingredients

For commoditizing a formulation or ingredient, the differentiation factors can be attached to the entire organization or a product or a group of product. Any product that is sold is to be considered as a holistic blend of product, service, and value. There have been many cases where the ingredient manufacturers, despite having the capability to bring new innovative products to the market, tend to drop products, once their margins start eroding. So, although customers may prefer this company for introducing new innovative products, they will start looking for alternate suppliers once this company drops its products. Hence, the companies are required to create a differentiation for themselves as "quick to launch new products company," so that customers stick with them. The benefits keep flowing in provided the manufacturer maintains this differentiation factor.

The main imperative of marketing is creating a brand, which in turn creates value. Companies need to identify various factors in order to differentiate their products, services, and marketing efforts from their competitors. Some of the differentiating factors include:

- *Overall strategy*: Developing strategies that define the value proposition to the customers even before entering the market can prove extremely beneficial in marketing. These strategies help us understand what we need to know but do not know. Different strategies to be considered for marketing are customer strategy, value strategy, R&D and product development strategy, pricing strategy, and retail strategy.
- *Strategy formulation*: Once the strategies are finalized, we need to meticulously formulate each strategy, in order to deliver the desired value proposition. While formulating the strategies, the product mix along with product specifications, packaging, price stamping, label design, claims, and so on should be articulated. Various other factors such as regulatory aspects, distribution, and accessibility affordability need to be addressed.
- *Business and marketing plan*: Articulating an organizational strategy as well as the structure of organization is essential from the point of view of making the marketing successful. Prioritizing of the segment, market, and distribution mix and planning of feasibility, viability, scalability, and sustainability along with brand creation are other important factors to be addressed while developing a business and marketing plan.

THE WAY FORWARD

The Movement from Pharma to Food

Over the last few years, pharmaceutical companies have been shifting toward the nutraceutical business. The nutraceutical sector is viewed by pharmaceutical companies as an extension of the healthcare sector where they have an opportunity to leverage their brand equity. There are many reasons for pharmaceutical firms to shift to the nutraceutical space. One example is that it is a fast-growing market that requires identical distribution capability as the pharmaceutical industry. In some sense, it also requires the same set of skills such marketing, packaging, and more. Also, in today's scenario, many pharmaceutical companies are under pressure in terms of profitability as a result of governmental price control of several drugs. Additionally, many drugs are going off the market because people are just not interested in using them anymore. This dryness of molecules is causing pharmaceutical companies to shift their focus to nutraceuticals, where there is a better chance of profitability and independence in pricing.

With respect to consumers, due to increasing awareness and the desire to maintain health and remain fit, during the last 2–3 years, there has been an evident shift toward prevention from cure. There has also been a great change in the healthcare scenario worldwide; it has changed from just food being consumed to satisfy hunger and stay alive to foods having natural functional benefits to human beings to the use of food in the treatment of diseases via medical foods.

Thus, the entire gamut of healthcare is shifting toward the prevention of diseases and the maintenance of health at large.

DEVELOPING THE NUTRACEUTICAL INDUSTRY THROUGH THE ECOSYSTEM

The nutraceutical industry can be developed in a holistic manner by understanding and developing the industry ecosystem. The concept of ecosystem involves a community working together and interacting with surrounding systems to create a new entity.

In the emerging markets, there are many small players entering the market, and since the industry and regulations are not well developed, they face a lot of problems like difficulty to invest in capital-intensive facilities such as cold stores, warehouses, and quality control laboratories. Therefore, these problems can be collectively handled in an ecosystem as the main infrastructure is shared by all the companies that are a part of the ecosystem. A hypothetical ecosystem is illustrated in Figure 8.3.

A well-developed ecosystem offers end-to-end control right from raw material procurement to storage, testing and transportation facilities, preservation, refrigeration, and so on. The main components of a nutraceutical or food ecosystem are the Primary Processing Centers (PPCs), Collection Centers (CCs), and Central Processing Center (CPC). The processing and manufacturing units guarantee supply of raw materials in the larger part of year, which becomes one of the key success factors. The layout and design of the ecosystem should be such that the procurement centers are established near the villages where the raw materials are produced; this forms the backward linkage. The collection centers should be well connected to processing centers. The forward linkage involves marketing- and supply-related aspects such as the retailers, traders (wholesale), super- and hypermarkets, and exporters.

The ecosystem can help fuel import of new technologies and products from international markets. They can also help in innovation and research with adequate resource funding, delivering safe and quality products/ingredients, achieving higher investments, and so on. It will also aid in timely delivery of the processed food products. Due to the size, the ecosystem can also expect to attract a large number of marketing tie-ups from national as well as international companies.

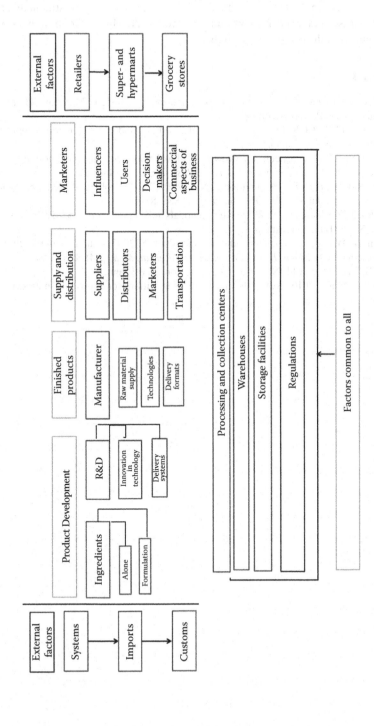

FIGURE 8.3 Nutraceutical ecosystem model. (Conceptual model by Interlink Knowledge Cell.)

Such ecosystems or nutraceutical or food parks can be based on public–private partnerships, wherein the government makes a certain amount of investment and the private enterprises make a certain amount of investment. This will definitely propel the nutraceutical industry toward growth.

REFERENCES

An overview of Indian nutraceuticals market, Pharmabiz Bureau, Mumbai, Thursday, February 16, 2012, Saffron media.

ASSOCHAM and RNCOS. Indian nutraceuticals, herbals, and functional foods industry: Emerging on a global map.

Basu, S.K. et al. 2007. Prospects for growth in global nutraceutical and functional food markets: A Canadian perspective. *Aust. J. Basic Appl. Sci.*, 1(4): 637–649.

Dahanukar, S.A., Kulkarni, R.A., and Rege, N.N. 2000. Pharmacology of medicinal plants and natural products, *Ind. J. Pharmacol.*, 32: S81–S118.

Nuffoods Spectrum. August 17, 2015. Nutraceuticals industry to touch $262.9 billion by 2020: Study. Bangalore, India.

Patwardhan, B., Warude, D., Pushpangadan, P., and Bhatt, N. 2005. Ayurveda and traditional Chinese medicine, *Evid. Based Complement. Alternat. Med.*, 2(4): 465–473.

Smarta, R.B. December 2014. Nuffoods spectrum: Food ecosystem.

Smarta, R.B. January 2016. Nuffoods Spectrum: Five pillars for growth of nutraceutical business.

9 Science to Business Viability

R. B. Smarta

CONTENTS

INTRODUCTION

In many different ways, science is linked to innovations and further to business firms as well. The advances in science were the reason for the pharmaceutical industry in the postwar period and the chemical industry in the late nineteenth and twentieth centuries to grow. This connection between business and science has always been there. Numerous companies like Xerox, DuPont, and Kodak had corporate laboratories that pursued science on a serious level largely in the twentieth century. There have been crucial changes in the nature of connection that exists between both science and business.

SCIENCE AND BUSINESS IMPERATIVES

Science and business are believed to be comprised in separate worlds on physical and philosophical levels. Similar to a differentiation between the state and the church, the boundary is more approximate rather than being precise between science and business. But, on another level, both business and science are linked with distinct norms and institutions. It would not be wrong to say that in much of the twentieth century, that science survived under the purview of the university and the actual application of the science or development was done in business enterprises. To state it in Stokes's words, "As pure science was being provided with an institutional home in the universities, the sense of separation of pure from applied was being heightened by the institutionalization of applied science in industry" (Stokes, 1997).

An absolutely unique class of entrepreneurial firms emerged in the biotech, nanotech, and even energy sectors in recent times, which were well rooted in science. There was a great risk and high level of uncertainty in the research conducted by these firms much before they thought of gaining a profit. Basically, their purview was the business of science. But they were not the only ones who thought of making a profit using science.

Universities seriously thought of gaining monetary returns through licensing and spin-offs. So, they have been vital not only in the pursuit of science but in its business as well. Since they are from two different worlds that have their own time horizons, risks, expectations, and norms, there are completely new challenges in science-based businesses. A great amount of knowledge has been generated with science, which is just simple but certainly very powerful.

Since its birth in the seventeenth century, modern science has changed the world beyond recognition and overwhelmingly for the better. But the success can breed complacency. Modern scientists are trusting too much and not verifying enough—to the detriment of the whole of science and of humanity (How Science Goes Wrong, October 2013).

Even now, science wields great respect. But based only on its strength to be right most times and ensure corrections if anything goes wrong does it get this privileged status? Scientists in every generation are sure to be busy working as there obviously would be no shortage or real mysteries. The ignominious research has created a big barrier that cannot be overlooked because of the false trails.

SCIENCE-BASED BUSINESS AND BIOTECHNOLOGY

There has been some serious organizational experimentation in the method of how science is created, diffused, and thereafter commercialized. Improved economic growth and better welfare can be achieved through advancements in science of energy, life, and materials. But organizational and institutional innovation will not be possible to achieve if the lessons of Chandler are neglected.

There was a change in the manner of connection between science and business. The downfall of the central corporate research laboratory was the first change. The kind of active role the universities played in ensuring financial gain through intellectual property was the second trend.

The establishment of specialized *science-based businesses* mostly in nanotechnology, life sciences, and the energy sector was the last change. It can be said that a science-based business is an organization that not only involves the creation and advancement of science but also aims at getting financial returns from it. This is because they are not just contributors but users of science too. So, a biotech science–based business now has to begin research that would have conventionally been under the domain of a university.

It is important to point out that science-based businesses differ greatly from the traditional *high-technology* businesses that come from the United States. When involved in science, a science-based business faces a greater risk profile as well as long-term time horizons.

THE NUTRITION TRANSITION

There has been a difference in the basic food habits because of a number of reasons such as using excessive technology, the fast pace of life, and a variety of easily available packaged, ready-made food unlike before when there was a major reliance on crops.

More and more people are now very health conscious due to the change in lifestyle. But it is essential to remember that there is a great evolution in their food habits, timings, and nutrition content as well. This evolution is called nutrition transition (NT). The result of this NT is seen in many people by the way of obesity or even numerous diseases due to nutrition imbalance.

It is evident that there is a shift from healthy to unhealthy with regard to food consumption. This has to be monitored and reversed as early as possible. The harmful lifestyle diseases resulting from NT can be curbed only through awareness and education. In countries that are not as affluent, the lower- and middle-class populations are at a high risk. This situation of undernutrition where there is a deficiency of micronutrients and fiber and overnutrition where there is an excess of salt, sugar, fats, and others occurs because of food that is inexpensive, nutrient-deficient, and energy intense. There is an epidemic of diabetes and obesity because of the double burden of over- and undernutrition. As the healthcare costs of tackling this situation are high, some serious measures should be undertaken.

The nutraceutical market is one of the most promising ones all over the world. It has a great potential as people worldwide are now more aware of the need to be in the pink of health always. But this market is not without its share of challenges. One of the most important fields of focus today is the need to have *evidence-based nutraceuticals*. These are also referred to as the third-generation nutraceuticals. The market for these third-generation nutraceuticals is very different from the conventional market that stands at ~8500 crores. When deriving evidence-based nutra products, it is vital that they be studied scientifically, supported on the clinical level, and contain standardized new ingredients derived from plants, foods, and so on.

Thus far, nutraceuticals have lagged behind because of the lack of the much needed scientific data for standardization. For a nutraceutical company to maintain consistency and abide by the quality standards, it should have access to high-quality ingredients. Today, this is one big challenge for any nutra company as getting nutra ingredients of a consistent quality and at the right time is not always possible.

The earlier method of cultivation of plants and foods did not always yield the necessary quantity for companies to get the adequate amount of ingredients. So, it was not possible to keep the costs low when pricing nutraceutical products. But this challenge was resolved with the introduction of new techniques for production, which was successful in resolving supply shortage and costing woes. This is because the new techniques ensure improved supply and minimize the cost of procuring the raw materials.

Just as the new techniques resolved the previous challenges, they brought along new ones. Most importantly, the new techniques adopted the use of pesticides, heavy metals, mycotoxins, and so on. This only added to the gravity of the issue and the questions regarding the quality of natural products. It is well known that the crucial factors when launching a new nutraceutical product are timing, communication, vigilance, and the right quality management. Constantly changing suppliers would mean changes in the specifications needed, chalked-out processes, and the level of contaminants anticipated. So, the product manufacturers would not be able to maintain a standardized product. Ensuring clear communication with the raw material supplier about the manufacturer's needs and good management is of great importance when re-sourcing raw materials. Thus, it can be concluded that to extract the best ingredients for nutraceutical products, there need to be good-quality raw materials.

THREE FUNDAMENTAL PROBLEMS

The economic growth potential that technological progress creates can be achieved through complementary innovation in managements, organizations, and institutions. There is a large scope for advancement owing to the progress in the field of science, with respect to energy, agriculture, medicine, and advanced materials. But without having the right design for managerial, organizational, or institutional models, its full potential will not be utilized. The right model for a science-based business has still not been found.

Three fundamental economic problems are created by an advancing science, namely, managing risk, integration, and learning. A lucrative avenue for innovation would be the hybrid organizational forms that have mixed elements of markets and hierarchies. These network organizations are not the same as those *strategic alliances* that have been talked about in academic as well as popular press for the past two decades. One of the most important elements of innovation is *management technology*, which is essential for a science-based business as well (Chandler, 1977).

A science-based business faces three basic challenges:

1. The risk management challenge, wherein there is a need to motivate and reward risk-taking over longtime horizons
2. The integration challenge, wherein there is a necessity of integrating knowledge with greatly diverse disciplinary bodies
3. The learning challenge that talks of the need for cumulative learning

It is noteworthy that even though these challenges prevail in almost every business setting in varying degrees, in a science-based business, they have a greater force and are simultaneously present. There is no question of which challenge, be it risk, learning, or integration, to worry about in a science-based business. One has to be capable of managing all of these together.

THE RISK PROBLEM IN NUTRA

Going by the definition, science has the power of predictions. In the case of a mature science, it is possible to make predictions because of the amount of data such as supporting empirical evidence, principles, and accumulated cause–effect theories. A perfect example, is the science of aerodynamics. It has matured to a point where companies such as Boeing develop airframe designs through computer models. Further, a computer can check the performance and characteristics of a plane that has been designed. Having predictive models ensures low risks. But the prediction power would be lacking if it is a less mature science. There is a lack of understanding about the knowledge of the cause–effect relationship. In such a scenario, the R&D has to be iterative.

One crucial element of a science-based business, wherein the nature of R&D is iterative, is that the time horizon required to resolve any uncertainty is very long. Thus, financial cost being high is not the only issue to be thought about but also the technical uncertainties.

Today, science itself poses as a big question. Can science give us enough knowledge through evidence to make a certain claim?

In the pharmaceutical industry, it is possible to make claims as there is sufficient evidence-based knowledge to prove the claim to be the right one. Pharmaceuticals can be called an evolved science that involves R&D, brand development, brand marketing, and others along with postmarket surveillance as well.

In nutraceuticals, evidence for an ingredient needs to be converted into a combination of ingredients that comparatively needs to be evaluated. If we want to derive at the evidence for a specific usage of particular plantlike Triphala, then it is impossible to claim for a specific indication on a few parameters and with specific concentrations. As per the FDA rules, if one claims that a molecule mitigates an indication, then it is a drug. In such a case, there is a dilemma. If you abide by the claims prescribed for nutraceuticals, the composition allows you to go by nutraceuticals.

If claims are made, then the evidence available has to be clearly defined. The regulatory mechanism is evolving in medical foods.

THE INTEGRATION PROBLEM IN NUTRA

Recombination and integration of the different bodies of knowledge that already exist would be able to create breakthrough innovations (Fleming, 2001). This has happened in the nutra industry. There are nutrition bars, atta, and many other forms where the recombination and integration of the food and nutraceutical industries has been done. A good example here would be of toothpaste. Now, medicated toothpastes are easily available over the counter unlike in the past. Colgate did not offer medicated toothpastes like Colgate Sensitive as they do now. For those who had sensitive teeth, Sensodyne was available. So, integration and recombination is done in many fields of science. Food and nutrition are also not far behind in this race.

THE LEARNING PROBLEM IN NUTRA

In any science, there is a need to know the customer's needs. A hypothesis has to be derived from there further to derive at the learning. There is a need to have a standardized form. For instance, in nutraceutical products, there has to be a food form to market the product developed. The learning in nutraceuticals is very specific as there are numerous disciplines involved, such as developing, branding, and marketing of the product. It is absolutely crucial to be able to capture customer insights through these learnings. The key to having a successful science to business would involve how to get the right form, in what way should one capture the evolving demographics, and so on. By meeting these challenges, success can be achieved.

MEDICAL ISSUES IN NUTRA

TREATMENT OF MEDICAL PROBLEMS WITH NUTRITION-BASED PRODUCTS

There are three types of diseases to be considered. The first is metabolic syndromes, which account for the disorders that add to the risk of cardiovascular problems or diabetes. Second in line is gastrointestinal health, which involves the problems that occur in the intestinal tract. The third and last is the most challenging. There is evidence coming forth that cognitive decline can be managed well with good nutrition.

After extensive research Fruitflow—an extract from tomatoes—was launched recently. It can be added to yogurts, beverages, and other food products. It is the only functional food ingredient addressing platelet aggregation by keeping them smooth, thereby avoiding aggregation in the blood vessels (Cowland, 2013).

Another notable example of nutrition for improved health is that of ubiquinol. It is a safe, cost-effective ingredient and key to male infertility. Ubiquinol or coenzyme Q10 has now been used in a wide range of nutraceuticals either alone or in combination with other substances to create *all-round* fertility products (Daniells, 2013).

BUSINESS MODEL CREATION

When developing a business model, ensure the beliefs in the products, ideas, or services sold by the company reach the likely buyers. For this purpose critical analysis of the existing infrastructure and core capabilities should be done. The traditional structures as well as infrastructures already exist in the country with regard to nutraceuticals. But here, having the vital capabilities is essential to create the right products, be for plantation, processing, R&D, and so on. Partners are needed in bringing about the commercialization of the innovation, so a company must analyze the partner network. If there is no difference between the product created and the ones already existing, then configuration of value or differentiation for the product cannot be done.

A company has to build a value proposition, which develops a link and graduates to a relationship with the customer. It is necessary to have a cost structure of a particular amount along with surplus so that revenue streams could be characterized especially in the case of new business creation of a value proposition that is needed in such a case. A business model does not have any identity unless a value proposition is created as it does not require a regular stream.

VALUE PROPOSITION

It may happen that a customer sees just the price and does not give a glance to the sales pitch due to the need to reduce costs. Therefore, making the customers realize the true value of the offerings is vital.

Organizations would certainly need the following (Anthony et al., 2008):

- The customer value proposition that defines the product(s) and/or the service offering(s) an enterprise delivers to its customers at a given price
- The profit system or company value proposition that an enterprise employs to deliver economic value to its stakeholders
- The key resources a company deploys to create value
- The critical processes that guide and shape operations and how the company organizes and acts to create and deliver the value proposition to the customer and itself (Smarta, 2012)

Is there a need to have a business model?

Yes, a good business model is needed and a company must have a *cutting edge.* One lesson to be learned here is that being number 1 may not mean you have achieved success.

The most basic element of success is to communicate the features of the company's product, service, or idea to its likely buyers. Ultimately, it is the complexity that matters for the consumer to make a decision.

So, to summarize what was said earlier, a business model involves the value a company has to offer to its different customers and showcases the capabilities as well as the partners needed for developing, marketing, and delivering the value created; it also involves the relationship capital with the thought of ensuring profits and substantial revenue streams.

An apt example of a science business being formed is Genentech in 1976. It was the first biotech company and was formed to capture the recombinant DNA technology, which uses a technology to engineer cells that produce human proteins. Besides proving that it is quite possible to create drugs through biotechnology, the company also developed a model that drew nonintellectual property. This has been an influencing force in how the biotechnology industry is and how it performs as well.

In Pisano's words, this model developed by Genentech consists of three interrelated elements, which are

1. Technology transfer from universities to the private sector by creating new firms rather than selling to existing companies
2. Venture capital and public equity markets that provide funding at critical stages and reward the founders—investors, scientists, and universities—for the risks they have taken
3. A market for know-how in which young companies provide their intellectual property to established enterprises in exchange for funding (Pisano, 2006)

Genentech made an agreement with the big pharmaceutical company Eli Lilly in 1978. With this agreement, for the marketing and manufacturing rights of recombinant insulin to Lilly, they would pay for developing the product along with giving Genentech the royalties for the sales. This agreement has resolved the major issue that new firms faced when they want to enter a pharma business of huge costs that are needed to develop a drug over a period. The fact is that a pharmaceutical company totally outsourced a proprietary R&D program, for the very first time to a for-profit enterprise. This is how as almost every biotechnology firm began, that is by having a contractual partnership with at least one well established pharmaceutical company.

It would seem that the biotech industry has retreated from its previous position, which was at a more risky and radical end of the R&D spectrum. There has been a remarkable change in the strategies adopted by start-ups as well as the venture capitalist's preferences since the time of the genomics bubble burst in 2001. Instead of having a molecule to market company where the first product's revenue would not be cashed in before a decade, investors and businesses prefer to choose a model that involves low risks and fast paybacks such as simply licensing the already existing products from another company and working to refine it further.

THE NEED FOR A NEW DESIGN

To deal with profound uncertainty and high risks, allow closely interdependent problem solving, and harness the collective experience of disciplines throughout the sector, biotech needs a new anatomy—one that involves a variety of business models, organizational forms, and institutional arrangements (Pisano, 2006). There is a great difference in the approaches that require more innovative drugs compared to less innovative ones. It is certainly not the case of one size fits all. Some of the elements that a good design must have are as follows:

Added vertical integration: Vertical integration, believed to have been discontinued, would be very important for the pharma industry's future. It would prove pivotal when looking at scientifically innovative drugs. A degree of scale is needed for vertical integration. To facilitate this, pharma companies that are established should be positioned well as integrators. But for this purpose, some change is required. Many pharma companies have drawn a line as far as creating their expertise goes within the corporate boundaries. This problematic practice is the real reason for the poor R&D productivity. To truly become integrators, pharma companies will have to have new internal structures, processes, and systems so that there is a link between both the technical and functional domains of expertise.

Long durational alliances: For internal R&D, alliances will be an important factor. It is not possible to venture into all areas of R&D, even for big firms. So, expertise from outside parties, be it universities and small biotech firms, is necessary when looked at from the point of view of the fast technological changes. But such alliances would differ greatly in form and number from the ones that dominate the sector today.

Forming few and deeper alliances is more sensible for technologically innovative projects. In the larger scheme of things, signing one deal in 5 to 6 years for a long duration is better than signing 40 deals in just 1 year. This is because such an alliance would involve more sharing of propriety information and acquiring bigger, better, and productive investment and joint learning.

Handful of independent biotech companies: Even though small entrepreneurial biotech companies remain on the scene, there would be just a few handful of independent public firms. This is because companies that have earnings and allow investors to judge their prospects would be able to use the publicly held model.

Quasi-public corporations: This is another alternative to having a public company. Such a company's shares are traded publicly but the major stake is owned by a large company that has a strategic interest of a long duration in the biotech firm's success. In this case, it would be possible to have better oversight over the firm than in the case of general public corporations. There would also be assured funding from the long-term perspective, which is important in the case of drug R&D. This would facilitate companies to be more independent as well as offer stock options and such incentives to retain as well as attract entrepreneurs. A perfect example of this today is Genentech, where the majority stakeholding is owned by Roche. It is noteworthy that Genentech is one of the most profitable companies to have one of the most productive R&D programs and sustained growth along with having an entrepreneurial and science-based culture.

Science can definitely be a business if organizational forms and institutional arrangements exist.

CONCLUSION

BRIDGING THE GAP BETWEEN SCIENCE AND BUSINESS

In this commercial world, there is a need to commercialize scientific knowledge into viable initiatives. Bridging the gap between science and business is crucial in order to commercialize science. The process of conversion of science to business drives growth, which in turn adds value to the business. By investing in the process of science to business, the companies in turn invest in themselves—and the returns are definitely high. Having a strong conversion process ensures that the final products/offerings manufactured are safe for all those involved from users to manufacturers, service personnel, and so on.

For now, we can certainly hope that a good model will be derived through upcoming science-based businesses. Just as the case with the pharmaceutical industry and the way it has evolved, there is a need to have a distinct anatomy—something that would take into account both the needs of science and business. Only then would a successful business model for a science-based business emerge in the nutra industry.

REFERENCES

Anthony, S., Johnson, M.W., Sinfield, J.V., and Altman, E.J. 2008. *The Innovator's Guide to Growth: Putting Disruptive Innovation to Work*. Innosight LLC, Boston. August 26, 2016.

Chandler, A.D. 1977. *The Visible Hand: The Managerial Revolution in American Business*. Harvard University Press, Cambridge, MA.

Cowland, D. November 2013. Heart-healthy Fruitflow for sport performance. Retrieved from *Nutraceuticals World*. http://www.nutraceuticalsworld.com/ (November 28, 2013).

Daniells, S. January 2013. CoQ10 may boost "semen parameters": Study. Retrieved from NUTRAingredients-usa.com. http://www.nutraingredients-usa.com/ (November 28, 2013).

Fleming, L. 2001. Recombinant uncertainty in technological search. *Manag. Sci.*, 11: 117–132.

Problems with scientific research: How science goes wrong. October 2013. *The Economist*. Accessed July 4, 2016.

Pisano, G.P. 2006. Can science be a business? *Harv. Bus. Rev.*, 10: 1–12.

Smarta, R.B., Ghosh, D., Das, S., and Bagchi, D. 2012. Market-focused innovation in food and nutrition. In *Innovation Healthy & Functional Foods*, p. 616. CRC Press, Boca Raton, FL.

Stokes, D.E. 1997. *Pasteur's Quadrant: Basic Science and Technological Innovation*. Brookings Institution Press, Washington, DC.

Section IV

Regulatory Perspective

10 The Role of Nanoparticles in Both Nutraceutical and Pharmaceutical Products

Dilip Ghosh

CONTENTS

INTRODUCTION

Nanotechnology is defined as creation, utilization, and manipulation of materials, devices, or systems in the nanometer scale (smaller than 100 nm). Nanoencapsulation as an important field of nanotechnology is a process that involves entrapping bioactive agents within carrier materials with a dimension in nanoscale (Fathi et al., 2014). Currently, the market of nanotechnology products in the food industry is approaching $1 billion (most of this on nanoparticle coatings for packaging technologies, health-promoting products, and beverages) and has the potential to grow to more than $20 billion in the next decade (Chau et al., 2007). Recent reviews present an excellent summary of the research groups and private and government organizations that have been spearheading the field of food nanotechnology (Chau et al., 2007; Chen et al., 2006; Sanguansri and Augustin, 2006). Most of the work that these research groups have generated over the last 5 years on nanoparticle vehicles has concentrated on developing production methods inspired on pharmaceutical drug delivery systems

(Sanguansri et al., 2006). The challenge in developing such production methods has been to replace some of the polymers and surfactants used in the pharmaceutical industry with food-grade alternatives.

Nanotechnology generally refers to a range of techniques for directly manipulating materials, organisms, and systems at a scale of 100 nm or less—1 nm—being a billionth of a meter. Nanotechnologies provide new and more powerful means to engage with, manipulate, and control nature and materials at the level of atoms, molecules, genes, cells, and bits of information—what we refer to as the "nanoatomic level of engagement with nature."

Nanotechnology can be understood not so much as a separate and distinct technoscientific field, but rather as a new technoscientific platform, whereby a range of existing disciplines—such as molecular biotechnology, chemistry, materials science, and information technologies—are able to shift their focus down to the molecular level (ETC Group, 2003). Within the food system, this is achieved via the development of nanochemical technologies, nanobiotechnologies, and nanoinformation technologies.

Food nanotechnology has its history from pasteurization process introduced by Pasteur to kill the spoilage bacteria (1000 nm), which made the first step of revolution in food processing and improvement in quality of foods. Later, Watson and Crick's model of DNA structure that is about 2.5 nm opened the gateway of applications in biotechnology, biomedical, agricultural, and production processes. Further, the invention of carbon nanotubes *buckyball fullerene*, which is 1 nm in size, served as the cutting-edge discovery to the world of innovation and led to the era of nanoscience (Pray and Yaktine, 2009). Carbon shows an enormous potential in all fields, including food sectors.

In summary, the novel (unusual) properties of engineered nanoparticles are attributable to their (Nel et al., 2006)

- Small size, resulting in a relatively large surface area (and distribution in sizes)
- Chemical composition, that is, purity, crystallinity, and electronic properties
- Surface structure, that is, surface reactivity, surface groups, and inorganic or organic coatings
- Solubility, shape, and aggregation

Table 10.1 shows the summary of techniques use to characterize nanoparticles.

NANOTECHNOLOGY IN DRUGS AND PHARMACEUTICALS

The most common problem associated with the natural extract is their poor solubility/stability in the aqueous medium, which is essential for the biological applications. Most anticancer drugs have limitations in clinical administration due to their poor solubility and other unfavorable properties. They usually require the aid of adjuvants or excipients, which often cause serious side effects. Moreover, intravenous injection and infusion are unavoidably associated with considerable fluctuation of drug concentration in the blood. Therefore, the drugs can be administered only in limited doses and over limited time periods. Their efficacy is far from

TABLE 10.1

Summary of the Techniques Used to Characterize Nanoparticles

Parameters	Techniques
Physicochemical characterization—particle size and size distribution	Photon correlation spectroscopy
Chemical composition	Energy dispersive x-ray spectroscopy; chemical analysis
Surface change	Zeta-potential capillary electrophoresis, laser Doppler anemometry
Surface hydrophobicity	Water contact angle measurement
Surface chemical analysis	Secondary ion mass spectrometry microscopy; x-ray photoelectron spectroscopy; Fourier transform infrared spectroscopy
Morphology	Scanning electron microscopy
In vitro performance; drug release studies	In simulated gastric and intestinal fluids, with and without enzymes
Blood contact properties	Whole blood clotting time; hemolysis; plasma protein adsorption; platelet aggregation/activation; complement activation
Cell-based assays	Cytotoxicity; phagocytosis; transepithelial electrical resistance; cell/fluorescence staining
Mucoadhesion	Various in-house techniques
Blood concentrations of drug over time	Drug/particle permeation across the *ex vivo* intestine; pharmacodynamic measurements
In vivo performance; toxicological studies	Systemic toxicity; oral toxicity; genotoxicity
Bioavailability and efficacy	Animal models of disease

Source: Adapted from Rekha, M.R. and Sharma, C.P., *Peptide and Protein Delivery*, ed., Van Der Walle, C., Elsevier, 2010, pp. 166–194.

satisfactory and the quality of life of the patients greatly deteriorates. Our aim is to develop techniques to fabricate polymeric nanoparticles and liposomes for better clinical administration, which will not use any harmful adjuvants and can realize a controlled and targeted form of chemotherapy. Paclitaxel (Taxol), which is one of the best antineoplastic drugs found in nature, is currently used as a prototype drug in this lab. It has excellent therapeutic efficacy for a wide spectrum of cancers, especially for ovarian and breast cancer. Due to its poor solubility, however, an adjuvant called Cremophor EL has to be used in its current clinical administration, causing serious side effects, including hypersensitivity reaction, nephrotoxicity, neurotoxicity, and cardiotoxicity. Nanoparticles of biodegradable polymers and other bioadhesive materials as well as liposomes could be an ideal solution to prevent these problems. A few key techniques are being developed in this lab to make the product of desired therapeutic properties. For example, one of our contributions is to use natural emulsifiers such as phospholipids, vitamins, and cholesterol in particle processing, as this greatly improves the drug encapsulation efficiency and its pharmacokinetic and pharmacodynamics properties. Nanoparticles and liposomes of various compositions, produced under various preparation conditions, are characterized by state-of-the-art techniques such as laser light scattering for size and size distribution, scanning electron microscopy (SEM), and atomic force microscopy (AFM) for surface morphology, differential scanning calorimetry (DSC) for the physical status of the drug in the polymeric matrix, zeta-potential measurement for surface charge, and Fourier transform infrared spectroscopy (FTIR) and x-ray photoelectron spectroscopy (XPS) for surface chemistry. *In vitro* release is carried out for a best design of the product. Cell line experiments and animal tests are done before clinical trials. The product is expected to make significant contribution to the economy and healthcare.

Oral delivery of anticancer drugs will be a revolution in the history of chemotherapy. It can bring great convenience and improve the patient's quality of life. Moreover, oral delivery can achieve a prolonged exposure to the drug as opposed to intermittent intravenous injections. This will greatly increase the efficacy and decrease the side effects of the anticancer drug. Unfortunately, oral delivery of anticancer drugs has not been achieved thus far. This is because the oral anticancer drugs would be eliminated from the first-pass extraction of cytochrome P450–dependent metabolic process and the overexpression of plasma membrane transporter P-glycoprotein (Pgp). Oral anticancer drugs are thus not bioavailable. This problem is currently under intensive investigation worldwide. The general medical idea is to apply Pgp/P450 inhibitors such as cyclosporin to suppress the elimination process. The interaction mechanism between the drug and the cell as well as between the nanoparticles and the cell will be investigated so as to design an appropriate nanoparticles system for oral delivery of anticancer drugs. Many chemotherapeutic agents like paclitaxel are water-insoluble compounds and, as such, pose significant drug delivery challenges to solid tumors due to the solubilizing agent, which can be toxic. ABI-007 leverages the attributes of nanotechnology by encapsulating paclitaxel in an albumin-based paclitaxel nanoparticle. This technology can be used to replace solvents, such as the chronopher that is used to solubilize paclitaxel in current formulations, which we are now beginning to understand, which may pose drug availability issues in addition to their toxicity.

Drug carrier systems are now as important as the drug itself. Controlled release provides prolonged delivery of a drug while maintaining its blood concentration within therapeutic limits. Drug delivery systems can thus influence the pharmacological activity by modulating its release from the carrier. Other advantages include increased patient compliance (given a reduction in the frequency of administration), noninvasive routes of administration, minimized local and systemic side effects, and thus a reduced toxicity profile. Nanosized, controlled drug delivery systems can deliver the drugs to the site of action in a predesigned manner, thereby minimizing side effects as well as enhancing the bioavailability of these drugs (Farokhzad and Langer, 2006; Janes et al., 2001; Langer, 2003).

Increasing the bioavailability of orally administered therapeutic peptides and proteins is still a challenging and unachieved goal (Rekha and Sharma, 2010). By virtue of their small size and high surface area, nanoparticle-mediated oral peptide delivery is believed to enhance the bioavailability of these proteinaceous drugs. The purpose of this chapter is to review the different nanoparticulate matrices, the stability of nanoparticles and the encapsulated peptides/proteins, the issues related to the bioavailability, biocompatibility and toxicity of the nanoparticles, and other related topics such as techniques used to characterize the delivery systems and clinical applications.

The potential applications of nanotechnology in various therapeutics and diagnostics areas with special emphasis on key frontiers in angiogenesis modulation using naturally driven drug targets including compounds that modulate oxidative stress and inflammatory pathways for the potential treatment of vascular, cancer, inflammatory, and ocular disorders (Mousa et al., 2007). Also, recent advances in the nanotechnology-mediated gene delivery will be described in this chapter.

NANOTECHNOLOGY IN FOOD AND NUTRITION

Enormous demands for production of functional food with higher nutritional value, lower doses of synthetic preservatives, and better organoleptic features lead to innumerable applications of nanoencapsulation in food processing. For example, this technology has been used to enhance the stability of sensitive compounds during production, storage, and ingestion (e.g., vitamins [Khayata et al., 2012]), decrease evaporation and degradation of volatile bioactives (e.g., aromas [Donsi et al., 2011]), mask unpleasant tastes (e.g., polyphenols [Fathi and Varshosazb, 2013]), or limit exposure to oxygen, water, or light (e.g., unsaturated fatty acids [Bouwmeester et al., 2007; Nedovic et al., 2011]). The encapsulating carrier material must be food-grade, biodegradable, and stable in food-systems during processing, storage, and consumption. The most suitable nanoscale carrier materials for food applications are carbohydrate-, protein-, or lipid-based.

There are two basic approaches to generate nanoparticle systems; one is the *top-down* approach, whereby small particles are produced through different size reduction (mechanical) processes, and the other approach is the *bottom-up* approach, where the nanoparticle is produced by the self-assembly of smaller molecules such as lipids and proteins (chemical processes) (Sanguansri and Augustin, 2006; Shimomura and Sawadaishi, 2001). However, there is a growing trend to combine bottom-up and top-down approaches to produce nanoparticle systems (Horn and Rieger, 2001).

CARBOHYDRATE-BASED NANO- AND MICROENCAPSULATION

Natural and modified polysaccharides are promising vehicles for nano- and microencapsulation of active food ingredients. Polysaccharide-based delivery systems are suitable for many industry applications since they are biocompatible and biodegradable and possess a high potential to be modified to achieve the required properties. In contrast to lipid carriers, carbohydrate-based delivery systems can interact with a wide range of bioactive compounds via their functional groups, which makes them versatile carriers to bind and entrap a variety of hydrophilic and hydrophobic bioactive food ingredients. On the other hand, they are considered as a suitable shell under high-temperature processes due to their temperature stability in comparison to lipid- or protein-based delivery systems that might be melted or denatured. Generally, carbohydrate-based delivery systems are conveniently categorized according to their biological origins: plant origin

TABLE 10.2
Some Modified Carbohydrates Used for the Delivery of Bioactive Ingredients

Biopolymer	Encapsulant	Aim/Outcome
Starch	Meat flavor, gallic acid	To produce amphiphilic starch, increase hydrophibicity
Cellulose	Insulin, nifedipine, *Lactobacillus reuteri*	To increase acid and heat resistance and hydrophobicity
Pectin	Doxorubicin	To enhance biological and anticancer effect of pectin
Guar gum	Bovine serum albumin	To decrease burst release
Chitosan	Mint oil, salmon calcitonin, monoclonal antibody	To increase emulsifying ability, enhance particle stability, and increase solubility in neutral pH
Alginate	Bovine serum albumin, human hemoglobin, *Helicobacter pylori* urease	To produce amphiphilic alginate
Dextran	DNA, doxorubicin	To increase biocompatibility, hydrophobicity, and target selectivity to tumor cells
Cyclodextrin	Lysozyme, quinine, triamcinolone acetonide	To improve targeted delivery and increase pH sensitivity and loading capacity

(e.g., starch, cellulose, pectin, and guar gum), animal origin (e.g., chitosan), algal origin (e.g., alginate and carrageenan), and microbial origin (e.g., xanthan, dextran, and cyclodextrins) (Eliasson, 2006). Table 10.2 shows some modified carbohydrates used for the delivery of bioactive ingredients in the food and nutrition industry.

METHODS USED IN ENCAPSULATION

A wide range of different methods have been utilized for assembling carbohydrate-based nanocapsules (Jones and McClements, 2010; Matalanis et al., 2011). Some of the mostly widely used techniques for encapsulating food bioactives are presented in Table 10.3.

PHENOLIC PHYTOCHEMICALS: A UNIQUE EXAMPLE OF NANOPARTICLE DELIVERY SYSTEMS

Phenolic phytochemicals represent a variety of compounds that are the largest category of phytochemicals and more than 8000 phenolic phytochemicals have been reported to exist in different fruits and vegetables (Crozier et al., 2009). Phenolic phytochemicals have been of particular interests in food and pharmaceutical fields because they have the potential to reduce the incidences of coronary heart disease, diabetes, cancers, and other chronic diseases. Although the positive effects of phenolic phytochemicals on human health have been confirmed by a variety of studies, low absorption rates and limited bioavailability of phenolic phytochemicals have also been also reported (Table 10.4). Naturally low aqueous solubility, poor gastrointestinal stability, passive diffusion, and active efflux of phenolic phytochemicals in the gastrointestinal tract result in such low absorption.

TABLE 10.3
Some Common Methods for Nanoencapsulation

Method	Description	Applied Materials
Reverse micellar method	Prepare reverse micelles in nonpolar organic solvents. The aqueous solution is then mixed with encapsulant with cross linking agent. The organic solvent is then evaporated to obtain the transparent dry mass. The supernatant solution, which contains the encapsulant-loaded nanoparticles, is segregated	Dextran–doxorubicin conjugates using chitosan
Emulsion-droplet coalescence method	A stable emulsion containing aqueous acetic acid solution of chitosan along with encapsulant and oil phase is produced and then, another stable emulsion containing chitosan aqueous solution of NaOH is added under high-speed stirring. Droplets of each emulsion are collided and coalesced and therefore precipitating of chitosan droplets to give small size particles is occurred	Chitosan
Emulsification/ solvent evaporation method	Emulsification of the polymer solution (polymer + encapsulant + organic solvent) followed by homogenization process. During the second step solvent is evaporated and polymer precipitation as nanospheres is occurred	Ethyl cellulose, cellulose acetate phthalate
Salting-out method	Separation of a water-miscible solvent to be done from aqueous solution via a salting-out effect. Next step, biopolymer and hydrophobic encapsulant to be added to get an aqueous gel containing the salting-out agent and a colloidal stabilizer. By adding sufficient volume of water, loaded nanocarriers is formed.	L-Lactide-co-glycolide
Ultrasonication	By cavitation process, ultrasound energy can be transferred to the particles. Ultrasonication therefore is a useful process to couple with other nanoencapsulation methods for breaking up the aggregates of particles formed through the hydrogen bonds, thereby reducing the size of nanoparticles.	Waxy maize starch, alginate–dextran sulfate
High-pressure homogenization	High-pressure homogenization to be performed in several cycles to form nanoparticles based on mechanical stress.	Chitosan, starch

Source: Adapted from Fathi, M. et al., *Trends Food Sci. Technol.*, 39, 18, 2014.

TABLE 10.4
Absorption Rate of Selected Phenolic Phytochemicals

Phenolic Phytochemicals	Sources	Absorption Rate (%)
Anthocyanins	Berries	<1
Flavan-3-ols or procyanidins	Tea, chocolate, and grape seed extract	<5
Isoflavones	Soy	<1
Flavonols (quercetin)	Plant food	3–7
Flavanones (hesperidin)	Citrus	3–9
Stilbenes (resveratrol)	Grapes and wine	<1
Hydroxycinnamic acids	Coffee, tomatoes, and cereals	1–25

Source: Adapted from Li, Z. et al., *Food Hydrocoll.*, 43, 153, 2015.

Nanoparticles can interact with phenolic phytochemicals by hydrogen bonds and hydrophobic interactions to encapsulate phenolic phytochemicals in nanoparticles, which can enhance aqueous solubility of phenolic phytochemicals. Nanoparticles also can prevent against oxidation/degradation of phenolic phytochemicals encapsulated in the gastrointestinal tract. More importantly, nanoparticles can be taken directly up by epithelial cells in the small intestine, which significantly increases absorption and bioavailability of phenolic phytochemicals (Li et al., 2015).

BIOAVAILABILITY AND TOXICITY

Bioavailability is defined as the fraction of unchanged bioactive components that absorb and eventually reach the systemic circulation (Naidu et al., 2008). During the GI process nanoparticles pass through the mouth, stomach, small intestine, and colon, and undergo different changes (e.g., size, surface charge, and physicochemical properties). For example, particles might be swelled, eroded, flocculated (association of nanoparticles), or digested (shrinkage or dissociation of nanoparticle). It is therefore important to monitor carbohydrate nanocarriers throughout the gastrointestinal tract. Due to poor water solubility and short biological half-life of most food bioactives (e.g., water-insoluble or acid-sensitive components), their bioavailabilities are almost low (Hoppe et al., 2013; Yang and McClements, 2013). Nanoencapsulation of bioactives using biocompatible and biodegradable carbohydrates may lead to the improvement of their bioavailability as the result of an increase in water solubility of encapsulated hydrophobic components within the particles (due to the interfacial free energy effect), protection against gastrointestinal conditions, and an increase in the resident time in the gastrointestinal media (due to the ability of the nanoparticles to penetrate into the negatively charged mucous layer) (Acosta, 2009; McClements, 2013). An increase in bioavailability has been reported for drug-loaded β-cyclodextrin (Skiba et al., 1995) and chitosan (Rajera et al., 2013). Some studies also revealed the enhancement of the bioavailability of food bioactives as the result of nanoencapsulation (Arunkumar et al., 2013; Hoppe et al., 2013; Sessa et al., 2014; Yang and McClements, 2013). There is agreement that formulating nanostructured delivery systems yields an increase in drug uptake; however, the mechanisms by which this occurs are not well understood. These mechanisms may involve increasing the apparent solubility of the active ingredient, increasing the rate of mass transfer, increasing the retention time, or increasing the absorption via direct uptake of the nanoparticle carrier (Hussain et al., 2001).

NANOTECHNOLOGY PRODUCTS ON THE MARKET

Food products containing nanotechnologies are penetrating the market, albeit currently predominantly outside the EU (e.g., Japan, China, and the United States). It is widely anticipated that they will appear on the EU market in the next few years. Currently, many nanoproducts are globally available a.o. due to sales via the Internet. But not all applications and not all nanoparticles (NPs) are alike and thus they do not share the same hazard or risk profile. A ranking of risks given the application and type of NPs should be made. An integrated inventory of applications of nanotechnologies and NPs in food has been made. This inventory has been

TABLE 10.5

Summary of the Number of Products per Class of Application in the Inventory

Class of Application	Number of Products
Nanosensors	2
Pesticides	5
Water purification/soil cleaning	5
Food processing and storage	10
Food packaging	7
Food commodities, inert particles	9
Food commodities, delivery systems	19
Food commodities, others	9

Source: Bouwmeester, H. et al., Health impact of nanotechnologies in food production, Report 2007.014, RIKILT and RIVM, Wageningen, the Netherlands, 2007.

made using Google™ 3, the database of consumer products of the Nanotechnology Project (www.nanotechproject.org), by the Woodrow Wilson International Center for Scholars, the Global New Products Database of Mintel (www.gnpd.com), the Nanotechnology Product Directory (www.nanoshop.com), and the report of nanoforum (www.nanoforum.org). The results of this inventory can be found in Annex I of the background document. As stated earlier, applications can be found throughout food production. Products claiming to contain nanotechnology are used in food processing and storage and applied directly in food commodities (Table 10.5).

CONSUMER ACCEPTANCE

Nanotechnology is an emerging technology that will have a great impact on product innovation in the coming years. Currently, the technology is already used in innovative cosmetic and medical products. In the food industry, there is a clear potential for product and process innovation using nanotechnology and nanoparticles. This has already been exemplified by the availability of food products developed by making use of nanotechnology.

It is however the societal responsibility of industry, governments, and researchers to get into potential risks of the application of this evolving technology. The smaller the particles are, the closer they come to the size/structure of natural barriers in nature and our body. Since we currently do not know what this means for the natural barrier functions, we cannot simply extrapolate our knowledge on the safety of micro- and macrostructures and delivery systems to their nanosized equivalents.

Consumer acceptance of new products or products produced with new technologies has had serious dents in recent years with the introduction of food irradiation technology and genetic modification technology. Consequently, both risk evaluation and consumer perception are important issues to be addressed in parallel with the development and application of new technologies. Disregarding these aspects could have a dramatic negative aspect not only on the introduction of nanotechnology but also more in general on public perception of new technologies and product innovation (Bouwmeester et al., 2009).

Although potential beneficial effects of nanotechnologies are generally well described, the potential (eco)toxicological effects and impacts of NPs have so far received little attention.

The high speed of introduction of NP-based consumer products observed nowadays prompts the need on generate a better understanding about the potential negative impacts that NPs may have on biological systems. Some recent studies have shown that indeed there are reasons to suspect that NPs may display toxicological effects on biological systems (Donaldson and Seaton, 2007; Nel et al., 2006; Oberdorster et al., 2007). As nanofood-related products are already on the market and uncertainty about potential risks is high (Morgan, 2005), the need for science-based adaptation of the regulatory frameworks is high.

CONCLUSION

Polymeric nanoparticles have advantageous features for the encapsulation and oral delivery of peptides and proteins, including controlled/sustained release properties and protection from endogenous enzymes. The focus of several research groups appears to be moving from *in vitro* cell culture models and data toward animal models of disease and the assessment of bioavailability. Much work has yet to be performed to determine the exact mechanism of nanoparticulate uptake and subsequent clearance, the associated potential for *in vivo* nanotoxicology, tissue-specific targeting (whether or not this actually improves therapeutic efficacy), and modulation of GI transit; to date, no commercial formulations exist. Despite this, steady, albeit modest, improvements in bioavailability look increasingly promising, and standardization of storage and dosage reconstitution should be relatively straightforward. It is hoped that emerging methods for the analysis of nanosystems and increasing commercial interest in nanotechnologies will provide strong drivers, such that in the near future a nano-based oral peptide or protein formulation will emerge successfully.

The field of food nanotechnology is experiencing significant growth due to the confluence of interests of industry, government, and academia. In the area of nutrient and nutraceutical delivery, there have been important advances made in nanoparticle formulations designed to improve the bioavailability of poorly water-soluble ingredients. However, very little has been done on the improvement of the uptake of hydrophilic compounds such as some soluble minerals (like calcium and iron) and soluble antioxidants (such as isoflavones). Most researchers have worked under the assumption that improvement in bioavailability comes from improvement in apparent solubility and have neglected the impact that mass transfer issues and direct nanoparticle uptake play to enhance bioavailability. More fundamental studies on nanoparticle-mediated nutrient and nutraceutical transport are needed to understand this technology and engineer new nanoparticle delivery systems.

In addition to the potential technological impact of nanoparticle delivery systems in the food industry, there are also concerns about unforeseen side effects of the technology. The fact that these carriers are designed with food-grade ingredients does not mean that they might not cause undesired effects such as transporting or depositing active ingredients or excipients in tissue that they are not supposed to or enhancing the absorption of substances that they are not meant to transport but that are present in the food matrix. Regulations on food nanotechnology are a likely development in the near future that may have a significant impact on the methods of preparations, dosages, and ingredients used in these systems.

Nanomedicine has the potential for diagnosing, treating, curing, and preventing disease and traumatic injury, relieving pain, and preserving and improving human health, using molecular tools. Nanomedicine is not a substitute in most cases for current medicine but rather complementary. It is about moving the technology up in the chain and solving bigger problems.

REFERENCES

Acosta, E. 2009. Bioavailability of nanoparticles in nutrient and nutraceutical delivery. *Curr. Opin. Colloid Interface Sci.*, 14: 3–15.

Arunkumar, R., Harish Prashanth, K.V., and Baskaran, V. 2013. Promising interaction between nanoencapsulated lutein with low molecular weight chitosan: Characterization and bioavailability of lutein in vitro and in vivo. *Food Chem.*, 141: 327–337.

Bouwmeester, H., Dekkers, S., Maryvon, Y. et al. 2009. Review of health safety aspects of nanotechnologies in food production. *Regul. Toxicol. Pharmacol.*, 53: 52–62.

Bouwmeester, H., Dekkers, S., Noordam, M. et al. 2007. Health impact of nanotechnologies in food production. Report 2007.014. RIKILT and RIVM, Wageningen, the Netherlands.

Chau, C.F., Wu, S.H., and Yen, G.C. 2007. The development of regulations for food nanotechnology. *Trends Food Sci. Technol.*, 18: 269–280.

Chellarama, C., Murugaboopathib, G., Johna, A.A. et al. 2014. Significance of nanotechnology in food industry. *APCBEE Procedia*, 8: 109–113.

Chen, H., Weiss, J., and Shahidi, F. 2006. Nanotechnology in nutraceuticals and functional foods. *Food Technol.*, 60: 30–36.

Crozier, A., Jaganath, I.B., and Clifford, M.N. 2009. Dietary phenolics: Chemistry, bioavailability and effects on health. *Nat. Prod. Rep.*, 26: 1001–1043.

Donaldson, K. and Seaton, A. 2007. The Janus faces of nanoparticles. *J. Nanosci. Nanotechnol.*, 7: 4607–4611.

Donsìa, F., Annunziatab, M., Sessaa, M. et al. 2011. Nanoencapsulation of essential oils to enhance their antimicrobial activity in foods. *LWT—Food Sci. Technol.*, 44: 1908–1914.

Eliasson, A.C. 2006. *Carbohydrates in Food*, 2nd edn. Taylor & Francis Group, Boca Raton, FL.

ETC Group. 2003. The Big Down. Atomtech: Technologies converging at the nano-scale. Action Group on Erosion, Technology and Concentration, Ottawa, Ontario, Canada.

Farokhzad, O.C. and Langer, R. 2006. Nanomedicine: Developing smarter therapeutic and diagnostic modalities. *Adv. Drug Deliv. Rev.*, 58: 1456–1459.

Fathi, M. and Varshosazb, J. 2013. Novel hesperetin loaded nanocarriers for food fortification: Production and characterization. *J. Funct. Foods*, 5: 1382–1391.

Fathi, M., Martın, A., and McClements, D.J. 2014. Nanoencapsulation of food ingredients using carbohydrate based delivery systems. *Trends Food Sci. Technol.*, 39: 18–39.

Hoppe, J.B., Coradini, K., Frozza, R.L. et al. 2013. Free and nanoencapsulated curcumin suppress β-amyloid-induced cognitive impairments in rats: Involvement of BDNF and Akt/GSK-3b signalling pathway. *Neurobiol. Learn. Mem.*, 106: 134–144.

Horn, D. and Rieger, J. 2001. Organic nanoparticles in the aqueous phase—Theory, experiment, and use. *Angew. Chem. Int. Ed.*, 40: 4330–4361.

Hussain, N., Jaitley, V., and Florence, A.T. 2001. Recent advances in the understanding of uptake of microparticulates across the gastrointestinal lymphatics. *Adv. Drug Deliv. Rev.*, 50: 107–142.

Janes, K.A., Calvo, P., and Alonso, M.J. 2001. Polysaccharide colloidal particles as delivery systems for macromolecules. *Adv. Drug Deliv. Rev.*, 47: 83–97.

Jones, O.G. and McClements, D.J. 2010. Functional biopolymer particles: Design, fabrication, and applications. *Compr. Rev. Food Sci. Food Saf.*, 9: 374–397.

Khayataa, N., Abdelwaheda, W., and Chehnaa, M.F. 2012. Preparation of vitamin E loaded nanocapsules by the nanoprecipitation method: From laboratory scale to large scale using a membrane contactor. *Int. J. Pharm.*, 423: 419–427.

Langer, R. 2003. Where a pill won't reach. *Sci. Am.*, 288: 50–57.

Li, Z., Jiang, H., Xu, C. et al. 2015. A review: Using nanoparticles to enhance absorption and bioavailability of phenolic phytochemicals. *Food Hydrocoll.*, 43: 153–164.

Matalanis, A., Jones, O.G., and McClements, D.J. 2011. Structured biopolymer-based delivery systems for encapsulation, protection, and release of lipophilic compounds. *Food Hydrocoll.*, 25: 1865–1880.

McClements, D., Nedovica, V., Kalusevica, A. et al. 2011. An overview of encapsulation technologies for food applications. *Procedia Food Sci.*, 1: 1806–1815.

McClements, D.J. 2013. Edible lipid nanoparticles: Digestion, absorption, and potential toxicity. *Prog. Lipid Res.*, 52: 409–423.

Morgan, K. 2005. Development of a preliminary framework for informing the risk analysis and risk management of nanoparticles. *Risk Anal.*, 25: 1621–1635.

Mousa, S.A., Bharali, D.J., and Armstrong, D. 2007. From nutraceuticals to pharmaceuticals to nanopharmaceuticals: A case study in angiogenesis modulation during oxidative stress. *Mol. Biotechnol.*, 37: 72–80.

Naidu, R., Semple, K.T., Megharaj, M. et al. 2008. Bioavailability: Definition, assessment and implications for risk assessment. In *Developments in Soil Science*, Vol. 32, pp. 39–51, Chapter 3. Elsevier, Amsterdam, the Netherlands.

Nel, A., Xia, T., Madler, L. et al. 2006. Toxic potential of materials at the nanolevel. *Science*, 311: 622–627.

Oberdorster, G., Stone, V., and Donaldson, K. 2007. Toxicology of nanoparticles: A historical perspective. *Nanotoxicology*, 1: 2–25.

Pray, L. and Yaktine, A. 2009. Nanotechnology in food products: A workshop summary, Food Forum, Food and Nutrition Board, pp. 13–19. http://www.nap.edu/catalog/12633/nanotechnology-in-food-products-workshop-summary.

Rajera, R., Nagpal, K., Singh, S.K. et al. 2013. Toxicological study of the primaquine phosphate loaded chitosan nanoparticles in mice. *Int. J. Biol. Macromol.*, 62: 18–24.

Rekha, M.R. and Sharma, C.P. 2010. Nanoparticle mediated oral delivery of peptides and proteins: Challenges and perspectives. In *Peptide and Protein Delivery*, (ed) Van Der Walle, C., pp. 166–194, Chapter 9. Elsevier Inc.

Sanguansri, P. and Augustin, M.A. 2006. Nanoscale materials development—A food industry perspective. *Trends Food Sci. Technol.*, 17: 547–156.

Sessa, M., Balestrieri, M.L., Ferrari, G. et al. 2014. Bioavailability of encapsulated resveratrol into nanoemulsion-based delivery systems. *Food Chem.*, 147: 42–50.

Shimomura, M. and Sawadaishi, T. 2001. Bottom-up strategy of materials fabrication: A new trend in nanotechnology of soft materials. *Curr. Opin. Colloid Interface Sci.*, 6: 11–16.

Skiba, M., Morvan, C., Duchene, D. et al. 1995. Evaluation of gastrointestinal behaviour in the rat of amphiphilic β2-cyclodextrin nanocapsules, loaded with indomethacin. *Int. J. Pharm.*, 126: 275–279.

Yang, Y. and McClements, D.J. 2013. Encapsulation of vitamin E in edible emulsions fabricated using a natural surfactant. *Food Hydrocoll.*, 30: 712–720.

11 A Regulatory Perspective of Nutraceuticals and Phytomedicines in India

R. B. Smarta

CONTENTS

INTRODUCTION

The establishment of safety for human consumption is very crucial for nutraceuticals and functional foods as these products are directly consumed by consumers, and if these products are mishandled or are of poor/substandard quality, then they can have adverse effects on consumers.

The main objective of regulating food and other consumable products is ensuring safety of the consumer's health. Apart from this, the regulations also help to bring about fair trade, harmonization, uniformity in practices, price control, and more. Thus, regulations are important holistically.

THE NUTRACEUTICAL SCENARIO IN INDIA

The Indian scenario is quite complex in the area of nutrition. It is really a nutritransition. People are shifting toward functional foods and nutraceuticals.

NUTRITRANSITION

In earlier days, food was traditionally being viewed as a means of satisfying hunger, normal growth, and development but with the advancement of science and research, food and medicine now go hand in hand. The new self-care paradigm promotes the co-existence of traditional medical approaches to disease treatment and the health benefits obtained from food. Thus, consumers have learned that food has a greater value and impact on health than was previously known.

The Indian consumer, especially the middle class, relies heavily on traditional wisdom to achieve complete nutrition. These consumers prefer to use natural extracts of medicinal plants and herbs for their health and nutrition as opposed to products readily available on the market.

The concept of nutritransition is complex with having a malnourished population that includes an undernourished, overnourished, and not fed population in India. This situation makes the transition difficult in India, yet India needs to take the challenge of nutritransition.

Undernourishment is the lack of adequate consumption of nutrients or food. According to the Food and Agriculture Organization (FAO), about 18% of India's population was undernourished in 2012. Today, although the number of people in India suffering from chronic hunger has dropped by around 6.5% to 21.38 Cr. from 22.86 Cr. in 2008–2012, there are still 21.38 Cr. who suffer from hunger and 18% who are undernourished.

Overnutrition is the overconsumption of nutrients or food to a point where it adversely affects a person's health. In India, approximately 11% of the population is overnourished, consuming extra or the wrong calories.

Nutritransition, which can be alternatively referred to as a nutritional paradox, is very much the reality of the nutritional status of India. Certain measures need to be taken in order to maintain the balance of nutrition or the nutritional status in India.

REGULATIONS IN INDIA

In India, the regulatory body that legalizes nutraceutical products is the Food Safety and Standards Authority of India (FSSAI), which was established under the Food Safety and Standards Act, 2006. FSSAI was created to develop science-based standards for food articles and to regulate their manufacture, storage, distribution, sale, and import to ensure the availability of safe and wholesome food for human consumption. The Ministry of Health and Family Welfare, Government of India, is the administrative ministry for the implementation of FSSAI. Some of the global food and nutrition policy–related bodies include WHO (World Health Organization), Codex Alimentarius (or Codex), WTO (World Trade Organization), and FAO (Food and Agriculture Organization) (Figure 11.1).

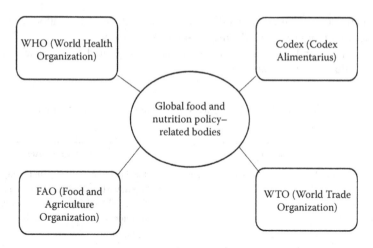

FIGURE 11.1   Global food policy representative model.

Every country has its own regulations and nomenclature for nutraceuticals. When considering the entry into the global nutraceuticals market, understanding these varying regulations becomes quintessential. Some countries have notification-based approaches for market entry (Mexico, Chile), while some have registration-based approaches (India, Brazil, Colombia, and Argentina).

VARIATIONS ACROSS THE WORLD

Some countries consider nutraceuticals in the category of foods, while others consider them in the category of drugs.

Here are some examples:

1. In the United States, the Food and Drug Administration (FDA) regulates nutraceuticals under a different set of regulations when compared with those for "conventional" foods and drug products. According to the Dietary Supplement Health and Education Act (DSHEA) of 1994, it is the manufacturer's responsibility to ensure that a nutraceutical is safe before it is marketed.
2. The FDA is authorized to take action against any unsafe product after it reaches the market. Manufacturers have to ensure that the information on the product label is truthful and not misleading, but they are not obliged to register their products with the FDA or get FDA approval before producing or selling nutraceuticals.
3. In Europe, the food legislation is largely under the umbrella of the European Food and Safety Authority (EFSA). This legislation focuses on "food supplements," which are defined as concentrated sources of nutrients (e.g., proteins, minerals, and vitamins) and other substances with a beneficial nutritional effect.
4. New products from Europe are presumed to have passed stringent European development and quality requirements. As a result, European nutraceutical

companies, which are generally considered leaders in innovation, enjoy a perception of producing the highest-quality products.

5. In Canada and Australia, nutraceuticals are regulated more closely as a drug than as a food category.

The table below illustrates regulatory acts and issues of various countries.

	Regulatory Act	Regulatory Issues
India	The Food Safety and Standards Act (FSSA), 2006	Manufacturing, selling, or importing novel foods, GMFs, irradiated food, organic food, and food for special dietary uses, functional food, nutraceuticals, and health supplements
	The Food Safety and Standards Authority of India (FSSAI) being the single reference point for all matters relating to food safety and standards	
	Revised—Food Safety and Standards Rules and Regulations, 2009	More emphasis on science-based and participatory decisions
	Revised—The Food Safety and Standards Authority of India (FSSAI), 2010	Implemented
Japan	Food for Specified Health Use, 1991	Focuses on health claims for specific products
	Food with Health Claims (FHC), 2001	Category of products expanded to include capsules and tablets
	Foods with Nutrient Function Claims, 2005	Restricted to the specified nutrients having nutritional function claims in FHC
China	State Food and Drug Administration of China (SFDA), 2003	Oversees and coordinates the health, food, and drug agencies
	State Food and Drug Administration (SFDA), 2005	Guidelines for registration of functional foods being promulgated
	State Council Legislative Office (SCLO), 2009	Regulates foods that have functional or health claim associated with their use
United States	Nutrition Labeling and Education Act ,1990	Nutrition labeling of most foods regulated by the agency
	Nutrition labeling of most foods regulated 48	
	Dietary Supplement Health and Education Act (DSHEA), 1994	Describes the role of a nutrient or a dietary ingredient in the normal structure or function of the human body
	Food and Drug Administration Modernization Act, 1997	Federal Food, Drug, and Cosmetic Act relating to the regulation of food, drugs, devices, and biological products
	Food Safety Modernization Act (FSMA), 2011	Ensures safe U.S. food supply by preventing contamination

(*Continued*)

	Regulatory Act	**Regulatory Issues**
European Union	Functional Food Science in Europe (FUFOSE), 1996	Establishes a science-based approach for concepts in functional food science
	Regulation (EC) No 258/97,1997	Applies to GMP, foods, and food ingredients
	Regulation (EC) No 1831/2003	For the authorizations of probiotics used as additives
	Directive 2004/24/EC	Medicinal claims made based on its traditional use of herbs
	Regulation (EC) No 1924/2006	Establishes rules in the labeling, presentation, and advertising of foods
	Regulation (EC) No 353/2008	Establishes implementing rules for health claims in Regulation (EC) No 1924/2006
	Regulation (EU) No 383/2010	Authorizes food that reduces disease risk and children's health
Brazil	National Sanitary Surveillance Agency, ANVISA, 2002	Checks natural or synthetic substances having a demonstrated and physiologic activity
Canada	Canadian Food and Drugs Act and Regulation, 1953	Presented the definition of food
	Food Directorate of the Health Protection Branch of Health Canada, 1996	Nutraceutical generally sold in medicinal forms not usually associated with food
	Canadian Food and Drugs Act, 2001	Describes foods with health benefits beyond basic nutrition
	Natural Health Product Directorate (NHPD), 2003	Defines nutraceutical
Australia and New Zealand	Food Standards Australia New Zealand (FSANZ), 1991	Develops food standards to cover the food industry in Australia and New Zealand
	Australian Capital Territory—Food Regulations Act, 2002	Modification made in food act available in parliamentary counsel
	Queensland—Food Act, 2006	Ensures food for sale is safe and suitable for human consumption
	New South Wales Government—Food Regulation, 2010	Regulation in food safety for food business

The FSSA consists of 12 chapters; of these, Chapter 4, Section 22 of the Food Safety Standard Act, 2006, addresses the regulations related to the manufacture, distribution, selling, or importing of novel food, genetically modified articles of food, irradiated food, organic foods, foods for special dietary uses, functional foods, nutraceuticals, health supplements, proprietary foods, and such other articles of food (Figure 11.2).

WHY IS FOOD REGULATION IMPORTANT?

All living organisms need to consume food in order to survive, as it provides essential nutrients required for the daily functioning of the body. Food is the greatest source of nutrients to our body; food when consumed in balanced

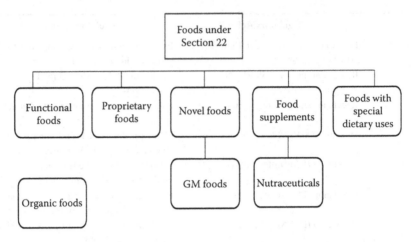

FIGURE 11.2   Foods under Section 22 of the Food Safety and Standards Authority of India.

amount is the principal factor for good health. However, when food is mishandled, underprocessed, or of poor quality and if such food is consumed, it can lead to various foodborne illnesses, which may have adverse effects or may even lead to death.

For this reason and to ensure the safety of humans, it is essential that food be regulated, whether it is in raw form, processed form, or supplement form.

BEFORE THE FSSA

In India before the establishment of FSSA 2006, there were a number of different acts for different types of foods or other related products.

Previously, nutraceuticals were regulated under the act of Prevention of Food Adulteration (PFA). Later, the PFA was replaced by the FSSA. The various acts repealed by FSSA 2006 are

- Prevention of Food Adulteration Act, 1954
- Fruit Products Order, 1955
- Meat Food Products Order, 1973
- Vegetable Oil Products (Control) Order, 1947
- Edible Oils Packaging (Regulation) Order, 1988
- Solvent Extracted Oil, De-Oiled Meal and Edible Flour (Control) Order, 1967
- Milk and Milk Products Order, 1992

Since there were several different earlier acts, the FSSA aims to establish a single reference point for all matters relating to food safety and standards, by moving from multilevel, multidepartmental control to a single line of command. To this effect, the act has established an independent statutory authority—the Food Safety and Standards Authority of India.

The Food Safety and Standards Regulations 2011 notified in the Gazette of India came into force on August 5, 2011, to regulate the manufacture, distribution, and sale of nutraceuticals, functional foods, and dietary supplements in India. The regulations with respect to licensing and registration of food business, labeling and packaging, food additives and others, have been issued by the FSSAI. The acts, rules, and regulations have been implemented starting August 5, 2011. Thus, there is now one single legislation and specified authority to regulate the manufacture, distribution, and selling of nutraceuticals, functional foods, and dietary supplements in India.

Benefits of the FSSA

The FSSA unifies the earlier eight different laws; this has been a step toward harmonization, alignment of international regulations, science-based standards, and clarity and uniformity on novel food areas and also helps to curb corruptions.

THE PRODUCT APPROVAL SYSTEM THROUGHOUT THE WORLD

The product approval process varies across the world (Figure 11.3).

Some countries have a registration-based system, others have a notification-based system, while some do not require any prior product approval.

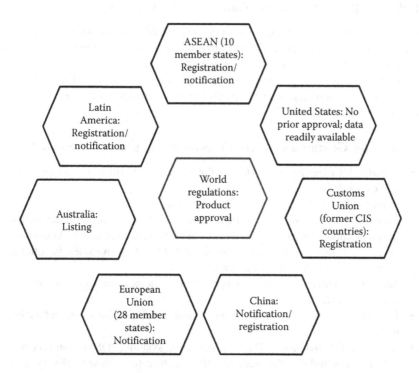

FIGURE 11.3   Representative model of product approval system in the world.

CURRENT REGULATORY SCENARIO IN INDIA

India saw maximum turmoil on the regulatory front from 2013 to 2014. On the one hand, there was imposition of new rules and regulations causing a lot of distress for the importers of nutraceutical products in India, while on the other hand, there was improved product approval process and online registration with FSSAI. FSSAI launched the online FSSAI Product Approval System (FPAS) to make product approval and registration easier.

In order to attract investments, the Ministry of Food Processing Industries, Government of India, has already taken up initiatives such as approving a number of food parks and coming up with schemes for the development of food processing to address the constraints in the food processing sector.

THE NEED FOR CHANGE AND REFORM

Currently, all the different categories are listed under one section, that is, Section 22 of the FSSAI. With the increasing market of each segment/category, it would be better if each category is mentioned separately. So there is a need for a viable and clear categorization in terms of rules and regulations for each of the segment in India as well as globally. The current framework as provided by the FSSAI includes functional foods, foods/nutraceuticals/dietary supplements, traditional medicines, and medicine.

THE ROLE OF REGULATIONS IN THE GROWTH OF THE INDUSTRY

Regulations play a very important role in the growth of industry, through its policies and regulations. In order for the industry to grow, it is very essential that the government and regulations are business-friendly and supportive.

The industry associations, special platforms, manufacturers, and marketers are making their efforts to give a shape to this industry; in addition, governmental support is needed.

HOW CAN THE GOVERNMENT OF THE COUNTRY AID IN INDUSTRY GROWTH?

- *Import and export*—Reduction in the basic and additional customs duty and excise levy
- *Import*—Strengthen the import laws and policies
- *Research and development*—Subsidies for research and development activities and initiatives. For the growth of the nutraceutical industry, innovation is essential; thus, some tax benefits for R&D would prove quite beneficial to the nutraceutical industry at large
- *Investors*—Develop loans and investment schemes for local as well as foreign investors
- *Industry in general*—Government should develop substantial industrial policies
- *Supply and distribution*—Public distribution system (PDS) for nutraceutical products and development of infrastructure for quicker delivery and better connectivity within the country

CHARACTERISTICS OF GOOD OR IDEAL REGULATIONS

The regulations should be such that they support and provide real value to the consumers and also facilitate the growth of the industry and should be business-friendly. Some of the characteristics of good regulations are as follows:

- Developed with all relevant groups in society
- Supported by good science
- Developed on a risk-based approach
- Backed by industry
- Enforceable
- Able to promote public health
- Capable to protect consumers
- Qualified to stimulate innovation and research
- Competent to stimulate economic growth

THE NEED TO MAKE THE NUTRACEUTICAL INDUSTRY VIABLE FOR GROWTH IN INDIA

For the development of a nutraceutical industry, there is a need for a conducive business environment and infrastructure, that is, an industry ecosystem comprising of all stakeholders' right from the investors, manufacturers, marketers, suppliers and distributors, research and development, and customers to government support. Apart from the integration of the stakeholders, there is a need to consider the 3 As, that is, the affordability, accessibility, and accuracy of the nutraceutical products. This basic formula of 3 A's is required for the general population of India to avail the benefits of nutraceuticals.

AFFORDABILITY

During recent years, there has been an increase in quality of life and income; this phenomenon is observed mainly in urban areas, whereas in rural areas, the condition is more or less the same. Around 70% of India's population lives in rural areas, so if we want nutraceuticals to penetrate there, the products need to be priced accordingly; that is, they need to be made affordable for rural population.

ACCESSIBILITY

The availability of nutraceuticals in rural areas is relatively low as compared to urban parts. Most nutraceutical manufacturers are currently looking to penetrate only tier 2 and tier 3 cities. Additionally, traditional retail stores, even in urban centers, have limited nutraceutical products on their shelves, with a bulk of the distribution focused on pharmacies and modern retail outlets. So the distribution and availability of nutraceuticals on the whole is still not well developed.

ACCURACY

The way to promote nutraceuticals is different from that of drugs; nutraceutical products are promoted directly by targeting consumers, whereas drugs are promoted via doctors. Since the nutraceutical products come in to direct contact with consumers, accuracy of the products in terms of safety as well as efficacy is of utmost importance.

CONCLUSION

Regulations are essential from the point of view of consumers as they ensure their safety, but at the same time, the regulations should promote industry and business as well.

In India, with the regulatory guidelines falling into place, it would be critical to understand what this would mean to the industry. Increased health consciousness and increasing disposable incomes of the general population would continue to be crucial drivers of nutraceutical business.

If the regulations are business-friendly, then the manufacturers and marketers feel it relatively easier to get their products launched; in India now, since the regulations are falling in place and the environment is moving toward becoming business-friendly, it is a good time for the foreign companies to enter the nutraceutical market.

For the future the industry needs to focus on marketing strategy concentrating on health benefit claims so that it is easier for consumers to use the products in their daily lives by reviewing the label claims. The industry is expected to focus on disease-specific and overall wellness–related products. The nutraceutical industry currently and in the future is going to be driven by consumer benefits and demands.

With the positive change in regulatory system, increased awareness among consumers now and in the coming years is perfect for the nutraceutical industry to prosper.

REFERENCES

Food Safety and Standards Authority of India, http://www.fssai.gov.in/AboutFssai/Introduction. aspx?RequestID=0kSe4hme1sStsU0emMK_doAction=True. Accessed July 5, 2016.

Keservani, R.K. 2014. *Nutraceutical and Functional Food Regulations in the United States and Around the World*, ed., Debasis Bagchi, Nutraceutical and functional food regulations in India, Chapter 19, Elsevier, pp. 439–444. http://www.researchgate.net/publication/261007048_Ch_19_Nutraceutical_and_Functional_Food_Regulations_in_India.

Smarta, R.B. Nuffoods spectrum, budget—Way forward, eds., Jagdish Patankar, Milind Kokje, February 2015a. Accessed July 5, 2016.

Smarta, R.B. Nutraceuticals: India entry (regulatory and commercialization), iPHEX, Mumbai, May 13, 2015b.

Smarta, R.B. Regulatory perspectives for global opportunities in nutraceuticals, iPHEX, Mumbai, May 13, 2015c.

Section V

Underpinning Science

12 Vitamin E in Health and Wellness
What Would Be the Ideal Therapeutic Dosage?

Dilip Ghosh and Rohit Ghosh

CONTENTS

INTRODUCTION

Evans and Bishop (1922) founded the concept of "substance X," better known today as vitamin E, almost a century ago in relation to the postfertilization placental development in rats. Later work in the 1950s and 1960s (Granados and Dam, 1950; Harris and Embree, 1963; Sondergaad and Dam, 1966), demonstrated the effect of greens or wheat germ oil concentrates containing vitamin E on rancidity of fat present in the experimental rodent diet. In the late 1960s, Klaus Schwarz (1961) rediscovered vitamin E as a cellular antioxidant system, and subsequently numerous scientists proved its effectiveness in preventing cellular lipid peroxidation and other oxidative stress outcomes.

A wide variety of consumers in different age brackets frequently use antioxidant vitamins, including vitamin E complex, for a variety of conceptual and unsupported health benefits—from aging retardation to improving memory and enhancing cardiovascular health. The well-publicized images of antioxidant vitamins with safe and well-tolerated research support (Kappus and Diplock, 1992) are motivating many healthcare professionals to consider routine use of vitamin E isoforms as a potential preventive tool in many diseases.

The Centers for Disease Control and Prevention (2012) estimates that >10% of the population may have nutritional deficiencies. These deficiencies may result from inadequate consumption of nutrient-rich foods; lack of absorption in the digestive tract; illness and disease; interactions among prescription medications, over-the-counter medicines, and dietary supplements; and following "fad" diets that limit the intake of a variety of foods.

OBJECTIVE

The main objective of this review is to assess the efficacy of vitamin E complex in the treatment of health alignments, particularly related to antioxidative and anti-inflammatory effects. This review also includes two other important issues: the bioavailability and the effects of high therapeutic dose of vitamin E stereoisomer for human use.

METHODS

SELECTION CRITERIA FOR CONSIDERING STUDIES

Search Strategy

The following strategy was used in the search:

> [{intervention} AND {outcome/disease}] AND/OR [{safety}]
> {Intervention}:<[MeSH terms/all subheadings] vitamin E OR tocopherol
> OR tocotrienols OR tocochromanol
> AND
> {Outcome/disease}: [MeSH terms/all subheadings] Antioxidant OR
> Anti-inflammatory OR Cardiovascular*
> AND/OR
> {Safety}: safety OR bioavailability

The asterisk (*) was used as a truncation symbol.

Types of Interventions

Any dosage of vitamin E or any of its isomers, tocopherols or tocotrienols, is included in this review. Coadministration of another drug with vitamin E was also considered in this review. We concentrated mainly on randomized double-blinded, placebo-controlled trial, but other clinical trials are also included. High level of randomized animal and *in vitro* studies are also considered for elucidation of mechanism of action. All primary and secondary outcome measures are considered during assessment of study quality had to derive from validated, published scales.

Search Methods for the Identification of Studies

Four Internet sources were used to search for appropriate papers that satisfied the study purpose. These sources included the National Library of Medicine, Washington, DC (MEDLINE–PubMed), the Cochrane Central Register of Controlled Trials (CENTRAL), EMBASE (Excerpta Medica Database by Elsevier), and ScienceDirect (by Elsevier). For this comprehensive search, all four databases were searched for eligible studies up to December 12, 2013. The structured search strategy was designed to include any published paper that evaluated the effect of assessment of methodological quality.

Search Results

Four database searches yielded 366,867 references without any limits. Exclusion of duplicates and irrelevant references left 645 citations. After further evaluation, we excluded 540 studies because they were not good-quality clinical trials or did not fulfill our inclusion criteria. The remaining 105 were finally considered for writing this review. Of these, only 13 studies were able to provide data for our evidence summary analyses (see detail in Figure 12.1).

CHEMISTRY AND BIOCHEMISTRY

The label of "vitamin E" is recommended for all tocol and tocotrienol derivatives that expresses the qualitative biological activity of alpha-tocopherol (IUPAC-IUB, 1982) as the generic descriptor. Tocopherols, the powerful lipid-soluble antioxidants, have a series of related benzopyranols (or methyl tocols) structures that occur in plant tissues and vegetable oils. The basic difference between these two derivatives is in the tocopherols, the C-16 side chain is saturated, whereas three *trans* double bonds are found in the tocotrienols. Together, these two groups are termed the tocochromanols. The tocopherols have a 20-carbon phytyl tail (including the pyranol ring), whereas the tocotrienols carry a 20-carbon geranylgeranyl tail with double bonds at the 3′, 7′, and 11′ positions attached to the benzene ring. The four main constituents of the two classes are termed "alpha" (5,7,8-trimethyl), "beta" (5,8-dimethyl), "gamma" (7,8-dimethyl), and "delta" (8-methyl) (Figure 12.2).

Although the whole "vitamin E" complex (the individual tocopherols are "vitamers") comprises essential components of the human diet, these compounds are only synthesized by plants and other oxygenic, photosynthetic organisms. In plants, there is a wide range of tocochromanol contents and compositions, and photosynthetic plant tissues contain 10 to 50 µg tocochromanols per g fresh weight. Tocopherols are present in all photosynthetic organisms, with α-tocopherol often constituting as the main tocochromanol in leaves; however, the tocotrienols are found only in certain plant families. Seed oils are a major source for the human diet and the compositions of tocopherols in some unrefined oils are listed in Table 12.1.

AVAILABILITY OF VITAMIN E IN PLASMA AND TARGET ORGANS

The lipid-soluble vitamin E isoforms are easily absorbed from the intestinal lumen by biliary and pancreatic secretions after dietary intake via breakdown micelles (Brigelius-Flohe and Traber, 1999; Yap et al., 2001; Traber et al., 1998).

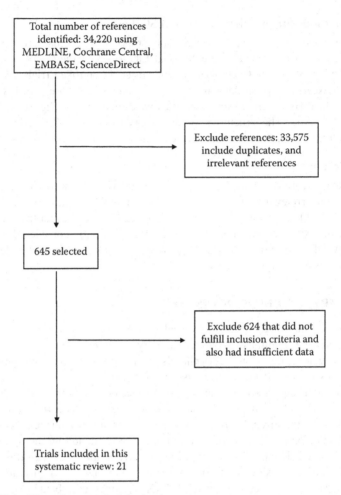

FIGURE 12.1 Flow diagram of trial selection.

The chylomicron-incorporated vitamin E isomers are then secreted into the circulation and transported to the liver through the help of various lipoproteins. Plasma α-tocopherol concentrations in humans range from 11 to 37 μmol/L, whereas γ-tocopherol are between 2 and 5 μmol/L. The regulation of α-tocopherol levels is centrally controlled by the liver through distribution, metabolism, and excretion of this vitamin (Hacquebard and Carpentier, 2005). The most important hepatic regulatory protein, α-tocopherol transfer protein (α-TTP), facilitates secretion of α-tocopherol from the liver into the bloodstream. The α-tocopherol promptly associates with the different nascent lipoproteins (Horiguchi et al., 2003; O'Byrne et al., 2000) before delivering its biological effect.

Tocopherol concentrations vary with age, sex, and demographics. Ford et al. (2006) demonstrated that the mean human serum concentrations in U.S. Caucasian populations for α-tocopherol and γ-tocopherol were 30.1 and 5.7 μM, respectively. Lower serum concentrations of α-tocopherol is very common for African- and

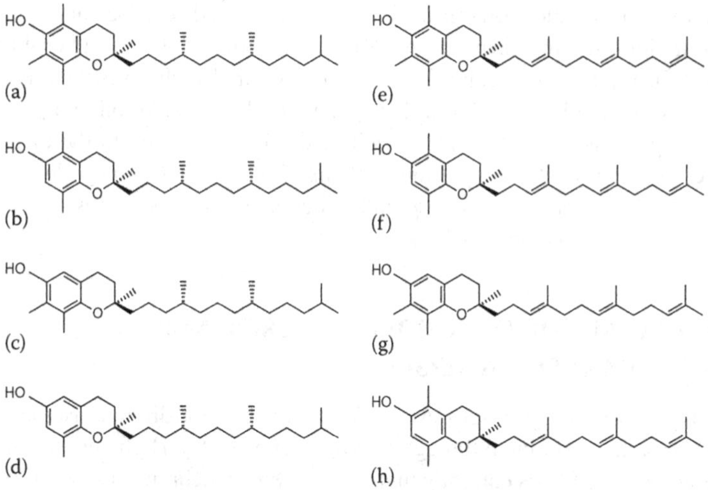

FIGURE 12.2 Molecular structure of vitamin E congeners: α-tocopherol (a), β-tocopherol (b), γ-tocopherol (c), δ-tocopherol (d), α-tocotrienol (e), β-tocotrienol (f), γ-tocotrienol (g), and δ-tocopherol (h). α-Tocopherol is the most abundant and well-studied vitamin E molecule. (Adapted from Joshi, Y.B. and Pratico, D., *BioFactors*, 38, 90, 2012.)

TABLE 12.1

Top 10 Food Sources of Vitamin E (α-Tocopherol, Except Palm Oil)

Source	Milligram (mg) per Serving	Percent DV[b]
Palm oil, 1 tea cup	93.76[a]	100
Wheat germ oil, 1 tablespoon	20.3	100
Sunflower seeds, 1 ounce	7.4	37
Almond, 1 ounce	6.8	34
Safflower oil, 1 tablespoon	4.6	25
Hazelnuts, 1 ounce	4.3	22
Peanut butter	2.9	15
Corn oil, 1 tablespoon	1.9	10
Spinach, boiled, ½ cup	1.9	10
Broccoli, chopped, boiled, ½ cup	1.2	6

Source: Adapted and modified from Office of Dietary Supplements, NIH.

[a] Sum of tocopherols and tocotrienols.

[b] Daily value.

Mexican-Americans and therefore they are potentially predisposed to greater risks from oxidative stress-linked diseases, such as few types of cancers, cardiovascular disorders, and inflammatory diseases (e.g., arthritis, atherosclerosis, IBD).

Plasma concentration of vitamin E depends completely on the absorption, tissue delivery, and excretion rate. The estimated half-life of γ-tocopherol (~15 hours) is much shorter than α-tocopherol (~48–60 hours) in plasma of healthy individuals.

During interventions, these kinetic data must be considered because non-α-tocopherol isoforms of vitamin E are cleared very fast from blood, while α-tocopherol levels are maintained in a steady-state condition. The carboxyethyl-hydroxychromans (CEHC), a short chain metabolite of vitamin E is generated by β-oxidation and glucuronide conjugation processes in cytochrome P450 and finally excreted in the urine or bile (Traber et al., 2005). The unique metabolism of α-tocopherol keeps low excretion level of α-CEHC, whereas ingested γ- and δ-tocopherol may be almost quantitatively excreted out in urine as their CEHCs.

ANALYTICAL METHODS FOR TOCOPHEROL AND TOCOCHROMANOL ANALYSES

The development of a highly selective analytical method for different isomers of vitamin E is one of the major breakthroughs in vitamin chemistry. High-performance liquid chromatography (HPLC) is currently in use to analyze tocochromanol, but several other methods (Ng et al., 2004; Panfili et al., 2003; Ryan et al., 2007) have been developed in the last decade using HPLC coupled with UV (usually 292 nm) and/or fluorescence detection (usually ex. = 295 nm, em. = 325 nm) at fixed wavelengths or electrochemical detection at a fixed oxidation/reduction potential. The downside of these fixed wavelengths is that the analysis does not permit exact quantification of the tocopherol and the tocotrienol isomers in the study material. New technological developments in this analytical field by coupling coulometric array electrochemical Detector (ECD) with HPLC revolutionized the qualitative and quantitative analysis of vitamin E stereoisomers, and as a result, the tocochromanol isomers can be detected in animal and plant samples (Colombo et al., 2009; Roy et al., 2002) without any extra chemical treatment.

SAFETY

The traditional cellular antioxidant effects of various tocopherols and tocotrienols are not consistent with their *in vivo* activities and have raised several controversies in recent years. A few recent mechanistic and human studies identified other "out-of-box" effects such as metabolic and signaling properties. Due to a relatively narrow "window of efficacy" (approximately threefold to fourfold variation), the effective health benefits from tocopherols might not require consumption of "megadoses"; and henceforth the toxicity from overconsumption is uncommon (Wells et al., 2010). Table 12.2 describes the recommended dietary allowance (RDA) and tolerable upper intake level (TUIL) of vitamin E.

The bioabsorption of most of the antioxidant nutrient supplementation compounds in human gastrointestinal tract is a saturable process with low returns. In real-life situation, low doses of vitamin C are absorbed nearly completely, but with higher doses absorption rate drops to ~16%. Similarly, vitamin E (α-tocopherol), at the recommended doses of ~20%–40%, is absorbed satisfactorily with a fractional drop in absorption at higher doses. Orally administered vitamin E after ingestion reaches a plateau in the plasma by 24 hours but it takes ~1 week to distribute evenly to all biological compartments, which is consistent with its calculated half-life (Vaule et al., 2003).

TABLE 12.2
Recommended Dietary Allowance, Tolerable Upper Intake Level, Experimental Doses, and Regimen of Vitamin E

RDA[a]					
Man	Women	TUIL	Experimental Doses	Median Doses	Regimen
15 mg	15 mg	1000 mg[b]	10–5000 mg	400 mg	Daily or on alternate days

Sources: Adapted from Bjelakovic, G. et al., *Cochrane Database Syst. Rev.*, 2, 2008a; Bjelakovic, G. et al., *Aliment. Pharmacol. Ther.*, 28, 689, 2008b.

TUIL, tolerable upper intake level, is the highest level of daily nutrient intake that is likely to pose no risk of adverse health effects in almost all individuals.

[a] RDA, the recommended dietary allowance is the average daily intake level that is sufficient to meet the nutrient requirement of nearly all (97%–98%) healthy individuals in a particular life stage and gender group.

[b] The EC Scientific Committee on Food published its opinion on the tolerable upper intake level of vitamin E (SCF, 2003). The TUIL was established as 270 mg for adults, rounded to 300 mg.

The dose-related toxicity and biological activity of tocopherols are species-specific and depend on the cell type and the chemical isoforms.

Extensive regulatory toxicology and pharmacological studies have been done on animals. From subchronic toxicity studies in rats with tocotrienol, the EFSA scientific panel (EFSA, 2008) recommended the NOAEL for male rats as 120 and 130 mg/kg bw/day for female rats. A meta-analysis of 54 trials with vitamin E used either singly or in combination with other antioxidants showed no significant effect on mortality (RR 1.02, 95% CI 1.00–1.05). They found differences in morbidity in low-bias and high-bias risk trials. Interestingly in 37 low-bias risk trials, vitamin E significantly increased mortality (RR 1.04, 95% CI 1.01–1.06), whereas in 17 high-bias risk trials, the opposite effect (reduced mortality, RR 0.92, 95% CI 0.85–0.99) was reported. No significant effect on morbidity was found when vitamin E was given singly in high (more or equal to 1000 IU) or low dose (less than 1000 IU).

HIGH-DOSAGE VITAMIN E SUPPLEMENTATION

There is a strong commercial trend to use high dose of vitamers (such as 1000 mg of tocotrienol per softgel capsule per day). This would result in a daily intake of 17 mg tocotrienols/kg bw/day for a 60 kg person, which is equivalent to seven times below the NOAEL of the rat study and slightly higher than the dose demonstrated to be without adverse effects in human studies.

Few animal and *in vitro* studies suggest that high doses of alpha-tocopherol supplements can cause hemorrhage and interrupt blood coagulation by inhibiting platelet aggregation. Several randomized trials have largely demonstrated no significant health benefit of vitamin E supplementation (at high dose) on the management of CVD or cancer (Table 12.3). Recent meta-analyses demonstrated no overall efficacy of vitamin E on survival (Miller et al., 2005; Vivekananthan et al., 2003), although the authors did not consider dose–response relationships. The results from a large meta-analysis

TABLE 12.3

Clinical Trials of High-Dose Vitamin E Supplementation and Risk for All-Cause Mortality, Ordered by Dosage of Vitamin E

Study, Year (Reference)	Country	Population	Mean Age (Years)	Vitamin E Dosage (IU/day)
HOPE, 2000 (Yusuf et al., 2000)	19 countries	High risk for CVD events	66	400
AREDS, 2001 (AREAD Report, 2001)	United States	Well-nourished older adults	68	400
PPS, 1994 (Greenberg et al., 1994)	United States	Recent history of large-bowel adenoma	61	440
VECAT, 2004 (McNeil et al., 1998)	Australia	Healthy older adults	66	500
CHAOS, 1996 (Stephens et al., 1996)	United Kingdom	Angiographic evidence of CAD	62	400 or 800
REACT, 2002 (European American Cataract Trial, 2002)	United States, United Kingdom	Early age-related cataracts	66	660
MRC/BHF HPS, 2002 (MRC/BHF trial, 2002)	United Kingdom	High risk for CVD events	Range, 40–80	660
SPACE, 2000 (Boaz et al., 2000)	Israel	Dialysis patients with CVD	65	800
WAVE, 2002 (Waters et al., 2002)	United States, Canada	Postmenopausal women with CAD	65	800
ADCS, 1997 (Sano et al., 1997)	United States	Alzheimer disease	73	2000
The Women's Health Study (WHS) 2005 (Lee et al., 2005)	United States	CVD and cancer	55	600
DATATOP, 1998 (Mortality in DATATOP, 1998)	United States, Canada	Early Parkinson's disease	62	2000

Source: Adapted from Miller, E.R. et al., *Ann. Intern. Med.*, 142, 37, 2005.
ADCS, Alzheimer's Disease Cooperative Study; AREDS, Age-Related Eye Diseases Study Group; CHAOS, Cambridge Heart Antioxidant Study; DATATOP, Deprenyl and Tocopherol Antioxidative Therapy of Parkinsonism; HOPE, Heart Outcomes Prevention Evaluation; MRC/BHF HPS, Medical Research Council/British Heart Foundation Heart Protection Study; PPS, Polyp Prevention Study; SPACE, Secondary Prevention with Antioxidants of Cardiovascular Disease in End Stage Renal Disease; VECAT, Vitamin E, Cataracts, and Age-Related Maculopathy; WAVE, Women's Angiographic Vitamin and Estrogen.

of 19 clinical trials involving 135,967 participants using dosages of vitamin E ranging from 16.5 to 2000 IU/day (median, 400 IU/day) were very convincing (Miller et al., 2005). Nine of 11 trials testing high-dosage vitamin E (>400 IU/d) showed increased risk (P = 0.035) of all-cause mortality in comparison with low vitamin E (P > 0.2) and controls. A statistically significant dose–response relationship between vitamin E and all-cause mortality was demonstrated with higher risk at dosages greater than 150 IU/day.

VITAMIN E: PHARMACOLOGICAL AND THERAPEUTIC EFFECTS

It has been almost a century since the birth of vitamin E; still a large number of investigators are attempting to fully explore its role in a variety of pathophysiological contexts. The antioxidant property of vitamin E has been at the center of all research since its discovery, and as a result, there is a strong belief that vitamin E complex, as a lipophilic antioxidant, protects membranes from being oxidatively damaged by free radicals (Wolf, 2005). However, several lines of investigation have recently revealed that vitamin E has biological roles unrelated to its antioxidant properties. Among these roles, gene regulator for signal transduction and gene expression, redox sensor, and modulator of specific cell functions were advocated. Based on these emerging hypotheses, it is clear that vitamin E is a complex molecule with varied and pleiotropic effects (Rimbach et al., 2002; Roy et al., 2002; Traber and Atkinson, 2007; Zingg, 2007).

ANTIOXIDANT AND ANTI-INFLAMMATORY ACTIVITY

Traditional as well as epidemiological evidence indicates that a dietary antioxidant trio, for example, vitamins A, C, and E, may be a contributing factor in human and animal health maintenance (Sen et al., 2007; Yoshida et al., 2003).

Some early epidemiologic data have indicated the inverse relationship of high plasma concentrations of vitamin E with a lower risk of cardiovascular disease and certain types of cancer. A randomized, double-blinded, placebo-controlled study using a mixture of α-, β-, γ-, and δ- tocotrienols and α-tocopherol on human cellular DNA damage suggested a possible relationship between the molecular mechanisms involved in formation and the repair of breaks in the DNA with vitamin E mixture supplementation (Siok-Fong et al., 2008).

One of the largest French randomized, double-blind, placebo-controlled primary prevention trial "Supplementation en Vitamines et Mineraux Antioxidants (SU.VI.MAX)" study (Malvy et al., 2001) on 13,017 adults with a median follow-up time of 8 years was conducted with a combination of antioxidant vitamins and minerals at nutritional doses. Study results indicated the low-dose antioxidant supplementation reduced the total cancer incidence in men only. Similar conclusions were found in a few other human studies also (Hercberg et al., 1999; Kesse-Guyot et al., 2009).

Recent *in vitro* and *in vivo* findings demonstrate that tocotrienols act as UV filters by reducing UVB-induced inflammatory gene and protein expression, particularly cyclooxygenase-2/COX-2, interleukin/IL-1b, IL-6, and monocyte chemotactic protein-1, but did not show any significant effect on PGE_2 (Pedrelli et al., 2012).

In our evidence summary (Table 12.4), most of the trials (Arlt et al., 2012; Dahlan et al., 2012; Hernandez et al., 2013; Luliano et al., 2001; Melhem et al., 2005;

TABLE 12.4

Evidence Summary Table: Antioxidant and Anti-Inflammatory Effects

Health Platform	Reference	Study Design	Tocopherol or Tocotrienol Isomers Studied	Subject Characteristics	Treatment Regimen Including Dosage	Treatment Outcome	Strength of Evidence	Original Author Recommendations and Conclusions
Antioxidant	Arlt et al. (2012)	Open label	None specified but α-tocopherol indicated	23 mild-to moderate-stage Alzheimer's disease patients with current cholinergic treatment	Supplementation with 400 IU vitamin E per day at lunch and 1000 mg vitamin C given in two doses (morning and evening); continued cholinergic treatment	Overall, no significant clinical effects observed between the supplemented and control groups Biochemically, the supplemented group saw a reduced oxidizability of the CSF lipoproteins after 1 month	Medium level High-bias risk Low power, open label study	Combined vitamin E and C supplementation of AD patients increases CSF vitamin concentration and reduces *in vitro* CSF lipoprotein oxidation after 1 month. No slowing of cognitive decline *(Continued)*

TABLE 12.4 (*Continued*)
Evidence Summary Table: Antioxidant and Anti-Inflammatory Effects

Health Platform	Reference	Study Design	Tocopherol or Tocotrienol Isomers Studied	Subject Characteristics	Treatment Regimen Including Dosage	Treatment Outcome	Strength of Evidence	Original Author Recommendations and Conclusions
Cellular protection	Dahlan et al. (2012)	Randomized	Tocotrienol extract (TRF) containing of α, β, δ-tocotrienol, and α-tocopherol	Peripheral venous blood from healthy individuals of 39–50 years (young) and >50 years old (old)	Pretreatment of lymphocytes with 50,100 or 200 μg/mL TRF for 25 hours prior to 1 mM H_2O_2 exposure for 6 hours; also posttreatment 6 hours after 1 mM H_2O_2 exposure with TRF (50, 100, or 200 μg/mL) for 24 hours	Pretreatment with <400 μg/mL resulted in no effect on cell death. Pretreatment with 400–1000 μg/mL caused a 12% reduction in cell viability Posttreatment with TRF increased cell viability with dose Reversal of protein downregulation by TRF treatment is applied, making this less evident in older groups	High with mechanistic evidence	Younger group more prone to externally induced changes to protein expression compared to older group. No clear dose–response relationship between protein changes and TRF dosage. TRF reversed down-regulation of peroxiredoxins, indicating increased cellular ability to resist oxidative damage *(Continued)*

TABLE 12.4 (Continued)
Evidence Summary Table: Antioxidant and Anti-Inflammatory Effects

Health Platform	Reference	Study Design	Tocopherol or Tocotrienol Isomers Studied	Subject Characteristics	Treatment Regimen Including Dosage	Treatment Outcome	Strength of Evidence	Original Author Recommendations and Conclusions
Antioxidant	Melhem et al. (2005)	Open label	Multiple antioxidants including α-tocopherol	50 Chronic hepatitis C patients; mean age 53.3 years	Bidaily orally given combination of seven antioxidants for 20 weeks; concurrent intravenous treatment twice weekly with four different preparations for the first 10 weeks; dosage constant	Large decreases in circulating alanine aminotransferase (ALT) were observed. Fifty percent of patients with previously elevated ALT had normalized ALT at the end of treatment. Serum hepatitis C viral RNA reduced in around 25% of patients Some improvement in hepatic histology was observed	Medium level, high risk bias, no controls. Combination study with several known hepatoprotective agents	Antioxidative therapy had a positive outcome on chronic hepatitis C virus patients possibly due to favorable antioxidative effects on viral-induced inflammation. Further double-blind studies are required

(Continued)

TABLE 12.4 (Continued)
Evidence Summary Table: Antioxidant and Anti-Inflammatory Effects

Health Platform	Reference	Study Design	Tocopherol or Tocotrienol Isomers Studied	Subject Characteristics	Treatment Regimen Including Dosage	Treatment Outcome	Strength of Evidence	Original Author Recommendations and Conclusions
Anti-inflammatory	Hernandez et al. (2013)	Randomized, double-blinded, crossover	γ-Tocopherol (γT)	Male F344/N rats, 9–10 weeks of age, and 13 healthy human subjects, mean age of 26	Rats, 30 mg/kg body weight γT in tocopherol, stripped corn oil by oral gavage for 4 consecutive days; humans, γT-enriched tablet (50 mg d-α-tocopherol, 240 mg d-β tocopherol plus d-d-δ-tocopherol, 540 mg d-γ-tocopherol) for 7 days	In rats, oral γT treatment saw reduced LPS-induced BALF neutrophil counts similar to controls. γT shown to reduce tissue infiltration and airway neutrophil accumulation imposed by LPS challenge AND Humans—Decreased levels of 5-nitro-γT during γT treatment period. γT treatment reduced the increase of induced sputum neutrophils during LPS challenge, no change in placebo	Medium level; Low risk bias Some carryover effects observed Small sample size	γT supplementation reduced neutrophil recruitment to the airway. Decreased 5-nitro-γT during treatment period indicating reduced nitrosative stress. Supplementation with γT may be beneficial for neutrophilic airway inflammatory disease

(Continued)

TABLE 12.4 (Continued)
Evidence Summary Table: Antioxidant and Anti-Inflammatory Effects

Health Platform	Reference	Study Design	Tocopherol or Tocotrienol Isomers Studied	Subject Characteristics	Treatment Regimen Including Dosage	Treatment Outcome	Strength of Evidence	Original Author Recommendations and Conclusions
Antioxidant	Pedrelli et al. (2012)	A single-center, open, placebo-controlled intra-individual study	Monoderma-ET10, a commercial topical combination containing active agents, tocopherols (at concentration of 10%), and tocotrienols (at concentration of 0.3%)	30 volunteers; mean age 45.07 years; phototype 6.7% with II, 90% with III, and 3.3% with IV, with a clinical history of photosensitivity	Selected fields (field size 2 × 2 cm) on non-sun-exposed gluteal skin being irradiated with UVB doses ranging from 0.06 to 0.50 J/cm², one of which was treated with the antioxidant formulation (in quantities of 2 mg/cm²) for 30 minutes, whereas the other field (control) did not undergo any treatment	The pretreatment with the vitamin E formulation highly protects against photosensitivity, and all reactions to irradiation were significantly lower in the areas treated with the topical vitamin E formulation compared to those treated with the simple vehicle or vitamin A	Medium level. Small sample size and non-randomized trial	The use of a new topical formulation containing significant concentrations of tocotrienols and tocopherols represents a promising strategy to reduce the photo-induced skin damage

(Continued)

TABLE 12.4 (Continued)
Evidence Summary Table: Antioxidant and Anti-Inflammatory Effects

Health Platform	Reference	Study Design	Tocopherol or Tocotrienol Isomers Studied	Subject Characteristics	Treatment Regimen Including Dosage	Treatment Outcome	Strength of Evidence	Original Author Recommendations and Conclusions
Cellular protection	Luliano et al. (2001)	Randomized	Vitamin E (not specified)	20 healthy Italian subjects	300 mg/day vitamin E on an empty stomach or during dinner for 15 days	The lipid-peroxide scavenging ability of plasma increased in those taking the supplement after eating but was not affected in the control group	Low, small sample size No explanation on mechanism	Plasma vitamin E concentration and plasma antioxidant activity in oral supplement is affected by food intake. Maximal absorption is if vitamin E is given during meals

Pedrelli et al., 2012) showed some promising strategy to reduce oxidation-induced damages, but convincing conclusions are yet to come.

Several recent meta-analyses (Bjelakovic et al., 2007, 2008b) suggest antioxidant supplements may not convey health benefits in both primary and secondary points of view. Since variations in the response of different individuals was one of the key determining factors for convincing outcome measures, all these negative conclusions were most likely due to this factor.

CARDIOVASCULAR DISEASE

Again, traditional evidence and epidemiological studies indicated the effectiveness of vitamin E supplementation in reducing atherosclerosis progression. However, large interventional clinical trials in the last decade (Lee et al., 2005; Lonn et al., 2005; Mustad et al., 2002) have not shown cardiovascular benefits by vitamin E supplementation (Table 12.5). Although few studies showed increased levels of serum tocotrienols in plasma, there is no measurable beneficial effect on cardiovascular disease risk factors. Nevertheless, Rasool et al. (2008) showed some positive effects on arterial compliance with a mixture of tocotrienol and α-tocopherol in a randomized, placebo-controlled, double-blinded end point clinical study. Schurks et al. (2010) contradicted this effect in their meta-analysis of nine randomized trials totaling 118,765 participants. They demonstrated the risk for hemorrhagic stroke was increased by 22% and the risk of ischemic stroke was reduced by 10% from vitamin E supplementation, which is in well agreement with other negative studies. However, some cardiovascular deaths in recent supplemented groups raised demands of further large and long-term clinical research.

THE REGULATORY POSITION OF VITAMIN E AROUND THE WORLD

The Scientific Committee on Food (SCF), after evaluation of vitamin E intake, has established a tolerable upper intake level (UL) as d-α-tocopherol for adults of 300 mg α-tocopherol/equivalents day. The Joint Expert Committee on Food Additives (JECFA) of WHO/FAO and the scientific opinion of the EU panel have formulated and recommended an acceptable daily intake (ADI) of 0.15–2.0 mg/kg bw/day calculated as α-tocopherol (EC Directive, 2008, 2009). The recent European Directive (EC Directive, 2008) recommended a revised RDA value for vitamin E as 12 mg. This regulation shall be binding in its entirety and directly applicable in all Members States (EC Directive, 2009).

In Australia, NHMRC recommended an adequate intake (AI) rather than an estimated average requirement (EAR) for vitamin E for both healthy populations with no apparent vitamin E deficiency (http://www.nrv.gov.au/nutrients/vitamin%20e. htm, accessed on August 8, 2013). Based on the U.S. NOAEL (540 mg/day) value (Meydani et al., 1998), the upper limit (UL) for vitamin E was therefore established as 270 mg/day for Australian and New Zealand adults (rounded to 300 mg/day). The ULs for other age groups were developed on the basis of relative body weight.

TABLE 12.5
Evidence Summary Table: Cardiovascular

Health Platform	Reference	Study Design	Tocopherol or Tocotrienol Isomers Studied	Subject Characteristics	Treatment Regimen Including Dosage	Treatment Outcome	Strength of Evidence	Original Author Recommendations and Conclusions
Cardiovascular	Lee et al. (2005)	Randomized, double-blind, placebo controlled	Vitamin E, α-tocopherol specified	39,876 apparently healthy U.S. women with mean age 54.6 years	Capsules of low-dose aspirin (100 mg) AND 600 IU of α-tocopherol every second day OR placebo for 10 years	Non-significant risk reduction (7%) and significant death reduction (24%) in cardiovascular events in supplemented group compared to placebo. No effects on specific cardiovascular events. No changes in risk or deaths after treatment adjustment	Very high double-blind High power Low bias risk Varied sample characteristics	No support or recommendation of vitamin E supplementation as prevention for cardiovascular disease among healthy women. Some cardiovascular death reduction in supplemented group needs further research

(Continued)

TABLE 12.5 (*Continued*)
Evidence Summary Table: Cardiovascular

Health Platform	Reference	Study Design	Tocopherol or Tocotrienol Isomers Studied	Subject Characteristics	Treatment Regimen Including Dosage	Treatment Outcome	Strength of Evidence	Original Author Recommendations and Conclusions
Cardiovascular	Lonn et al. (2005)	Randomized, double-blind, placebo controlled	Daily dose of natural source vitamin E (400 IU) or matching placebo	3,994 patients of at least 55 years of age	Daily intake of natural source vitamin E (RRR-α-tocopheryl acetate) (400 IU/day) vs. placebo	After a median 7.0 years of follow-up for the entire study population no significant effect on myocardial infarction, stroke, cardiovascular death, unstable angina, revascularization, and total mortality	High. High number of patients for 2 years treatment and 7 years follow-up	In addition to lack of benefit for vitamin E in preventing major cardiovascular events, this study raises concern about an increased risk of heart failure related to vitamin E

(*Continued*)

TABLE 12.5 (Continued)
Evidence Summary Table: Cardiovascular

Health Platform	Reference	Study Design	Tocopherol or Tocotrienol Isomers Studied	Subject Characteristics	Treatment Regimen Including Dosage	Treatment Outcome	Strength of Evidence	Original Author Recommendations and Conclusions
Cardiovascular	Mustad et al. (2002)	Randomized, double-blind parallel	α-Tocotrienol γ-Tocotrienol P25-complex tocotrienol	68 healthy subjects (39 male, 29 female) aged 25–65 years old	Intake of tocotrienols was 200 mg/day over 28 days Capsules of either-mixed α-tocotrienol and γ-tocotrienol palm oil extract OR High γ-tocotrienol rice bran oil extract OR P25-complex extract from rice bran oil	Increased serum α-tocotrienol observed (up to ninefold) with the high γ-tocotrienol supplement Overall the LDL cholesterol increased with statistical significance in the combined α- and γ-tocotrienol supplement compared with P25-complex supplement	Medium with low risk bias	Increased serum tocotrienols indicate active components were absorbed Supplementation with the three tested commercially available 200 mg tocotrienol/day supplements has no beneficial effect on cardiovascular disease risk factors

(Continued)

TABLE 12.5 (Continued)
Evidence Summary Table: Cardiovascular

Health Platform	Reference	Study Design	Tocopherol or Tocotrienol Isomers Studied	Subject Characteristics	Treatment Regimen Including Dosage	Treatment Outcome	Strength of Evidence	Original Author Recommendations and Conclusions
Cardiovascular	Sesso et al. (2008)	Randomized, double-blind, placebo controlled factorial trial	Vitamin E as synthetic α-tocopherol and vitamin C as synthetic ascorbic acid	14,641 U.S. male physicians aged 50 years and older	Intake of 400 IU of vitamin E every other day and 500 mg of vitamin C daily for nearly 10 years	Although vitamin E intervention had no significant effect on total mortality (95% CI, 0.97–1), it was associated with an increased risk of hemorrhagic stroke	High. Long-term study with composite end point of major CVD outcome	Neither vitamin E nor vitamin C supplementation reduced the risk of major cardiovascular events
Cardiovascular	Malvy et al. (2001)	Randomized, double-blind, placebo controlled primary prevention study	Mixture of vitamins and minerals including vitamin E	12,735 general population	Daily supplementation of antioxidant vitamin and mineral tablet (1–3 times daily) for 2 years	The mean concentration of α-tocopherol is higher among men in the intervention group than women	High with larger number of participants, 8-year follow-up results	Authors predicted 8-year follow-up will improve incidence rate associated with such amounts of antioxidant agents

CONCLUSION

For over nearly a century, vitamin E has been explored and is in place for human use, but since then, scientists, manufacturers, regulators, and medical practitioners have been continuously debating its functional roles in human bodies. The tremendous advancement of isolation and identification techniques of the various types of tocopherols and tocotrienols has changed the whole gamut of vitamin E's scientific research and development. The enormous speed of new scientific discoveries is helping to establish its biological effects beyond traditional antioxidative action. New evidence has emerged to support vitamin E's new biological roles such as a physiological gene modulator of specific signaling pathways involved in metabolic and inflammatory events.

In general, there is a consistent agreement from series of human observational epidemiological studies with the hypothesis of health benefits of vitamin E consumption. In one recent nutrition cohort study (European Prospective Investigation into Cancer [EPIC] for development of EPIC Nutrient Database [ENDB]), the difference in overall intake of vitamin E evidenced by European region, that is, higher intake in the South, lower intake in the North. This may be due to the food sources of vitamin E, and in this case, the consumption pattern of vegetable oils is different. This unique trend may be the foundation of potential etiological links between the intake of vitamin E isomers and chronic disease risk in these countries (Jenab et al., 2009). All these well-publicized consumer message about the inverse relationship between vitamin E levels and intake with cognitive function, the risk of dementia and Alzheimer's-related disorders has been challenged at every level. Although the laboratory-based *in vitro* studies support the molecular mechanism of vitamin E isomers in mitigating the effects of disease pathophysiology, in reality, the majority of randomized clinical trials with vitamin E apparently do not fully support this pharmacokinetic and pharmacodynamic evidence.

The recent experts' opinion on this unconvincing clinical support to vitamin E's health benefits is mostly due to the failure of integration of novel aspects of vitamin E's biochemistry with analysis of epidemiological and interventional data sets. It is true, based on the available scientific information, that α-tocopherol is the most efficient and safest of the vitamin E isoforms because α-tocopheroxyl radical is relatively long-lived and converted easily by water-soluble antioxidants (Traber, 2013). The other non-α-tocopherol forms are readily metabolized into cytotoxic adducts by xenobiotic pathways. To reach a final conclusion better designed prospective interventional studies aimed at the uses and the dosage of different tocopherols and tocotrienols are urgently needed.

Furthermore, few recent studies conclusively showed the synergistic/combinational (Table 12.6) effects of combined tocotrienol isomers during treatment with other chemotherapeutic agents. They strongly suggested and showed a new therapeutic pathway that combination therapy may provide significant health benefits in the prevention and/or treatment of breast cancer in women, while at the same time avoiding tumor resistance or toxic effects associated with high-dose monotherapy (Sylvester et al., 2011).

TABLE 12.6

Evidence Summary Table: Combination Therapies

Health Platform	Reference	Study Design	Tocopherol or Tocotrienol Isomers Studied	Subject Characteristics	Treatment Regimen Including Dosage	Treatment Outcome	Strength of Evidence	Original Author Recommendations and Conclusions
Various	Galasko et al. (2012)	Randomized, double blind	α-Tocopherol	78 Mild to moderate Alzheimer's disease patients. Mean age 73.6 years old	800 IU/day of vitamin E plus 500 mg/day of vitamin C plus 900 mg/day of α-lipoic acid OR 400 mg of coenzyme Q 3 times/daily OR a placebo for 16 weeks	Drugs were well tolerated. No difference in CSF biomarkers observed except F2-isoprostane levels that decreased by 19% in the vitamin E supplemented group. MMSE score declined in the vitamin E supplemented group	Medium level Low bias risk	Antioxidants had no influence on amyloid or tau-related pathology. F2-isoprostane reduction indicates less oxidative stress brought about by vitamin E supplementation. Faster cognitive decline also observed in this group

(Continued)

TABLE 12.6 (Continued)
Evidence Summary Table: Combination Therapies

Health Platform	Reference	Study Design	Tocopherol or Tocotrienol Isomers Studied	Subject Characteristics	Treatment Regimen Including Dosage	Treatment Outcome	Strength of Evidence	Original Author Recommendations and Conclusions
Various	Pantzaris et al. (2013)	Randomized, double-blind, parallel	α-Tocopherol γ-Tocopherol	80 participants with relapsing-remitting multiple sclerosis. No recent relapses or prior immunosuppressant therapy	Treatments given orally once daily before dinner. A-Ω-3 and Ω-6 polyunsaturated fatty acids with minor quantities of unspecified fatty acids, vitamins A and E OR A with γ-tocopherol OR γ-tocopherol alone OR Placebo	Significantly reduced annual relapse rate in the group with combined omega fatty acids and γ-tocopherol as opposed to other three groups. Increased time to disability progression observed in the combined supplement group and probability of disability progression was 10% as opposed to 58% in placebo	Non-adherence rates and high dropout rates were addressed in results Low-bias risk	Combined supplementation significantly reduced the annual relapse rate and risk of disability progression. No serious adverse effects were observed. Larger studies needed to further assess efficacy and safety of the combined therapy

REFERENCES

AREAD Report. 2001. A randomized, placebo-controlled, clinical trial of high-dose supplementation with vitamins C and E and beta carotene for age-related cataract and vision loss: AREDS report no. 9. *Arch. Ophthalmol.*, 119: 1439–1452.

Arlt, S., Müller-Thomsen, T., Beisiegel, U. et al. 2012. Effect of one-year vitamin C- and E-supplementation on cerebrospinal fluid oxidation parameters and clinical course in Alzheimer's disease. *Neurochem. Res.*, 37: 2706–2714.

Bjelakovic, G., Nikolova, D., Gluud, L.L. et al. 2008a. Antioxidant supplements for prevention of mortality in healthy participants and patients with various diseases (Review). *Cochrane Database Syst. Rev.*, 2: 201–204.

Bjelakovic, G., Nikolova, D., Gluud, L.L. et al. 2007. Mortality in randomized trials of antioxidant supplements for primary and secondary prevention: Systematic review and meta-analysis. *JAMA*, 297: 842–857.

Bjelakovic, G., Nikolova, D., Simonetti, R.G. et al. 2008b. Systematic review: Primary and secondary prevention of gastrointestinal cancers with antioxidant supplements. *Aliment. Pharmacol. Ther.*, 28: 689–703.

Boaz, M., Smetana, S., Weinstein, T. et al. 2000. Secondary prevention with antioxidants of cardiovascular disease in end stage renal disease (SPACE): Randomised placebo-controlled trial. *Lancet*, 356: 1213–1218.

Brigelius-Flohe, R. and Traber, M.G. 1999. Vitamin E: Function and metabolism. *FASEB J.*, 13: 1145–1155.

Centers for Disease Control and Prevention, National Center for Environmental Health, Division of Laboratory Sciences. 2012. Second national report on biochemical indicators of diet and nutrition in the U.S. population 2012. www.cdc.gov/nutritionreport/pdf/Nutrition_Book_complete508_final.pdf (accessed April 12, 2013).

Colombo, M.L., Marangon, K., and Bugatti, C. 2009. CoulArray electrochemical evaluation of tocopherol and tocotrienol isomers in barley, oat and spelt grains. *Nat. Prod. Commun.*, 4: 251–254.

Commission Directive EC 2008/100. OJEU 2008, L 285/9-12.

Commission Regulation EC 1170/2009. OJEU 2009, L 314/36-42.

Dahlan, H.M., Karsani, S.N., Rahman, M.A. et al. 2012. Proteomic analysis reveals that treatment with tocotrienols reverses the effect of H_2O_2 exposure on peroxiredoxin expression in human lymphocytes from young and old individuals. *J. Nutr. Biochem.*, 23: 741–751.

European American Cataract Trial (REACT). 2002. A randomized clinical trial to investigate the efficacy of an oral antioxidant micronutrient mixture to slow progression of age-related cataract. *Ophthalmic Epidemiol.*, 9: 49–80.

Evans, H.M. and Bishop, K.S. 1922. On the existence of a hitherto unrecognized dietary factor essential for reproduction. *Science*, 56: 650–651.

Ford, E.S., Schleicher, R.L., Mokdad, A.H. et al. 2006. Distribution of serum concentrations of α-tocopherol and γ-tocopherol in the US population. *Am. J. Clin. Nutr.*, 84: 375–383.

Galasko, D.G., Peskind, E., Clark, C.M. et al. 2012. Antioxidants for Alzheimer disease: A randomized clinical trial with cerebrospinal fluid biomarker measures. *Arch. Neurol.*, 69: 836–841.

Granados, H. and Dam, H. 1950. On the histochemical relationship between peroxidation and the yellow-brown pigment in the adipose tissue of vitamin E-deficient rats. *Acta Pathol. Microbiol. Scand.*, 27: 591–598.

Greenberg, E.R., Baron, J.A., Tosteson, T.D. et al. 1994. A clinical trial of antioxidant vitamins to prevent colorectal adenoma. Polyp Prevention Study Group. *N. Engl. J. Med.*, 331: 141–147.

Hacquebard, M. and Carpentier, Y.A. 2005. Vitamin E: Absorption, plasma transport and cell uptake. *Curr. Opin. Clin. Nutr. Metab. Care*, 8: 133–138.

Harris, P.L. and Embree, N.D. 1963. Quantitative consideration of the effect of polyunsaturated fatty acid content of the diet upon the requirements for vitamin E. *Am. J. Clin. Nutr.*, 13: 385–392.

Hercberg, S., Preziosi, P., Galan, P. et al. 1999. The SU.VI.MAX. Study: A primary prevention trial using nutritional doses of antioxidant vitamins and minerals in cardiovascular diseases and cancers. Supplementation on Vitamines et Minéraux Antioxydants. *Food Chem. Toxicol.*, 37: 925–930.

Hernandez, M.L., Wagner, J.G., Kala, A. et al. 2013. Vitamin E, γ-tocopherol, reduces airway neutrophil recruitment after inhaled endotoxin challenge in rats and in healthy volunteers. *Free Radic. Biol. Med.*, 60: 56–62.

Horiguchi, M., Arita, M., Kaempf-Rotzoll, D.E. et al. 2003. pH-dependent translocation of alpha-tocopherol transfer protein (alpha-TTP) between hepatic cytosol and late endosomes. *Genes Cells*, 8: 789–800.

IUPAC-IUB Joint Commission on Biochemical Nomenclature (JCBN). 1982. Nomenclature of tocopherols and related compounds recommendations 1981. *Arch. Biochem. Biophys.*, 218: 347–348; *Eur. J. Biochem.*, 123: 473–475; *Mol. Cell. Biochem.*, 49: 183–185; *Pure Appl. Chem.*, 54: 1507–1510.

Jenab, M., Salvini, S., van Gils, C.H. et al. 2009. Dietary intakes of retinol, beta-carotene, vitamin D and vitamin E in the european prospective investigation into cancer and nutrition cohort. *Eur. J. Clin. Nutr.*, 63: S150–S178.

Joshi, Y.B. and Pratico, D. 2012. Vitamin E in aging, dementia, and Alzheimer's disease. *BioFactors*, 38: 90–97.

Kappus, H. and Diplock, A.T. 1992. Tolerance and safety of vitamin E: A toxicological position report. *Free Radic. Biol. Med.*, 13: 55–74.

Kesse-Guyot, E., Bertrais, S., Péneau, S. et al. 2009. Dietary patterns and their socio demographic and behavioural correlates in French middle-aged adults from the SU.VI.MAX. cohort. *Eur. J. Clin. Nutr.*, 63: 521–528.

Lee, I.M., Cook, N.R., Gaziano, J.M. et al. 2005. Vitamin E in the primary prevention of cardiovascular disease and cancer: The women's health study: A randomized controlled trial. *JAMA*, 294: 56–65.

Lonn, E., Bosch, J., Yusuf, S. et al. 2005. Effects of long-term vitamin E supplementation on cardiovascular events and cancer: A randomized controlled trial. *J. Am. Med. Assoc.*, 293: 1338–1347.

Luliano, L., Micheletta, F., Maranghi, M. et al. 2001. Bioavailability of vitamin E as function of food intake in healthy subjects: Effects on plasma peroxide-scavenging activity and cholesterol-oxidation products. *Arterioscler. Thromb. Vasc. Biol.*, 21: 34–37.

Malvy, D.J., Favier, A., Faure, H. et al. 2001. Effect of two years' supplementation with natural antioxidants on vitamin and trace element status biomarkers: Preliminary data of the SU.VI.MAX study. *Cancer Detect. Prev.*, 25: 479–485.

McNeil, J.J., Robman, L., Tikellis, G. et al. 1998. Assessment of the safety of supplementation with different amounts of vitamin E in healthy older adults. *Am. J. Clin. Nutr.*, 68: 311–318.

Melhem, A., Stern, M., Shibolet, O. et al. 2005. Treatment of chronic hepatitis C virus infection via antioxidants: Results of phase I clinical trial. *J. Clin. Gastroenterol.*, 39: 737–742.

Meydani, S.N., Meydani, M., Bluymberg, J.B. et al. 1998. Assessment of the safety of supplementation with different amounts of vitamin E in healthy older adults. *Am. J. Clin. Nutr.*, 68: 311–318.

Miller, E.R., Pastor-Barriuso, R., Dalal, D. et al. 2005. Meta-analysis: High-dosage vitamin E supplementation may increase all-cause mortality. *Ann. Intern. Med.*, 142: 37–46.

Mortality in DATATOP. 1998. A multicenter trial in early Parkinson's disease. Parkinson Study Group. *Ann. Neurol.*, 43: 318–325.

MRC/BHF. 2002. Heart protection study of antioxidant vitamin supplementation in 20,536 high-risk individuals: A randomised placebo-controlled trial. *Lancet*, 360: 23–33.

Mustad, V.A., Smith, C.A., Ruey, P.P. et al. 2002. Supplementation with 3 compositionally different tocotrienol supplements does not improve cardiovascular disease risk factors in men and women with hypercholesterolemia. *Am. J. Clin. Nutr.*, 76: 1237–1243.

Ng, M.H., Choo, Y.M., Ma, A.N. et al. 2004. Separation of vitamin E (tocopherol, tocotrienol, and tocomonoenol) in palm oil. *Lipids*, 39: 1031–1035.

O'Byrne, D., Grundy, S., Packer, L. et al. 2000. Studies of LDL oxidation following alpha-, gamma-, or delta-tocotrienyl acetate supplementation of hypercholesterolemic humans. *Free Radic. Biol. Med.*, 29: 834–845.

Panfili, G., Fratianni, A., and Irano, M. 2003. Normal phase high-performance liquid chromatography method for the determination of tocopherols and tocotrienols in cereals. *J. Agric. Food Chem.*, 51: 3940–3944.

Pantzaris, M.C., Loukaides, G.N., Ntzani, E.E. et al. 2013. A novel oral nutraceutical formula of omega-3 and omega-6 fatty acids with vitamins (PLP10) in relapsing remitting multiple sclerosis: A randomised, double-blind, placebo-controlled proof-of-concept clinical trial. *BMJ Open*, 3: e002170.

Pedrelli, V.F., Lauriola, M.M., and Pigatto P.D. 2012. Clinical evaluation of photoprotective effect by a topical antioxidants combination (tocopherols and tocotrienols). *J. Eur. Acad. Dermatol. Venereol.*, 26: 1449–1453.

Rasool, H.G., Rahman, A.R., Yuen, K.H. et al. 2008. Arterial compliance and vitamin E blood levels with a self emulsifying preparation of tocotrienol rich vitamin E. *Arch. Pharm. Res.*, 31: 1212–1217.

Rimbach, G., Minihane, A.M., Majewicz, J. et al. 2002. Regulation of cell signaling by vitamin E. *Proc. Nutr. Soc.*, 61: 415–425.

Roy, S., Lado, B.H., Khanna, S. et al. 2002. Vitamin E sensitive genes in the developing rat fetal brain: A high-density oligonucleotide microarray analysis. *FEBS Lett*, 530: 17–23.

Ryan, E., Galvin, K., O'Connor, T.P. et al. 2007. Phytosterol, squalene, tocopherol content and fatty acid profile of selected seeds, grains, and legumes. *Plant Foods Hum. Nutr.*, 62: 85–91.

Sano, M., Ernesto, C., Thomas, R.G. et al. 1997. A controlled trial of selegiline, alpha-tocopherol, or both as treatment for Alzheimer's disease. The Alzheimer's Disease Cooperative Study. *N. Engl. J. Med.*, 336: 1216–1222.

Schurks, M., Glynn, R.J., Rist, P.M. et al. 2010. Effects of vitamin E on stroke subtypes: Meta-analysis of randomised controlled trials. *BMJ*, 341: c5702.

Schwarz, K. 1961. A possible site of action for vitamin E in intermediary metabolism. *Am. J. Clin. Nutr.*, 9: 71–75.

Scientific opinion of the panel on food additives, flavourings, processing aids and materials in contact with food on a request from the commission on mixed tocopherols, tocotrienol tocopherol and tocotrienols as sources for vitamin E. 2008, Opinion of the Scientific Committee on Food on the Tolerable Upper Intake Level of Vitamin E. 2003. *EFSA J.*, 640: 1–34. SCF/CS/NUT/UPPLEV/31 Final.

Sen, C.K., Khanna, S., Rink, C. et al. 2007. Tocotrienols: The emerging face of natural vitamin E. *Vitam. Horm.*, 76: 203–261.

Sesso, H.D., Buring, J.E., Christen, W.G. et al. 2008. Vitamins E and C in the prevention of cardiovascular disease in men. The physicians' health study II randomized controlled trial. *JAMA*, 300: 2123–2133.

Siok-Fong, C., Noor Aini, A.H., Azian, A.L. et al. 2008. Reduction of DNA damage in older healthy adults by Tri E® tocotrienol supplementation. *Nutrition*, 24: 1–10.

Sondergaad, E. and Dam, H. 1966. Influence of the level of dietary linoleic acid on the amount of d-alpha-tocopherol acetate required for protection against encephalomalcia. *Z. Ernahrungswiss.*, 6: 253–258.

Stephens, N.G., Parsons, A., Schofield, P.M. et al. 1996. Randomised controlled trial of vitamin E in patients with coronary disease: Cambridge Heart Antioxidant Study (CHAOS). *Lancet*, 347: 781–786.

Sylvester, P.W., Wali, V.B., Bachawal, S.V. et al. 2011. Tocotrienol combination therapy results in synergistic anticancer response. *Front. Biosci.*, 17: 3183–3195.

Traber, M.G. 2013. Mechanisms for the prevention of vitamin E excess. *J. Lipid Res.*, 54: 2295–2306.

Traber, M.G. and Atkinson, J. 2007. Vitamin E, antioxidant and nothing more. *Free Radic. Biol. Med.*, 43: 3–15.

Traber, M.G., Burton, G.W., and Hamilto, R.L. 2005. Vitamin E trafficking. *Ann. N. Y. Acad. Sci.*, 1031: 1–12.

Traber, M.G., Elsner, A., and Brigelius-Flohe, R. 1998. Synthetic as compared with natural vitamin E is preferentially excreted as alpha-CEHC in human urine: Studies using deuterated alpha-tocopheryl acetates. *FEBS Lett.*, 437: 145–148.

Vaule, H., Leonard, S.W., and Traber, M.G. 2003. Vitamin E delivery to human skin: Studies using deuterated α-tocopherol measured by APCI LC-MS. *Free Radic. Biol. Med.*, 36: 456–463.

Vivekananthan, D.P., Penn, M.S., Sapp, S.K. et al. 2003. Use of antioxidant vitamins for the prevention of cardiovascular disease: Meta-analysis of randomised trials. *Lancet*, 361: 2017–2023.

Waters, D.D., Alderman, E.L., Hsia, J. et al. 2002. Effects of hormone replacement therapy and antioxidant vitamin supplements on coronary atherosclerosis in postmenopausal women: A randomized controlled trial. *JAMA*, 288: 2432–2440.

Wells, S.R., Jennings, M.H., Rome, C. et al. 2010. α-, γ- and δ-tocopherols reduce inflammatory angiogenesis in human microvascular endothelial cells. *J. Nutr. Biochem.*, 21: 589–597.

Wolf, G. 2005. The discovery of the antioxidant function of vitamin E: The contribution of Henry A. Matill. *J. Nutr.*, 135: 363–366.

Yap, S.P., Yuen, K.H., and Wong, J.W. 2001. Pharmacokinetics and bioavailability of alpha-, gamma-, and delta-tocotrienols under different food status. *J. Pharm. Pharmacol.*, 53: 67–71.

Yoshida, Y., Niki, E., and Noguchi, N. 2003. Comparative study on the action of tocopherols and tocotrienols as antioxidant: Chemical and physical effects. *Chem. Phys. Lipids*, 123: 63–75.

Yusuf, S., Dagenais, G., Pogue, J. et al. 2000. Vitamin E supplementation and cardiovascular events in high-risk patients. The Heart Outcomes Prevention Evaluation Study Investigators. *N. Engl. J. Med.*, 342: 154–160.

Zingg, J.M. 2007. Modulation of signal transduction by vitamin E. *Mol. Asp. Med.*, 28: 481–506.

13 Clinical Applications of Metabolites and Metabolomics

Dilip Ghosh

CONTENTS

INTRODUCTION

It is well known that diet is a modifiable risk factor for chronic disease; however, epidemiologic studies do not consistently support associations between specific foods or nutrients and disease end points. Most epidemiologic studies rely on self-reported dietary assessment methods that are subject to recall bias and measurement error (Ocke and Kaaks, 1997). Unlike drugs, very few nutritional studies depend on reliable end point measurements. There is a pressing need for dietary biomarkers to better capture exposure; however, few have been identified to date (Jenab et al., 2009).

Metabolomics, the measurement of small molecules in biofluids, may more precisely define dietary exposures and thus provide better estimates of disease risk in epidemiologic studies. Metabolites, the downstream components of metabolism or metabolic products of foods, may better reflect the "true exposure" of variability of metabolism because of lifestyle or genetics. Metabolites may also capture exposure to nonnutritive substances, such as pesticides and compounds generated by cooking (Jones et al., 2012), which may play an important role in disease etiology.

HOW METABOLOMICS SUPPORT BETTER CLINICAL OUTCOMES?

Metabolomics can give us information of the characterization of endogenous small molecules (referred to as metabolites) that are the products of biochemical reactions, revealing connections among different pathways that operate within a living cell (Wang et al., 2011). To develop targets for pharmacological/nutritional intervention by exploring the underlying cause(s) of disease, the metabolomics more specifically is able to uncover and evaluate biochemical differences within healthy and diseased organisms (Wang et al., 2012a,b). Metabolome analysis describes qualitatively and quantitatively the final products of cellular regulatory pathways and can be seen as the ultimate response of a biologic system to genetic factors and/or environmental changes (Cuperlović-Cul et al., 2010).

A cell metabolome can be defined as the set of all the metabolites present in cells and these metabolites can be used as the best indicator of an organism's phenotype (Nomura et al., 2011; Tautenhahn et al., 2012) and construct a "fingerprint" that can be unique to the individuals. Small-molecule metabolites as primary indicators have an important role in biological systems and represent attractive candidates to understand cell phenotypes (Riedelsheime et al., 2012; Tomita and Kami, 2012). To understand the molecular mechanism of disease progression, response, and resistance to therapeutics, cells are used extensively in disease research because cell applications are easier to control, less expensive, and easier to interpret than analysis of both animal models and human subjects. As a whole, it represents an untapped resource for identification of specific metabolite biomarkers that would help distinguish the normal and abnormal states, as well as response to drugs or stress agents.

Untargeted metabolomics, a new approach, has identified some novel potential dietary biomarkers in small dietary intervention and cohort studies (Wild et al., 2013). This approach has been successfully applied to small to medium dietary intervention trials (Beckmann et al., 2013; Lloyd et al., 2013; O'Sullivan et al., 2011). Traditionally, dietary biomarkers have been identified and validated in small feeding studies, but markers thus identified may not perform well as proxies for usual food intake in a large population study. If the biomarker has a short half-life or if the food of interest is consumed only infrequently, the levels detected at the time of actual biospecimen collection may not proxy usual intake. A recent metabolomics study demonstrated that groups of serum metabolites are associated with patterns of dietary intake, although the authors only investigated 127 metabolites, which were limited to acylcarnitines and choline-containing phospholipids (Floegel et al., 2013). An agnostic approach that measures hundreds of metabolites has the benefit of identifying novel findings that may not have been previously considered.

PLANT-DERIVED FUNCTIONAL METABOLITES IN DISEASE PREVENTION

In recent years several well-controlled nutrition studies have provided unambiguous evidence that a number of human health conditions such as chronic coronary thrombosis, hypertension, diabetes, osteoporosis, cancer, old age, and lifestyle-related diseases are associated with the diet. Although some human health disorders are often genetic, there is a definite interplay of disorders/disease with contributions arising from consumption of certain, commonly used foods (Desiere, 2004; Meydani, 2002; Rist et al., 2006). In fact, in some cases, beneficial as well as harmful effects that have nothing to do with genetic predisposition have been identified in humans. For instance, diseases classified as polygenic in nature such as epithelial cancers, diabetes, and heart disease seem to be reduced by the intake of dietary antioxidants, vitamins, and other phytonutrients. A gluten-free diet reverses the adverse health effects in celiac disorder (Niewinski, 2008; Pizzuti et al., 2004); diminishing intake of galactose helps in the control of galactosemia (Boonyawat et al., 2005). Wide dissemination of such information (with or without robust scientific evidence) has greatly helped to raise public awareness about the consumption of food promoting good health and containing active ingredients to combat nutritional and health disorders (Mattoo et al., 2009). Prevention and disease control by means of individualized diets and supplements seem conceivable but their content and dosage to ensure minimal side effects need to be evaluated on a scientific basis through nutrition trials on humans (Lavecchia et al. 2013).

Plants produce bioactive compounds that are classified as primary and secondary metabolites. Primary metabolites such as carbohydrates, lipids, and amino acids are necessary for the growth and basic metabolism in all plants, while secondary metabolites are not essential, but they may play crucial roles in plant well-being by interacting with the ecosystems. Compared to the main and most abundant molecules found in plants, the secondary metabolites often form less than 1%–5% of the dry weight. Some secondary metabolites are exploited for promoting public health as they provide health benefits in addition to basic nutrition (Diplock, 1999; Krzyzanowska et al., 2009; Wahle et al., 2009).

The field cultivation of medicinal plants is the alternative of production of plant secondary metabolites through chemical synthesis. However, plants originating from particular biotopes hardly ever succeed in growing outside their local ecosystems. It is often the case that common plants cannot withstand field cultivation due to their sensitivity to pathogens (Abang et al., 2005; Garrido et al., 2008; Kelly and Vallejo, 2004; Talhinhas et al., 2005). This difficulty has led scientists and biotechnologists to consider plant cell, tissue, and organ cultures as alternative ways of producing the corresponding secondary metabolites. Plants react against these external attacks, such as pathogens, by means of a protection mechanism, which leads to the production of secondary metabolites. But when such plant metabolites are used in manufacturing nutraceuticals, several other issues such as the dose, activity, and presence of contaminants are associated with the usages. Phytochemicals, if in excess, can result in undesirable effects; for example, high doses of carotenoids have been associated with an increased risk of lung cancer in smokers (Satia et al., 2009) and in alcohol drinkers (Ratnasinghe et al., 2000). Moreover, several products present on the market have little or no effect due to incorrect preparation and storage. In the enriched metabolic extracts, the presence of undesirable compounds is present frequently, such as the case of pesticides and heavy metals, or other toxic natural chemicals. For example, α-thujone, a natural monoterpene, is present as an active component in various herbal products such as the extracts of *Salvia officinalis* (Ozkan et al., 2009) and of *Artemisia absinthium* (Lopes-Lutza et al., 2008; Teixeira da Silva et al., 2005).

In the scientific literature, beneficial effects are reported for these plant extracts that possess antioxidant, bactericidal, and antimicrobial activities but α-thujone is also known for its psychoactive effects and its toxicity has become an important issue in recent years (Deiml et al., 2004; Haji Mahdipour et al., 2008; Kharoubi et al., 2009).

The growing interest of health-conscious consumers in the role nutrition plays on health is the primary driving force behind the success of healthy diets. People's

TABLE 13.1
Top Metabolites Associated with Dietary Nutrients

Category and Dietary Group	Metabolites
Fruit	
Citrus: oranges, orange juice, grapefruit	Stachydrine, chiro-inositol, *N*-methyl proline
Berries: strawberries	1-Palmitoylglycero-phospho-inositol
Apples, pears	13-HODE + 9-HODE
Melon: watermelon, cantaloupe	Pregnenolone sulfate
Bananas	γ-Tocopherol
Vegetables	
Cruciferous: broccoli, cabbage, Brussels sprouts, cauliflower, and others	α-CEHC glucuronide
Greens: lettuce, spinach, green peppers	CMPF
Yellow/orange vegetables: carrots, tomatoes, sweet potatoes, beets	Creatinine
Starchy vegetables: white potatoes, corn, peas	Cyclo (-Leu-Pro)
Alliums (garlic, onions)	CMPF
Meat/Fish	
Red meat	Indolepropionate
Poultry: chicken	Pyroglutamine
Fish (excluding shellfish)	CMPF, DHA, EPA,
Snack Foods	
Baked sweets	Glutamine
Chocolate	Theobromine
Chips	DHA
Beverages	
Dairy: milk	Homostachydrine
Coffee	Trigonelline, quinate, paraxanthine
Beer	16-hydroxypalmitate
Wine	Scyllo-inositol
Liquor	Ethyl glucuronide
Others	
Tofu	4-Ethylphenylsulfate
Eggs	Indolepropionate
Rice (white)	DHA

Source: Adapted from Guertin, K.A. et al., *Am. J. Clin. Nutr.*, 100, 208, 2014.

increasing desire to be more actively involved in optimizing their personal well-being is also an additional driving force for the nutraceutical and functional food markets.

Some nutraceutical compounds are of artificial origin but in recent years attention has been focused on natural compounds originating from plant secondary metabolism. Although much attention has been directed to create targeted nutrition and *in vitro* protocols for the mass production of secondary metabolites, little emphasis has been placed on nutraceutical activity and analysis. In recent years, a wide variety of biosensors applicable to the detection of pesticides, heavy metals, pollutants, and toxic compounds in food and in the cell cultures of secondary metabolites has entered the market. The most significant advancement in this area is to increase the sensitivity of detection limit. Now detection of metabolites at subnanomolar concentrations represents an important breakthrough by using all latest technologies.

Guertin et al. (2014) detected 412 metabolites of known identity and 231 metabolites of unknown identity. Among the 643 metabolites analyzed, the median percentage of individuals with nondetectable levels was 4%. Correlations between all 36 dietary groups and known metabolites are shown in Table 3; all significant correlations are shown, as well as the strongest, albeit nonsignificant, correlations for dietary groups with no significant findings. Guertin et al. identified 13 dietary groups correlated with known metabolites including citrus, green vegetables, red meat, fish, shellfish, butter, peanuts, rice, coffee, beer, liquor, total alcohol, and multivitamins. Most of the findings were for exogenous metabolites derived from their food sources. Table 13.1 represents the top metabolites associated with dietary nutrients.

METABOLITES VERSUS PARENT COMPOUNDS: PHENOLIC ACIDS AS AN EXAMPLE

Most of the phenolic acids after absorption from the gastrointestinal tract, passing through several metabolic changes such as conjugation reactions, cause several modifications in their initial structure and circulate in human plasma in their conjugated forms, such as glucuronide, methylated, and sulfated derivatives. These changes in their structures may increase or decrease the bioactivity of the initial phenolic acids (Heleno et al., 2015; Piazzon et al., 2012; Rechner et al., 2002).

Therefore, pharmacokinetic knowledge concerning the conjugative and metabolic events and resulting plasma levels following the ingestion of a polyphenol-rich diet is crucial for understanding their bioactivity (Rechner et al., 2002). Despite the presence of significant amount of data on the bioactivity of phenolic acids, only a few studies deal with the bioactive properties of their metabolites, especially as most of those molecules are not commercially available (Piazzon et al., 2012).

As mentioned earlier, phenolic acids represent a significant portion of polyphenols in our diet. Their bioactivity, especially antioxidant properties, are related to the phenolic hydroxyl groups attached to ring structures. These molecules can act as reducing agents, hydrogen donators, singlet oxygen quenchers, superoxide radical scavengers and metal chelators over hydroxyl and peroxyl radicals, superoxide anions, and peroxynitrites (Terpinc et al., 2011). Nevertheless, there has been some controversy about the bioactivity of polyphenols after metabolism. Once ingested, these molecules are metabolized and transformed into methylated, glucuronated, and sulfated metabolites (Manach et al., 2004). These conjugation reactions significantly reduce the polyphenols' antioxidant activity, since both sulfation and glucuronidation occur at the reducing hydroxyl groups in the phenolic structure.

Overall, the results from the antioxidant activities revealed that although ferulic and caffeic acids are extensively metabolized after absorption, their glucuronated metabolites can retain a strong antioxidant activity and might still exert a significant antioxidant action *in vivo*. These two phenolic acids are the most representative in the human diet, and after absorption, they are metabolized and circulate in human plasma in conjugated forms. Thus, the strong antioxidant activity exhibited by some of these metabolites might contribute to the increased plasma antioxidant activities measured after the intake of phenolic acid–rich foods (e.g., mushrooms) as described before.

Regarding the antimicrobial activity, the methylation reactions in the parental molecules have considerably increased the activity of CoA. However, the inclusion of acetyl groups increased the antifungal activity but maintained the antibacterial effects. In the case of HA and CA, the inclusion of methyl groups did not increase the antimicrobial activity; however, demelanizing activity of the parental compounds increased. Regarding the antitumor potential, in most of the cases, the substitution of the carboxylic group (in parental organic acids) for an ester (in methylated derivatives) increased the cytotoxicity of the parental compounds. Glucuronated protected derivatives showed an increase in cytotoxicity of the respective parental compounds due to the inclusion of acetyl molecules in the parental compound.

POTENTIAL APPLICATIONS

CANCER

There are many possible applications for cell metabolomics in a context of cancer based on targeted therapies. Apoptosis-inducing agents are currently considered as a powerful tool for cancer therapeutics. Metabolomic signatures might be used in the tests of efficacy of agents causing apoptosis in cell culture. Several metabolites indicated for apoptotic processes in cell culture, including aspartate, glutamate, methionine, alanine, glycine, propionyl carnitine, and malonyl carnitine, were identified, and metabolite identification and quantification were used to examine metabolic differences between the cell types. It demonstrated (Dewar et al., 2010) a clear difference in the metabolite profiles of drug-resistant and sensitive cells, with the biggest difference being an elevation of creatine metabolites in the imatinib-resistant MyL-R cells.

PATHOGEN INFECTIONS

Metabolic profiling demonstrated the differentiation of fatty acid biosynthesis and cholesterol metabolism during viral replication (Lin et al., 2010). Distinct effects of infection by each serotype were evaluated, and these differences were attributed to changes in levels of metabolites, including amino acids and dicarboxylic acids related to the tricarboxylic acid cycle. These studies demonstrated the application of metabolomics to improve understanding of the effect of dengue infection on endothelial cells' metabolome.

TOXICITY

Metabolomics can add new insights into the molecular basis of toxicity based on the combinatorial platform of novel cellular models with molecular profiling technologies and provide a rich source of biomarkers that are urgently required in a twenty-first-century approach to toxicology (Zhang et al., 2013). Metabolic profiling of RPTEC/TERT1 cells demonstrated the effect of chemical exposure on multiple cellular pathways producing different response profiles for the different compounds tested. The key findings would be useful in investigating the mechanism of action of toxins at a low dose.

OTHER APPLICATIONS

Emerging metabolomic tools can now be used to establish metabolic signatures of specialized circulating hematopoietic cells in physiologic or pathologic conditions and in human hematologic diseases, such as sickle cell disease. High-resolution NMR spectra demonstrated the changes in metabolites that are present at both the early undifferentiated and the late differentiated states of cells that become gluconeogenic.

METABOLOMIC AND DIETARY BIOMARKER STUDIES

Applications of metabolomics to identify novel dietary biomarkers have in general terms taken three approaches: (1) specific acute intervention to identify food markers, (2) search for biomarkers in cohort studies, and (3) analysis of dietary patterns in conjunction with metabolomic profiles to identify nutritypes and biomarkers. Approaches (1) and (2) form the basis of the studies described under biomarkers of specific foods, while approach (3) is discussed under dietary patterns. This issue is dealth with in detail in Chapter "Biomarkers in therapeutic intervention".

CONCLUSION

Metabolomics is a powerful tool for exploring the alterations in the metabolite abundance and metabolic pathways and networks, which are involved in various pathophysiological conditions, and offers the platform for identification of genotype–phenotype as well as genotype–envirotype interactions (Kumar et al., 2014; Peng et al., 2015). In preclinical and clinical drug development, the applications of metabolomics have a considerable scope for the pharmaceutical industry, almost at each step, right from drug discovery to clinical development. These include determination of drug target, potential safety and efficacy biomarkers and mechanisms of drug action, the validation of preclinical experimental models against human disease profiles, and the discovery of clinical safety and efficacy biomarkers (Kumar et al., 2014). Applications of discovery metabolomics in nutritional research can include three main areas: identification of dietary biomarkers, study of diet-related diseases, and identification of biomarkers of disease and application to dietary intervention studies as a tool to identify molecular mechanisms (Gibbons et al., 2015).

Metabolite levels were reproducible and stable over a year, indicating that metabolomics can be informative for nutritional epidemiologic studies. Moreover, the sample sizes needed to design an adequately powered study of metabolites and disease risk are realistically attainable.

In conclusion, the large number of correlations between self-reported diet and serum metabolites confirms that metabolomics can be applied to epidemiologic studies for identification of novel dietary biomarkers. There is a need for specific, reliable biomarkers that accurately reflect dietary intake and that can be applied to many populations. We emphasize, however, that although we appear to have uncovered objective biomarkers of diet, it should not yet be assumed that there should be a perfect balance between biomarker selection and self-report as a measure of usual dietary intake. Ultimately, whether a biomarker is a good measure of usual diet depends on the frequency of consumption of the food or nutrient, as well as the half-life of the metabolite. In addition, the identification of serologic metabolites reflects not only dietary intake but also metabolic processes, including the effects of genetic variation and the gut microbiota. Nevertheless, our metabolomic approach for identifying potential dietary biomarkers showed viable biomarkers for further investigation in feeding studies.

REFERENCES

Abang, M.M., Fagbola, O., Smalla, K. et al. 2005. Two genetically distinct populations of *Colletotrichum gloeosporioides* Penz. causing anthracnose disease of yam (*Dioscorea* spp.) *J. Phytopathol.*, 153: 137–142.

Boonyawat, B., Kamolsilp, M., and Phavichitr, N. 2005. Galactosemia in Thai patient at Phramongkutklao hospital: A case report. *J. Med. Assoc. Thai.*, 88: S275–S280.

Beckmann, M., Lloyd, A.J., Haldar, S. et al. 2013. Dietary exposure biomarker-lead discovery based on metabolomics analysis of urine samples. *Proc. Nutr. Soc.*, 72: 352–361.

Cuperlović-Culf, M., Barnett, D.A., Culf, A.S. et al. 2010. Cell culture metabolomics: Applications and future directions. *Drug. Discov. Today*, 15: 610–621.

Deiml, T., Hasenederc, R., Zieglgänsbergerb, W. et al. 2004. α-Thujone reduces 5-HT3 receptor activity by an effect on the agonist-induced desensitization. *Neuropharmacology*, 46: 192–201.

Desiere, F. 2004. Towards a systems biology understanding of human health: Interplay between genotype, environment and nutrition. *Biotechnol. Annu. Rev.*, 10: 51–84.

Dewar, B.J., Keshari, K., Jeffries, R. et al. 2010. Metabolic assessment of a novel chronic myelogenous leukemic cell line and an imatinib resistant subline by H NMR spectroscopy. *Metabolomics*, 6: 439–450.

Diplock, A.T. 1999. Scientific concepts of functional foods in Europe—Consensus document. *Br. J. Nutr.*, 81: 21–27.

Floegel, A., von Ruesten, A., Drogan, D. et al. 2013. Variation of serum metabolites related to habitual diet: A targeted metabolomic approach in EPIC-Potsdam. *Eur. J. Clin. Nutr.*, 67: 1100–1108.

Garridom, C., Carbúm, M., Fernández-Acero, F.J. et al. 2008. Isolation and pathogenicity of *Colletotrichum* spp. causing anthracnose of strawberry in south west Spain. *Eur. J. Plant Pathol.*, 120: 409–415.

Gibbons, H., O'Gorman, A., and Brennan, L. 2015. Metabolomics as a tool in nutritional research. *Curr. Opin. Lipidol.*, 26: 30–34.

Guertin, K.A., Moore, S.C., Sampson, J.N. et al. 2014. Metabolomics in nutritional epidemiology: Identifying metabolites associated with diet and quantifying their potential to uncover diet-disease relations in populations. *Am. J. Clin. Nutr.*, 100: 208–217.

Haji Mahdipour, H., Zahedi, H., Kalantari Khandani, N. et al. 2008. Investigation of α and β-thujone content in common wormwood from Iran. *J. Med. Plant.*, 7: 40–44.

Heleno, S.A., Martins, A., João M. et al. 2015. Bioactivity of phenolic acids: Metabolites versus parent compounds: A review. *Food Chem.*, 173: 501–513.

Jenab, M., Slimani, N., Bictash, M. et al. 2009. Biomarkers in nutritional epidemiology: Applications, needs and new horizons. *Hum. Genet.*, 125: 507–525.

Jones, D.P., Park, Y., and Ziegler, T.R. 2012. Nutritional metabolomics: Progress in addressing complexity in diet and health. *Annu. Rev. Nutr.*, 32: 183–202.

Kelly, J.D. and Vallejo, V.A.A. 2004. Comprehensive review of the major genes conditioning resistance to anthracnose in common bean. *HortScience*, 39: 1196–1207.

Kharoubi, O., Slimania, M., and Aouesa, A. 2009. The effect of wormwood (*Artemisia absinthium* L.) extract on brain region antioxidant system after intoxication by lead. *Toxicol. Lett.*, 189: 1S128.

Krzyzanowska, J., Czubacka, A., and Oleszek, W. 2009. Dietary phytochemicals and human health. In: Giardi, M.T., Rea, G., and Berra, B. (eds.), *Bio-Farms for Nutraceuticals: Functional Food and Safety Control by Biosensors*. Austin, TX: Landes BioScience; Release date: January 1, 2010.

Kumar, B., Prakash, A., Ruhela, R.K. et al. 2014. Potential of metabolomics in preclinical and clinical drug development. *Pharmacol. Rep.*, 66: 956–963.

Lavecchia, T., Rea, G., Antonacci, A. et al. 2013. Healthy and adverse effects of plant-derived functional metabolites: The need of revealing their content and bioactivity in a complex food matrix. *Crit. Rev. Food Sci. Nutr.*, 53: 198–213.

Lin, S., Liu, N., Yang, Z. et al. 2010. GC/MS-based metabolomics reveals fatty acid biosynthesis and cholesterol metabolism in cell lines infected with influenza A virus. *Talanta*, 83: 262–268.

Lloyd, A.J., Beckmann, M., Haldar, S. et al. 2013. Data driven strategy for the discovery of potential urinary biomarkers of habitual dietary exposure. *Am. J. Clin. Nutr.*, 97: 377–389.

Lopes-Lutza, D., Alvianob, D.S., Alvianob, C.S. et al. 2008. Screening of chemical composition, antimicrobial and antioxidant activities of Artemisia essential oils. *Phytochemistry*, 69: 1732–1738.

Manach, C., Scalbert, A., Morand, C. et al. 2004. Polyphenols: Food sources and bioavailability. *Am. J. Clin. Nutr.*, 79: 727–747.

Mattoo, A.K. 2009. Genetic engineering to enhance crop-based phytonutrients (nutraceuticals) to alleviate diet-related diseases. In: Giardi, M., Rea, G., and Berra, B. (eds.), *Bio-Farms for Nutraceuticals: Functional Food and Safety Control by Biosensors*. Austin, TX Landes BioScience; Release date: January 1, 2010.

Meydani, M. 2002. The boyd orr lecture: Nutrition interventions in aging and age-associated disease. *Proc. Nutr. Soc.*, 61: 165–171.

Niewinski, M.M. 2008. Advances in celiac disease and gluten-free diet. *J. Am. Diet. Assoc.*, 108: 661–672.

Nomura, D.K., Morrison, B.E., Blankman, J.L. et al. 2011. Endocannabinoid hydrolysis generates brain prostaglandins that promote neuro inflammation. *Science*, 334: 809–813.

Ocké, M.C. and Kaaks, R.J. 1997. Biochemical markers as additional measurements in dietary validity studies: Application of the method of triads with examples from the European Prospective Investigation into Cancer and Nutrition. *Am. J. Clin. Nutr.*, 65(Suppl.): 1240S–1245S.

O'Sullivan, A., Gibney, M.J., and Brennan, L. 2011. Dietary intake patterns are reflected in metabolomic profiles: Potential role in dietary assessment studies. *Am. J. Clin. Nutr.*, 93: 314–321.

Ozkan, G., Sagdic, O., Gokturk, R.S. et al. 2010. Study on chemical composition and biological activities of essential oil and extract from Salvia pisidica. *LWT—Food Sci Technol.*, 43: 186–190.

Peng, B., Li, H., and Peng, X-X. 2015. Functional metabolomics: From biomarker discovery to metabolome reprogramming. *Protein Cell*, 6: 628–637.

Piazzon, A., Vrhovsek, U., Masuero, D. et al. 2012. Antioxidant activity of phenolic acids and their metabolites: Synthesis and antioxidant properties of the sulfate derivatives of ferulic and caffeic acids and of the acyl glucuronide of ferulic acid. *J. Agric. Food Chem.*, 60: 12312–12323.

Pizzuti, D., Bortolami, M., Mazzon, E. et al. 2004. Transcriptional downregulation of tight junction protein ZO-1 in active coeliac disease is reversed after a gluten-free diet. *Dig. Liver Des.*, 36: 337–341.

Ratnasinghe, D., Forman, M.R., Tangrea, J.A. et al. 2000. Serum carotenoids are associated with increased lung cancer risk among alcohol drinkers, but not among non-drinkers in a cohort of tin miners. *Alcohol Alcohol.*, 35: 355–360.

Rechner, A.R., Kuhnle, G., Bremner, P. et al. 2002. The metabolic fate of dietary polyphenols in humans. *Free Radic. Biol. Med.*, 33: 220–235.

Riedelsheimer, C., Lisec, J., Czedik-Eysenberg, A. et al. 2012. Genome-wide association mapping of leaf metabolic profiles for dissecting complex traits in maize. *Proc. Natl. Acad. Sci. USA*, 109: 8872–8877.

Rist, M.J., Wenzel, U., and Daniel, H. 2006. Nutrition and food science go genomic. *Trends Biotechnol.*, 24: 172–178.

Satia, J.A., Littman, A., Slatore, C.G. et al. 2009. Long-term use of β-carotene, retinol, lycopene, and lutein supplements and lung cancer risk: Results from the vitamins and lifestyle (VITAL) study. *Am. J. Epidemiol.*, 169: 815–828.

Tautenhahn, R., Cho, K., Uritboonthai, W. et al. 2012. An accelerated workflow for untargeted metabolomics using the METLIN Database. *Nat. Biotechnol.*, 30: 826–828.

Teixeira da Silva, J.A., Yonekura, L., Kaganda, J. et al. 2005. Important secondary metabolites and essential oils of species within the anthemideae (*Asteraceae*). *J. Herbs Spices Med. Plants*, 11: 41–46.

Terpinc, P., Polak, T., Šegatin, N. et al. 2011. Antioxidant properties of 4-vinyl derivatives of hydroxycinnamic acids. *Food Chem.*, 128: 62–68.

Tomita, M. and Kami, K. 2012. Systems biology, metabolomics, and cancer metabolism. *Science*, 336: 990–991.

Wang, T.J., Larson, M.G., Vasan, R.S. et al. 2011. Metabolite profiles and the risk of developing diabetes. *Nat. Med.*, 17: 448–453.

Wang, X., Zhang, A., Han, Y. et al. 2012a. Urine metabolomics analysis for biomarker discovery and detection of jaundice syndrome in patients with liver disease. *Mol. Cell. Proteomics*, 11: 370–380.

Wang, X., Zhang, A., and Sun, H. 2012b. Future perspectives of Chinese medical formulae: Chinmedomics as an effector. *OMICS*, 16: 414–421.

Wahle, K.W.J., Rotondo, D., and Heys, S.D. 2009. Plant phenolics in the prevention and treatment of cancer. In: Giardi, M., Rea, G., and Berra, B. (eds.), Bio-*Farms for Nutraceuticals: Functional Food and Safety Control by Biosensors*. Austin, TX: Landes BioScience; Release date: January 1, 2010.

Wild, C.P., Scalbert, A., and Herceg, Z. 2013. Measuring the exposome: A powerful basis for evaluating environmental exposures and cancer risk. *Environ. Mol. Mutagen.*, 54: 480–499.

Zhang, A., Sun, H., Xu, H. et al. 2013. Cell metabolomics. *OMICS*, 17: 495–501.

Section VI

New Journeys through Categorization

14 Medical Foods
A New Domain in the Food–Drug Interphase

Dilip Ghosh

CONTENTS

INTRODUCTION

Recently, Nestlé Health Science, a subsidiary of Nestlé, bought another U.S. medical food company, Pamlab, which produces prescription medical foods that support patients with various conditions, such as dementia, diabetic peripheral neuropathy, high-risk pregnancies, and depression. Nestlé's strong commitment in this domain is justified by a series of other acquisitions which include Accera, a firm that produces medical foods for the dietary management of Alzheimer's patients; Vitaflo, which provides nutritional solutions for those affected by genetic disorders influencing how the body processes foods; and Prometheus Laboratories, a firm specializing in diagnostics and pharmaceuticals in gastroenterology and oncology.

Medical food or foods for special medical purposes are principally formulated food products intended to be used under the supervision of medical and other appropriate health professionals (e.g., dietitians, nurses, and pharmacists). This is required for the dietary management of individuals (including children) with ongoing chronic diseases, disorders, or medical conditions or during acute phases of illness, injury, or disease states.

This chapter will discuss current market dynamics, regulations, the latest breakthroughs in research, and everything you need to navigate this advancing sector.

THE FOOD AND DRUG ADMINISTRATION ON MEDICAL FOOD

The U.S. Food and Drug Administration (FDA, 2010) designated medical food as a category of substances intended for the clinical dietary management of a particular condition or disease. Specific criteria necessary to receive this FDA designation include that the product be

- Specifically formulated for oral or enteral ingestion
- Intended for the clinical dietary management of a specific medical disorder, disease, or abnormal condition for which there are distinctive nutritional requirements
- Made with ingredients that have "generally recognized as safe" (GRAS) status
- Designed in compliance with FDA regulations that pertain to labeling, product claims, and manufacturing

Medical food, a therapeutic category, is distinct from both drugs and supplements. The label must include "to be used under medical supervision." Medical foods are produced under rigid manufacturing practices and maintain high labeling standards. Tables 14.1 and 14.2 describe the differences between dietary supplements, nutraceuticals, and prescription medicines.

TABLE 14.1

How Do Medical Foods Differ from Dietary Supplements and Nutraceuticals?

	Medical Foods	Dietary Supplements and Nutraceuticals
Medical care	Physician's supervision is required (Rx or others).	Self-administered (OTC)
Intended use	Nutritional or dietary management of a specific disease or its metabolic processes should be implemented.	Maintenance of well-being, generally for healthy individuals
Safety	Ingredients must obtain GRAS status.	Reasonable safety profile evidenced from traditional use
Clinical/scientific support	Preapproval is not required. Convincing nutritional requirements of the specific disease and the product efficacy must be shown by well-designed clinical trials.	No specific requirements for premarket clinical support or scientific testing
Manufacturing/regulatory requirements	Good manufacturing practices (GMPs) are required.	Good manufacturing practices (GMPs) required

TABLE 14.2
How Do Medical Foods Differ from Prescription Medicine?

	Medical Foods	Prescription Medicine
Medical care	Physician's supervision is required (Rx or others).	Physician's supervision is required (Rx).
Intended use	Nutritional or dietary management of a specific disease or its metabolic processes should be developed.	Cure or treatment of a specific disease or symptoms must be given.
Safety	Ingredients must obtain GRAS status	Preapproval by the regulatory authority for safety is required.
Clinical/scientific support	Preapproval is not required. Convincing nutritional requirements of the specific disease and the product efficacy must be shown by well-designed clinical trials.	Preapproval of the product's required efficacy and disease-specific claims must be supported by high-level clinical and scientific studies.
Manufacturing/regulatory requirements	Convincing nutritional requirements of the specific disease and the product efficacy must be shown by well-designed clinical trials.	Current good manufacturing practices for drugs are required.

WHAT ARE THE MAJOR HEALTH CONDITIONS THAT ARE BEING TARGETED?

From a medical standpoint, an increasing prevalence of diseases such as metabolic syndromes, irritable bowel syndrome (IBS), lactose intolerance, Alzheimer's disease, and food intolerances is continuously being targeted by industries for the development of medical foods. Age-related digestive tract diseases as well as reduced general digestive and absorptive function are another health condition receiving attention for the development of medical foods (Georgiou et al., 2011).

Vladimir Badmaev, MD, PhD, Head of R&D, NattoPharma ASA, Oslo, Norway, said, "The most popular categories of medicinal food address aging populations and wasting conditions like muscle wasting or sarcopenia, bone rarefaction or osteoporosis, health conditions caused by insufficient status of vitamins and minerals, gastrointestinal dysbiotic conditions." Zak Dutton, President of Prismic Pharmaceuticals, Arizona, added that "there are now medical foods available for a wide range of medical conditions from osteoarthritis to Alzheimer's disease." The field of candidates for the development of medical foods is continuously expanding due to advances in the understanding of nutrition and disease, coupled with advances in food technology in increasing the number of products that can be formulated and commercialized. Over the past 3 years, SKIM, a Switzerland-based company, has been involved in over 30 market research projects in the medical food area to help treat or prevent a vast range of conditions—from more severe (diabetes, oncology) to less severe conditions (allergies, sarcopenia, loss of energy, etc.)—mostly for multinational companies.

WHAT NUTRIENTS ARE BEING USED
TO COMBAT HEALTH CONDITIONS?

The majority (51 of 82) of U.S. medical food products on the market are for metabolic diseases. Protein-based medical foods have the most common mechanism of action. Other nutrients such as omega 3, isoflavone, soluble fiber, vitamin D, chelated zinc, flavonoids (e.g., baicalin, catechin, pterostilbene), chromium picolinate, phytosterols, and L-arginine are being used as the leading ingredients in manufacturing medical foods. Also other vitamins and minerals such as pyridoxine, thiamine, and folic acid are being used in combination with the aforementioned nutrients (Eussen et al. 2011).

RECENT ACTIVITIES IN THE MEDICAL FOOD DOMAIN

Biostrategies Group accounts for a total of 23 firms with products on the U.S. medical food market, of which 4 are from larger companies, which also account for the bulk of revenue, and 19 are from smaller firms (NZbio, 2012). More manufacturers are bringing more products to the market that address issues from metabolic processes to probiotics. In 2006, Limbrel® (flavocoxid), the first medical food for the management of osteoarthritis, was launched. Axona was deemed by FDA in 2009 as a medical food, targeting metabolic deficiencies associated with Alzheimer's disease; the well-researched VSL #3, a probiotic for ulcerative colitis and ileal pouch, hit the market in 2002. NiteBite, a snack bar for the nutritional management of hyperglycemia, has been marketed since 1996. Other health platforms are designed to provide solutions for osteopenia/osteoporosis (Fosteum, Primus Pharmaceuticals), depression (Deplin, Pamlab), sleep disorders associated with depression (Sentra PM, Targeted Medical Pharma), and pain and inflammation (Theramine, Targeted Medical Pharma).

In recent years, Theramine, an amino acid formulation (AAF), has been developed and is used as a prescription medical food for the clinical dietary management of the metabolic processes associated with pain and inflammation (Shell et al., 2012). The formulation is GRAS-approved and designed to increase the production of serotonin, nitric oxide (NO), histamine, and gamma-aminobutyric acid by providing precursors to these neurotransmitters. The neurotransmitters addressed in this formulation have well-defined and specific roles in the modulation of pain and inflammation.

Deplin® (Pamlab, Inc.) or L-methylfolate is described by the manufacturer (Roman and Bembry, 2011) as "an orally administered prescription medical food for the dietary management of suboptimal folate levels in depressed patients."

New dietary options are needed to improve compliance with a low-phenylalanine diet and subsequent metabolic control for individuals with phenylketonuria (PKU) (Camp et al., 2012). A variety of acceptable, nutritionally complete products can be made from whey protein glycomacropeptide (GMP) with the potential to replace, or partially replace, the traditional amino acid–based medical foods currently used in PKU diets (Calcar and Ney, 2012). GMP-based medical foods represent a new paradigm to move current PKU diets from synthetic amino acids as the primary source of protein equivalents to a more physiologically normalized diet based on intact protein, which, as our research demonstrates, improves protein use and promotes satiety (Khamsi, 2013).

NuMe Health LLC is an advanced New Orleans–based biotechnology company developing evidence-based prebiotic supplements for specific health conditions. Proliant Health and Biologicals has announced recently self-affirmed GRAS status for the company's proprietary, IP-protected ingredient ImmunoLin (bovine globulin concentrate). "The market for food and nutrition products that support gut health and immunity are expanding rapidly," said Eric Weaver, Proliant Chief Scientific Officer. "The formal approval allows the use of ImmunoLin in products requiring GRAS such as functional foods and beverages, meal replacement, and medical foods."

Prismic Pharma's new product, NEUREPA™ (eicosapentaenoic acid [EPA]), is a prescription medical food intended for the dietary management of omega-3 deficiency in patients with schizophrenia, bipolar disorder, and depression. It is a proprietary, highly purified omega-3 triglyceride formulation containing not less than 92% eicosapentaenoic acid (EPA) per 1.0 g.

NattoPharma has developed up to 98% pure, natural vitamin K2, MK-7 (MenaQ7® brand), in the form of crystals to prevent osteoporosis and to support the cardiovascular health of postmenopausal women.

Another candidate product in this segment is alpha-cyclodextrin. The unique structure imparts fascinating health benefits to this dietary fiber that allows it to form a stable nondigestible complex with dietary fat. Just as the fiber–fat complex is nondigestible, it is also nonfermentable, thus eliminating messy side effects.

FBCx is a patented (Soho Flordis International, a Sydney-based natural medicine company) α-cyclodextrin-based soluble dietary fiber, with the unique ability to bind and eliminate nine times its own weight in dietary fat. Several positive clinical outcomes from randomized, placebo-controlled trials intensified its health benefits as that of a medical food (Grunberger et al., 2007; Kevin et al., 2011).

HERBS AND BOTANICALS AS POTENTIAL CANDIDATES

Herbs and botanicals are often proposed as functional ingredients in functional foods and dietary supplements. Also, medicines frequently contain ingredients derived from plant material. A product containing herbs or botanicals will be considered as a medicinal product when presented as having properties for treating or preventing diseases in humans or when it may be used in or is administered to humans with a view to restore, correct, or modify physiological functions by exerting a pharmacological, immunological, or metabolic action or to make a medical diagnosis (European Commission, 2004). It is the competence and responsibility of the member states to decide, on a case-by-case basis, whether a herbal or botanical product falls within the definition of a medicinal product. This may lead to a situation in which a product containing exactly the same bioactive ingredients and in the same dosage is considered a dietary supplement in some European member states but is registered as a medicine in others. Since the manner in which a product is being presented and its anticipated pharmacological, immunological, or metabolic action determine its classification as food or drug, it is also possible that herbs and botanicals are exploited both as a dietary supplement and as a medicine within a member state, depending on dosage and form. For example, in the Netherlands, the herbals *Ginkgo biloba*, Valerian, and St. John's Wort are sold both as foods and drugs. The distinction between a food item and a medicine is of great significance for legal practice, since medicines are more tightly regulated than foods. The recognized therapeutic active level of substances may be used as a cutoff point to differentiate between a food item and a medicine (Coppens et al., 2006). Products with a recommended daily intake level that is higher than this cutoff point would be classified as a medicinal product, whereas products with a recommended daily dosage that is lower than this cutoff point would be regarded as a dietary supplement. This is in agreement with the view taken by the European Court of Justice. According to the Court, the legislation on medicines applies only to a product that is, at its recommended dosage, capable of modifying human physiological functions by exerting a pharmacological, immunological, or metabolic action (Baeyens and Goffin, 2009). In the case of Hecht-Pharma, red rice capsules were judged to be classified as a food agent. Although the capsules contained monacolin K, which is identical to the prescription drug lovastatin, the recommended daily dosage (1.33–4 mg/day) was lower than what is considered effective for lovastatin (20–80 mg/day) (Bradford et al., 1994). Nevertheless, differences in the production process, auxiliary agents, and the ratio of active and auxiliary ingredients between food products and medicines may contribute to differences in effectiveness.

WHAT ARE THE CHALLENGES TO SUCCESS IN THE MEDICAL FOOD MARKET?

In 1988, the FDA made steps to encourage the development of an additional medical food category by awarding them orphan drug status. These regulatory changes reduced the costs and time associated with bringing medical foods to market, as earlier medical foods were treated as pharmaceutical drugs.

Zak Dutton of Prismic breaks the challenges into two broad categories. "The first relates to the development of a medical food. Unlike dietary supplements, medical foods require strong scientific support to meet the medical food criteria. What this means is that the benefit of the medical foods should be proven in clinical trials. The second is relative lack of awareness or understanding of medical foods in the medical community. Most doctors in the United States have not heard of the term 'medical food' and don't know that it is a distinct, FDA regulated category. As a result there is a tendency to think of medical food as either a drug or as a dietary supplement." Dr. Badmaev of NattoPharma also echoed the same view. He said, "The challenges to efficacious medicinal foods stem from regulatory obstacles that can be resolved by a solid research program, and formulation of the active ingredients, like vitamin K2, into a stable, nutritious and attractive form of food delivery." "Companies developing medical nutrition solutions as a part of the treatment and prevention of chronic diseases like diabetes, sarcopenia, HIV and obesity face several challenges," Benoît Gouhier, project director of SKIM consumer health, added. He also highlighted that "most health services and insurers currently don't cover the cost of nutritional products for disease prevention or management. As such, consumers and patients become the final decision makers regarding the purchase of these products, often guided by the advice and recommendations of healthcare professionals. The result is a complex and competitive environment and decision-making process that poses real challenges for marketers."

WHAT WILL THE MARKET LOOK LIKE IN 5 TO 10 YEARS FROM NOW?

The "medical foods" category is relatively well known in the United States, but less so elsewhere. Zak Dutton of Prismic Pharmaceutical said, "My expectation is that the category, in the United States, will grow significantly. There is simply too great a need from both the health benefit and cost of healthcare perspectives." "The trend in medicinal food started approximately 15 years ago and since then the body of clinical peer-reviewed papers on the subject has grown dramatically," Vladimir Badmaev of NattoPharma added.

The size of the medical food market is unclear. The FDA predicts strong growth, in light of the increasing use of medical foods in long-term care and the growing population of older individuals. Global sales have been projected at just under $9 billion (Global Industry Analysts, 2011; Kalorama, 2010). The lack of an industry association and the scarcity of public data make it difficult to estimate U.S. medical food revenue; the best estimate is $2.1 billion for the year 2011 growing at ~10%.

REGULATORY CHALLENGES THE INDUSTRY IS EXPERIENCING

In the United States, medical foods are a special product category regulated by the FDA. In Europe, a similar category called "foods for special medical purposes" (FSMPs) is covered by the foods for particular nutritional uses directive and regulated by the European Commission (EC).

Medical foods do not require preapproval from the FDA for marketing. Unlike nutritional supplements, which have no disease claim and are intended for healthy individuals, medical foods must make a disease claim and are intended for use in specific diseased populations.

Disease claims must be supported by sound scientific evidence substantiating claims of successful nutritional management of the disease. All ingredients must be approved food additives or classified as "generally recognized as safe" (GRAS). Reimbursement for medical foods is inconsistent and varies by product and by health plan. Like medical foods in the United States, FSMPs are intended for use only under medical supervision, but they must comply with EC regulations. In the European Union, there is harmonized legislation on health claims, while compounds, ingredients, and plants are still regulated only at the national level.

BUSINESS MODELS AND MARKET POSITIONING

Medical food marketers widely use varying call points by their sales force and the distribution channels for their products, often using a combination for each. The call points are primary care MDs and PAs, specialist MDs and prescribing nurses, registered dieticians, mail-order pharmacies, long-term care providers (corporate and/or local), hospitals (corporate and/or local), and home care services. Retail and mail-order pharmacies, doctors' offices, the Internet, hospitals, home care services, and specialized disease clinics are the main distribution channels.

Market positioning of medical foods is challenging. Most of the marketing gurus suggest the following steps for successful positioning:

1. Raise awareness of a new category among physicians, patients, and payers.
2. Successfully leverage "consumer pull" and "healthcare professional push" by building targeted strategies for disease-specific medical nutrition.
3. Create new adherability such as taste, smell, color, "mouth feel," and presentation to differentiate medical foods from prescription drugs. "Naturalness" of a medical food is also another key element in building a positioning statement.

ARE MEDICAL FOODS ALWAYS SAFE AS GENERALLY ASSUMED?

The popularity of food supplements and medical foods, resulting in a billion-dollar market in the United States, reflects not only the societal trend away from "artificial" pharmaceutical drugs toward "natural" ingredients but also the lack of satisfactory drugs that both effective and safe. Consumers are likely to assume that medical foods are safe, but some recent studies suggest that this may not always be true. Flavocoxid, which is marketed as a medical food, is a proprietary blend of purified, plant-derived bioflavonoids. It is believed to act as a dual inhibitor of cyclooxygenase and 5-lipoxygenase enzymes, therefore inhibiting the conversion of arachidonic acid into both prostaglandins and leukotrienes. These mechanisms make flavocoxid an interesting therapeutic alternative to nonsteroidal anti-inflammatory drugs. Because it is classified as a medical food, flavocoxid was marketed beginning in 2004 in the absence of any published randomized trial. Although two trials became available in 2009 and 2010, four cases of acute liver injury associated with flavocoxid have been reported so far (Chalasani et al., 2012). Many herbal products used as food supplements or medical food, as well as vitamins, antioxidants, fiber, trace elements, proteins, and amino acids, can also be associated with liver injury.

TECHNOLOGICAL CHALLENGES

The creation of a medical food with potential health benefits for a particular patient population is a surprisingly complex process. Fortunately, the developmental process for a specific medical food is not as rigorous or as tightly regulated as that of a pharmaceutical agent (Juan et al. 2011). However, numerous factors unique to the enteral formulation of a new product come into play, such as physical/chemical compatibility, pH, stability, bioavailability, decay, and even palatability (Ochoa et al., 2011). Additional considerations such as the strength of health benefit claims, packaging or presentation, and marketability determine the ultimate commercialization and whether a product ends up being released to the public. A full understanding of the development, substantiation, and commercialization of a medical food is necessary for important physiologic concepts in nutrition therapy to end up as part of the therapeutic regimen at the bedside of the critically ill obese patient.

CONCLUSION

Taking a nutrition product from the bench to the bedside is a long and complex endeavor.

However, to understand the effectiveness and safety of any healthcare intervention—drug, medical device, food supplement, or medical food—clinical evidence from well-designed randomized trials and observational studies will always be necessary. Given the widespread use and potential harm of medical foods and food supplements, the policy of marketing these products in the absence of clinical evidence may need to be reconsidered.

Research is limited on the medical properties of food, particularly in human clinical studies. More work is needed to understand the potential benefits of medical foods, specifically on the following:

- More prospective, controlled studies
- Larger subject populations
- Longer treatment durations

In addition to medical food, research is needed to advance the technology used to deliver certain medical foods such as tubing and pumps.

REFERENCES

Baeyens, A. and Goffin, T. 2009. European Court of Justice. ECJ 2009/01 Synthon BV v. Licensing Authority of the Department of Health, October 16, 2008 (C/452/06). *Eur. J. Health Law*, 16: 105–109.

BioStrategies Group medical food study. 2011. http://biostrategies.com/about/news.

Bradford, R.H., Shear, C.L., Chremos, A.N. et al. 1994. Expanded Clinical Evaluation of Lovastatin (EXCEL) study results: Two-year efficacy and safety follow-up. *Am. J. Cardiol.*, 74: 667–673.

Calcar, S.C. and Ney, D.M. 2012. Food products made with glycomacropeptide, a low-phenylalanine whey protein, provide a new alternative to amino acid–based medical foods for nutrition management of phenylketonuria. *J. Acad. Nutr. Diet*, 112: 1201–1210.

Camp, K.M., Lloyd-Puryear, M.A., and Huntington, K.L. 2012. Nutritional treatment for inborn errors of metabolism: Indications, regulations, and availability of medical foods and dietary supplements using phenylketonuria as an example. *Mol. Genet. Metab.*, 107: 3–9.

Chalasani, N., Vuppalanchi, R., Navarro, V. et al. 2012. Drug-induced liver injury network acute liver injury due to flavocoxid (Limbrel), a medical food for osteoarthritis. A case series. *Ann. Intern. Med.*, 156: 857–860.

Coppens, P., Delmulle, L., Gulati, O. et al. 2006. Use of botanicals in food supplements. Regulatory scope, scientific risk assessment and claim substantiation. *Ann. Nutr. Metab.*, 50: 538–554.

European Commission. 2004. Directive 2004/27/EC of the European Parliament and of the Council of 31 March 2004 amending Directive 2001/83/EC on the Community code relating to medicinal products for human use. http://eurlex.europa.eu/LexUriServ/LexUriServ.do?uri=OJ:L:2004:136:0034:0057:EN:PDF. Accessed November 13, 2015.

Eussen, S.R., Verhagen, H., and Klungel, O.H. 2011. Functional foods and dietary supplements: Products at the interface between pharma and nutrition. *Eur. J. Pharmacol.*, 668: S2–S9.

FDA. 2010. Medical Foods Guidance Documents and Regulatory. http://www.fda.gov/Food/GuidanceRegulation/GuidanceDocumentsRegulatoryInformation/MedicalFoods/. Accessed July 7, 2016.

Georgiou, N.A., Garssen, J., and Witkamp, R.F. 2011. Pharma–nutrition interface: The gap is narrowing. *Eur. J. Pharmacol.*, 651: 1–8.

Grunberger, G., Jen, C., and Artiss, J.D. 2007. The benefits of early intervention in obese diabetic patients with FBCx™—A new dietary fibre. *Diabetes Metab. Res. Rev.*, 23: 56–62.

Juan, B., Ochoa, J.B., Stephen, A. et al. 2011. Issues involved in the process of developing a medical food. *J. Parenter. Enter. Nutr.*, 35: 73S–79S.

Kalorama Information. 2011. *The World Market for Clinical Nutrition Products (Infant, Parenteral and Enteral Foods)*, 4th edn. http://www.kaloramainformation.com/Clinical-Nutrition-Products-6126530/.

Kevin, B., Comerford, K.B., Joseph, D. et al. 2011. The beneficial effects α-cyclodextrin on blood lipids and weight loss in healthy humans. *Obesity*, 19: 1200–1204.

Khamsi, R. 2013. Rethinking the formula. *Nat. Med.*, 19: 525–529.

Ochoa, J.B., McClave, S.A., and Saavedra, J. 2011. Issues involved in the process of developing a medical food. *J. Parenter. Enteral. Nutr.*, 35: 73S–79S.

Roman, M.W. and Bembry, F.H. 2011. L-Methylfolate (Deplin R): A new medical food therapy as adjunctive treatment for depression. *Issues Ment. Health Nurs.*, 32: 142–143.

Shell, W.A., Elizabeth H., Marcus, A. et al. 2012. A double-blind controlled trial of a single dose naproxen and an amino acid medical food theramine for the treatment of low back pain. *Am. J. Ther.*, 19: 108–114.

15 Probiotics
From Bench to Market

Dilip Ghosh

CONTENTS

INTRODUCTION

The health-promoting use of fermented milk products started long before the existence of microorganisms and lactic acid bacteria was discovered. The early written records go back to 76 BC when Roman historian Plinio (Plinius) described their use in the therapy of various gastrointestinal infections (Bertazzoni et al., 2013; Bottazzi, 1983). The scientific basis of the probiotic concept was put forward only at the beginning of the twentieth century (Metchnikoff, 1907) after the invention of the microscope and the discovery of bacteria and especially lactic acid bacteria (LAB) in the seventeenth, eighteenth, and nineteenth centuries, respectively. Metchnikoff postulated that consumption of fermented milk would suppress the growth of proteolytic bacteria and thereby reduce putrefaction in the gut, thus prolonging the life span of the host. Soon after his theory, strains of LAB and bifidobacteria were applied as supplements and over-the-counter drugs for the treatment of diarrhea (e.g., *Lactobacillus LB Lactéol* in 1907, *Escherichia coli* Nissle in 1917, and end of the 1920s) and in food products for the promotion of intestinal health and prevention of disease (e.g., *Lactobacillus acidophilus* L-92 in 1910, *Lactobacillus casei* Shirota in 1935).

Skyrocketing interest in probiotics and dietary supplements is evidenced in increasingly aging population and their eagerness to ensure continuing fitness and good health as long as possible. In addition, there has been wide coverage in the media in the recent years about the expiry of patents owned by the big pharma and companies' quests to expand their product pipeline by obtaining licenses in new biotech products. Some are now looking to extend their product range outside drugs with big and specialty pharmaceutical companies starting to expand into the probiotic field. As a result, this is becoming a growth market. Increased activity in this area has included, for example, Nestlé's €50 million investment in Swedish probiotic player BioGaia, Pfizer's acquisition of a Danish company, Ferrosan and Reckitt Benckiser's acquisition of Schiff Nutrition in the United States, and Soho Flordis International's acquisition of U.S. healthcare professional probiotic player ProThera a few years ago. Probiotics are regulated differently than drugs and so it is necessary to consider different factors when looking to acquire or obtain a license for such products.

WHAT ARE PROBIOTICS?

The term "probiotic" refers to live microorganisms, specifically probiotic bacteria, which are widely believed to provide a health benefit when consumed by humans. Subcategories of the general term "probiotic" include probiotic drugs (intended to cure, treat, or prevent disease), probiotic foods (which include foods, food ingredients, and dietary supplements), direct-fed microbials (probiotics for animal use), and designer probiotics (genetically modified probiotics). However, when considered in a legal context, the use of the term has different implications, especially regarding any health claims made for these products. Under European legislation, the term "probiotic" is considered to be an unauthorized health claim. The European Commission considers that the term implies that a product provides a health benefit, which could be misleading to consumers unless it can be substantiated. The regulations put in place by the commission provide that a health claim may be permitted only if it is based on generally accepted scientific evidence and is well understood by the average consumer. Currently, there are no approved health claims for probiotics, except for the very recent approval of limited health claims on Yakult products. This is despite submission of many applications to the European Food Safety Authority (EFSA).

MECHANISMS OF ACTION

The most common misconceptions include understanding the benefits of probiotics and their associated mechanisms. Historically, commensal and fermentation microorganisms belonging to several genera, including *Lactobacillus*, were labeled as probiotics (Hill, 2010). However, by definition, probiotics must confer proven health effects that must be considered to be strain-specific, unless otherwise demonstrated. Some groups have suggested using the term "pharmabiotics" (Shanahan et al., 2009) for strain-specific usefulness of probiotics. This term refers to live, dead, or components of organisms that are part of the natural microbiota. But the term "probiotic" encompasses only live microbes from any source (human, animal, or environmental) so long as they are safe for their intended use and have documented health effects. Probiotics are commonly marketed to promote gastrointestinal (GI) health by "balancing" the GI microbiota. The concept of microbial balancing is undefined, but some evidence exists suggesting that certain probiotic strains can stabilize the gut microbiota by reducing the change in fecal bacteria communities in response to specific stress or health conditions (Kubota et al., 2009) or by promoting the return to a

TABLE 15.1

Proposed Mechanisms of Action of Probiotics

Produce antimicrobial substances, such as organic acids or bacteriocins

Upregulate immune response (e.g., secretory IgA) to possible pathogens or to vaccines

Downregulate inflammatory response

Assist in the early programming of the immune system to result in a better balanced immune response
  and reducing risk of development of allergy

Improve gut mucosal barrier function

Enhance stability or promote recovery of commensal microbiota when perturbed

Modulate host gene expression

Deliver functional proteins (e.g., lactase) or enzymes (natural and cloned)

Decrease pathogen adhesion

Source: Adapted from Sanders, M.E., *Funct. Food Rev.*, 1, 3, 2009.

baseline microbial community following a perturbing event such as antibiotic therapy (Engelbrektson et al., 2009). The dosages required to achieve beneficial effects are commonly reported to be in the order of 1–10 billion CFU/day. However, effective doses are sometimes greater or less than this recommended amount. For example, administration of 100 million CFU/day of certain probiotic can reduce abdominal discomfort in irritable bowel syndrome (IBS) patients (Whorwell et al., 2006) and improve colicky symptoms in infants (Savino et al., 2007). But recent trend in probiotic is "megadose," that is, more than 10 billion CFU per dose. Thus, controlled studies must be performed to determine the appropriate dose, not a general dose, before probiotic enters clinical practices. Table 15.1 shows the potential mechanisms of action of probiotics.

FROM CLINIC TO MARKET: THE REGULATORY HURDLE

In both the United States and Europe, supermarkets and pharmacies are bombarded with probiotics—products containing live microorganisms—claiming they improve health. The availability of these products justifies the growing consumer demand for foods that improve or maintain health and wellness. While some of these claims may have scientific merits, others have not been substantiated. For a number of products, claims are based on insufficient research, underpowered studies, or mixed research results (Hoffmann, 2013). The U.S. and the European Union regulatory bodies have taken two different approaches on this regulatory spectrum.

Orally administered probiotics may be marketed as dietary supplements, conventional foods, medical foods, and drugs (biologics). At present, no probiotic product is licensed in the United States as a biological drug product used for the treatment, prevention, cure, mitigation, or diagnosis of a specific human disease. Foods and dietary supplements cannot carry these types of claims, which are marketed for the purpose of ameliorating or preventing a disease.

Because dietary supplements and foods differ from therapeutic agents in how they are regulated by the U.S. Food and Drug Administration (FDA) and other regulatory bodies around the world, these study agents are considered therapeutic agents or investigational new drugs.

The intended use of a product dictates how it will be regulated and the nature of the claims that can be made. Thus, a thorough understanding of the definitions of various products is critical to its proper regulation. A dietary supplement is an orally administered product intended to supplement the diet. By contrast, a drug is any article intended for use in the diagnosis, cure, mitigation, treatment, or prevention of a disease. A biological product is a type of drug defined as containing any virus, therapeutic serum, toxin, antitoxin, or analogous product (Public Health Service Act, 1944). The Center for Food Safety and Applied Nutrition (CFSAN) at the FDA regulates probiotic products under the broad category of food, including dietary supplements. CFSAN is primarily responsible for postmarketing surveillance. The manufacturer is responsible for ensuring that the food or supplement is safe before it is marketed and is further responsible for substantiating labeling claims. Limited labeling claims may be made for products regulated as foods and dietary supplements, such as "structure/function" or "health" claims. Structure/function claims focus on maintaining or supporting normal structures or functions of the body; for example, it helps maintain healthy intestinal microbiota, helps maintain regularity, relieves occasional constipation, or helps support immune function. Structure/function claims for foods do not need CFSAN approval or notification, but they must be truthful, not misleading, and substantiated by competent and reliable scientific evidence. However, dietary supplement companies must notify the FDA within 30 days of marketing a supplement that bears a structure/function claim. In addition, the structure/function claim must be accompanied on the label or labeling by the FDA disclosure statement that the agency has not evaluated the claim and that the product is not intended to be used in the diagnosis, mitigation, treatment, cure, or prevention of a disease.

A health claim can be distinguished from a structure/function claim by its focus on risk reduction of disease or a health-related condition (FDA, 2008). An example of this type of claim that would be relevant to probiotic effects might be a statement claiming that the product reduces the risk of traveler's diarrhea. However, under current interpretation of food law, this claim would likely not be considered appropriate because it addresses a short-term, acute condition, not a long-term, diet-related condition. All health claims require CFSAN authorization. The challenge is determining if there is sufficient scientific evidence in risk reduction to support petitioning the FDA to permit a health claim related to the relationship of a food or supplement containing a specific probiotic strain (FDA, 2009). There are currently no approved health claims in the United States for probiotic products.

The main legislation regulating the health claims made by probiotics in Europe is to ensure high levels of protection for consumers and to aid in facilitating their choice (No. 1924/2006, HC Regulations). The HC Regulations were introduced in response to the increasing number of foods labeled and advertised within the European Community with nutrition and health claims. Article 13 of the HC Regulations has proved to be particularly controversial among manufacturers in the probiotics industry. The article specifically addresses health claims describing or referring to the role of a nutrient or other substances in the growth, development, and functions of the body, psychological and behavioral functions, or slimming or weight control. These claims may be permitted if they are based on generally accepted scientific evidence and are well understood by the average consumer. The HC Regulations also provide a list of approved claims and state that any changes to the list will only be made based on scientific evidence after consultation with the EFSA. To introduce a new claim to the list, a manufacturer must provide the competent authority in its member state with an application for a new claim, which is then referred to the EFSA for scientific assessment.

Manufacturers have, so far, been unsuccessful in convincing the EFSA of the health claims for probiotic products. The EFSA has, since its establishment, published opinions on many claims, but has yet to accept any for a probiotic product. On December 14, 2012, the use of the term "probiotic" was banned under the HC Regulations, as not a single claim relating to the use of the term had been accepted by EFSA. This means that products cannot be sold in the EU claiming to be probiotics. Additional points to consider in any submission to the EFSA should include clear, defined end points, clearly characterized bacterial strains (through molecular typing), and clear links to a cause-and-effect relationship for the product.

On September 20, 2013, the European Commission introduced Regulation No. 907/2013 (the Generic Descriptors Regulation), which sets out the rules for applications concerning the use of generic descriptors. Generic descriptors are words that have traditionally been used to indicate a characteristic of a class of foods or beverages that could imply an effect on health such as "digestive." In the past, these words have been exempted from the ban under the HC Regulation; the Generic Descriptors Regulation provides that generic descriptors for food and beverage products, which could be construed as health claims, will be allowed only if they have been in use for the product for more than 20 years in a member state. When a company can demonstrate use of these descriptors prior to the passing of the Generic Descriptors Regulation, it is possible to apply for an exemption to the ban.

The Generic Descriptors Regulation has not been well received by the probiotics industry due to the argument of supplying robust additional requirements to show consumer understanding of the implied health effects, as well as the evidence that the consumer links the generic descriptors to the particular class of food or beverage which is difficult and expensive to provide. It is generally believed that most claims for probiotics will be unsuccessful because the term is too closely associated in the average consumer's mind with a health claim and there is insufficient history of the terms used in the EU marketplace (ISAPP, 2009). The word "probiotic" has not taken on the additional everyday meanings used by products such as "tonic" water.

There are two key regulatory problems that will be faced by companies wishing to deal in probiotics. In any commercial agreement, first, it is not mandatory that the distributor will be required to market the probiotic product, and second, an application for a health claim should be made before marketing. It is possible that the time and cost of preparing a claim and the fact that the EFSA is unlikely to accept a probiotic product will mean that companies may need to look at alternative ways of marketing their probiotic products.

THE APPLICATION OF PROBIOTICS IN FOOD PRODUCTS

Historically, the development of probiotics was very much oriented toward pharmaceutical applications such as treatment of diarrhea, prevention of antibiotic-associated diarrhea, management of stomach and gastrointestinal infections, and management of chronic inflammation. However, these effects are not easily extended to the category of functional foods that are destined for the generally healthy population. Although beneficial effects of specific probiotics have been substantiated in short-term clinical trials in the treatment and prevention of several health disorders, the remaining challenge is to demonstrate long-term effects of probiotic foods as presently required by health claim regulations in Europe and other parts of the world. As large trials of long duration are difficult to support, particularly for small- and medium-sized laboratories and food companies, there is an urgent need to better identify and validate risk factors of diseases and biomarkers of health (Neef and Sanz, 2013).

The ability of exogenous probiotics to improve clinical outcomes through modulation of the immune response has been demonstrated in subjects with chronic and acute diseases. For example, the probiotic mix VSL#3 was shown to reduce pouchitis relapse (Gionchetti et al., 2007) and to improve clinical scores in ulcerative colitis patients (Miele et al., 2009) through improvement of the inflammatory status of the patients. *Lactobacillus rhamnosus* (LGG) given to infants during episodes of acute rotavirus diarrhea resulted in greater increase in nonspecific antibody secreting cells and specific antirotavirus antibodies in the circulation than that seen in the placebo group and resulted in shorter duration of the diarrhea (Majamaa et al., 1995). In the absence of an efficient therapy with no side effects, well-selected probiotic strains might provide a valuable alternative, such as *B. infantis* 35624 for IBM symptoms reduction (O'Mahony et al., 2005), *B. animalis* DN-173010 for constipation (Guyonnet et al., 2007), or *L. reuteri* ATCC55730 for inborn colicky symptom treatment (Indrio et al., 2008). Positive impact of probiotics is progressively being demonstrated beyond the gut; these include the following: oral intake of *Lactobacillus rhamnosus* GR-1 and *Lactobacillus fermentum* RC-14 had a positive impact on vaginal health (Anukam et al., 2006), *Lactobacillus paracasei* ST11 improved recovery of skin immune homeostasis (Peguet-Navarro et al., 2008), and *Streptococcus salivarius* K12 improved oral malodor parameters (Burton et al., 2006).

SAFETY OF PROBIOTICS

The application of probiotic microorganisms in foodstuffs requires a thorough safety assessment. Several guidelines are available on how to assess the safety of probiotics used in food applications (FAO, WHO, 2002).

The European Food Safety Authority (EFSA) has developed the QPS (Qualified Presumption of Safety) approach as a tool for the safety assessment of microorganisms used in food. This is based on a documented history of use and knowledge of potential pathogenic or toxicogenic properties associated with a particular genus

TABLE 15.2

Comparison of Assessment Schemes Used in Foods by FDA GRAS and the EU EFSA QPS Systems

GRAS Guidelines	QPS Guidelines
Applies to food additives in general	Applies to microorganisms only
Determination by FDS and/or external experts	Determination by EFSA
Open list	Positive list
Based on common use	Based on history of use and adverse effects
Describes specific substance	Describes taxonomic unit (e.g., genus, species, or strain)
Case-by-case assessment	General assessment

Source: Adapted from Jankovic, I. et al., *Curr. Opin. Biotechnol.*, 1, 7, 2010.

and species. In the United States, probiotic microorganisms could be assessed via the Generally Recognized as Safe (GRAS) system. For example, *B. lactis* BB12, *L. rhamnosus* LGG, and *L. reuteri* DSM 17938 strains have over the recent years been accepted in the United States as GRAS for their intended use. The main differences between the two approaches are summarized in Table 15.2.

Parameters such as taxonomy and identification, phenotypic characterization, history of food use, and human exposure are generally considered important (Sorokulova, 2008). If no history of safe use can be demonstrated, extensive preclinical studies, including standard 90-day toxicity studies as defined in OECD Testing Guideline 408, should also be considered. Clinical studies should include parameters to demonstrate safety in use or tolerability in the target population(s).

Rare cases of adverse effects linked to probiotic administration have been documented in individuals having serious underlying disease. Thus, special care must be taken with particularly vulnerable target population(s) such as neonates, immunocompromised subjects, or critically ill/hospitalized patients (Snydman, 2008). Overall, the vast amount of available data and long history of use in foodstuffs have not indicated any safety concerns for currently used probiotics (mainly lactobacilli and bifidobacteria) in healthy populations.

WHAT IS NEXT?

Since GRAS does not apply to "drug" use and is not recognized by the CBER as a safety measure, several scientists (Klein et al., 2010) have advocated the necessity for conducting Phase 1 and 2 clinical trials, even for the existing products on the market. There is still a strong debate whether IND level research is required for probiotics as food supplements when the products are not intended to be marketed as drugs. Several recommendations related to probiotic research have emerged from different forums (Table 15.3).

TABLE 15.3

Recommendations Related to Probiotic Research

U.S. FDA

Follow the guidance for substantiation of structure/function claims and health claims for probiotic foods, dietary supplements, and medical foods.

Adhere to the guidance specific to IND applications for human studies investigating probiotic products.

Consider extending health claim status (i.e., reduction of risk of disease) to acute diseases and health conditions, not just chronic, diet-related diseases.

National Institutes of Health

Provide service to investigators to stimulate study rigor.

Give support to patient-oriented clinical trials of probiotics.

Probiotic Food and Supplement Manufacturers

Understand FDA labeling regulations.

Provide proper substantiation structure/function claims with appropriate claim wording.

Develop sufficient evidence to meet requirements to petition FDA for health claims.

Researchers

Go for an early consultation with FDA as regards concept development of clinical research.

Request a pre-IND application meeting if necessary.

Engage individuals with experience in IND application processes.

Know the characteristics, potency, purity, and stability, as well as safety, of their probiotic test agents.

Follow the CONSORT guidelines in reporting study results.

Source: Adapted from Klein, M. et al., *Ann. N.Y. Acad. Sci.*, 1212, E1, 2010.

CONCLUSION

The demonstration of the beneficial health effects of probiotics in generally healthy humans continues to be a challenging task due to the lack of validated biomarkers of health and risk factors of diseases and the need to undertake generally large and long-term human trials. An additional challenge lies in probiotic production in a cost-effective way that will ensure probiotic viability over shelf life. One should keep in mind that inclusion of probiotics in increasingly diverse food vehicles requires product and process modifications that may bear the risk of modulating the probiotic functionality, as suggested so far mostly by *in vitro* testing.

Therefore, research and development in the probiotic area should dedicate sustained efforts in the development and validation of biomarkers of health and disease, the design of functional assays with predictive value, and the identification of bioactive molecules in probiotic products. This will strongly depend on continuous efforts to identify mechanisms of action of probiotics. With these tools in hands, it will be able to rationalize and optimize selection of probiotic candidates and downstream processing and to evaluate potential effects of the food matrixes on probiotic functionality. This in turn should help to better design the human trials required for health claim substantiation.

REFERENCES

Anukam, K., Osazuwa, E., Ahonkhai, I. et al. 2006. Augmentation of antimicrobial metronidazole therapy of bacterial vaginosis with oral probiotic *Lactobacillus rhamnosus* GR-1 and *Lactobacillus reuteri* RC-14: Randomized, double-blind, placebo controlled trial. *Microbes Infect.*, 8: 1450–1454.

Bertazzoni, M.E., Donelli, G., Midtvedt, T. et al. 2013. Probiotics and clinical effects: Is the number what counts? *J. Chemother.*, 25: 193–212.

Bottazzi, V. 1983. *Other Fermented Dairy Products. Biotechnology.* Verlag Chemie, Weinheim, Germany, pp. 315–363.

Burton, J.P., Chilcott, C.N., Moore, C.J. et al. 2006. A preliminary study of the effect of probiotic *Streptococcus salivarius* K12 on oral malodour parameters. *J. Appl. Microbiol.*, 100: 754–764.

Engelbrektson, A., Korzenik, J.E., Pittler, A. et al. 2009. Probiotics to minimize the disruption of faecal microbiota in healthy subjects undergoing antibiotic therapy. *J. Med. Microbiol.*, 58: 663–670.

FDA. 2008. Guidance for Industry: Substantiation for Dietary Supplement Claims Made Under Section 403(r) (6) of the Federal Food, Drug, and Cosmetic Act. http://www.fda.gov/food/guidanceregulation/guidancedocumentsregulatoryinformation/dietarysupplements/ucm073200.htm.

FDA. 2009. Guidance for Industry: Evidence-Based Review System for the Scientific Evaluation of Health Claims. http://www.fda.gov/Food/GuidanceRegulation/GuidanceDocuments RegulatoryInformation/LabelingNutrition/ucm073332.htm.

Food and Agriculture Organization, World Health Organization, 2009. 2002. Guidelines for the Evaluation of Probiotics in Food. Food and Agriculture Organization of the United Nations and World Health Organization, London, Ontario, Canada, pp. 11–27.

Gionchetti, P., Rizzello, F., Morselli, C. et al. 2007. High dose probiotics for the treatment of active pouchitis. *Dis. Colon Rectum*, 50: 2075–2082.

Guyonnet, D., Chassany, O., Ducrotte, P. et al. 2007. Effect of a fermented milk containing *Bifidobacterium* animalis DN-173 010 on the health-related quality of life and symptoms in irritable bowel syndrome in adults in primary care: A multicentre, randomized, double-blind, controlled trial. *Aliment. Pharmacol. Ther.*, 26: 475–486.

Hill, C. 2010. Probiotics and pharmabiotics. *Bioeng. Bugs*, 1: 79–84.

Hoffmann, D.E. 2013. Health claim regulation of probiotics in the USA and the EU: Is there a middle way? *Benefic. Microbes*, 4: 109–115.

Indrio, F., Riezzo, G., Raimondi, F. et al. 2008. The effects of probiotics on feeding tolerance, bowel habits, and gastrointestinal motility in preterm newborns. *J. Pediatr.*, 152: 801–806.

ISAPP. 2009. Probiotics: A consumer guide for making smart choices (www.isapp.net). http://isappscience.org/wp-content/uploads/2016/02/Consumer-Guidelines-probiotic.pdf.

Jankovic, I., Sybesma, W., Phothirath, P. et al. 2010. Application of probiotics in food products—Challenges and new approaches. *Curr. Opin. Biotechnol.*, 21: 1–7.

Klein, M., Ellen, M., Tri, S.D. et al. 2010. Probiotics: From bench to market. *Ann. N.Y. Acad. Sci.*, 1212(Suppl. 1): E1–E14. doi: 10.1111/j.1749-6632.2010.05839.x.

Kubota, A., He, F., Kawase, M. et al. 2009. *Lactobacillus* strains stabilize intestinal microbiota in Japanese cedar pollinosis patients. *Microbiol. Immunol.*, 53: 198–205.

Majamaa, H., Isolauri, E., Saxelin, M. et al. 1995. Lactic acid bacteria in the treatment of acute rotavirus gastroenteritis. *J. Pediatr. Gastroenterol. Nutr.*, 20: 333–338.

Miele, E., Pascarella, F., Giannetti, E. et al. 2009. Effect of a probiotic preparation (VSL#3) on induction and maintenance of remission in children with ulcerative colitis. *Am. J. Gastroenterol.*, 104: 437–443.

Metchnikoff, E. 1907. *The Prolongation of Life. Optimistic Studies.* Butterworth-Heinemann, London, UK.

Neef, A. and Sanz, Y. 2013. Future for probiotic science in functional food and dietary supplement development. *Curr. Opin. Clin. Nutr. Metab. Care*, 16: 679–687.

O'Mahony, L., McCarthy, J., Kelly, P. et al. 2005. *Lactobacillus* and *Bifidobacterium* in irritable bowel syndrome: Symptom responses and relationship to cytokine profiles. *Gastroenterology*, 128: 541–551.

Peguet-Navarro, J., Dezutter-Dambuyant, C., Buetler, T. et al. 2008. Supplementation with oral probiotic bacteria protects human cutaneous immune homeostasis after UV exposure-double blind, randomized, placebo controlled clinical trial. *Eur. J. Dermatol.*, 18: 504–511.

Public Health Service Act of 1944, 42, U.S.C. 262. http://www.fda.gov/RegulatoryInformation/Legislation/ucm149278.htm.

Sanders, M.E. 2009. How do we know when something called "Probiotic" is really a probiotic? A guideline for consumers and health care professionals. *Funct. Food Rev.*, 1: 3–12.

Savino, F., Pelle, E., Palumeri, E. et al. 2007. *Lactobacillus reuteri* (American Type Culture Collection Strain 55730) versus simethicone in the treatment of infantile colic: A prospective randomized study. *Pediatrics*, 119: e124–e130.

Shanahan, F., Stanton, C., Ross, P., and Hill, C. 2009. Pharmabiotics: Bioactives from mining host-microbe-dietary interactions. *Funct. Food Rev.*, 1: 20–25.

Snydman, D.R. 2008. The safety of probiotics. *Clin. Infect. Dis.*, 1: S104–S111.

Sorokulova, I. 2008. Preclinical testing in the development of probiotics: A regulatory perspective with *Bacillus* strains as an example. *Clin. Infect. Dis.*, 46: S92–S95.

Whorwell, P.J., Altringer, L., Morel, J. et al. 2006. Efficacy of an encapsulated probiotic *Bifidobacterium infantis* 35624 in women with irritable bowel syndrome. *Am. J. Gastroenterol.*, 101: 1581–1590.

16 The Combination of Foods and Drugs
Advantages and Drawbacks

R. B. Smarta

CONTENTS

INTRODUCTION

Drugs have been long known to cure, treat, and prevent diseases. With the recent advent of nutraceuticals and other allied fields, people have become aware of the curative and preventive properties of foods and food components as well. Although both exhibit similar actions when combined, they interact with each other and can increase, decrease, or have no effect at all.

Since drugs/medications are a critical factor in any illness, their effect on the patient and subsequently the illness should be maximum and predictable and more or less similar for all patients; they should not have any negative effects. Once ingested, their effect should not alter from what it was meant to be. The same is true in the case of foods; we want them to provide us with adequate nutrition and not cause us any harmful effects. The drugs have components that interact with human body in different ways, and our lifestyle and diet have significant interactions and effects on the drugs. These interactions are termed as "food–drug interactions" or "drug–nutrient interactions."

Drug–nutrient/food interactions can be defined as physical, chemical, physiological, or pathophysiological relationships between a drug and a nutrient/food/food component. These interactions may occur accidently, due to lack of knowledge, due to negligence, and so forth. The interactions may increase, decrease, alter the effect, or have no effect at all on the therapy/effect of the drug. The causes of most clinically significant drug–nutrient interactions are usually multifactorial. Failure to identify and properly manage drug–nutrient interactions can lead to serious consequences and have a negative impact on patient outcomes and health.

There are three major types of food–drug interactions: drug interaction with a food, drug interaction with nutrients, and drug interaction with herbs or dietary supplements.

UNDERSTANDING THE MECHANICS OF INTERACTIONS

In order to avoid any potential harmful interactions or to boost positive interactions, it is important to understand the mechanisms of what a drug does to the body once ingested and how a body reacts to the ingested drug.

PHARMACOKINETICS AND PHARMACODYNAMICS

The study of the effects of drugs on the body as well as the effect of the body on the drugs consumed is essential. This study is important to understand the various aspects involved in the metabolism of drugs/medicines.

Pharmacokinetics

The study of how the body responds to a specific drug after its administration in the body is termed pharmacokinetics. The various aspects involved in this are absorption, distribution, metabolism, and excretion (ADME) from the body. For some drugs, there is an additional step, that is, liberation, which is different from absorption, so it is often termed LADME.

Absorption

The absorption phase involves the movement of a drug from the site of administration to its absorption in the bloodstream. This depends on the route of administration, the nature and chemistry of the drug and its ability to cross membranes, the rate of gastric emptying (for oral drugs), GI movement, and the quality of the product. Food, food components, and nutritional supplements can interfere with absorption, especially if the drug is administered orally.

Distribution

After absorption in the bloodstream, the drug leaves the systemic circulation and circulates through the various parts of the body. Once in the bloodstream, drug molecules are often bound to plasma proteins and only unbound drugs can leave the blood and affect target organs. Low serum albumin levels can increase the availability of drug in the bloodstream and can enhance its effects. Also, certain food components can affect the distribution of drugs to the target organ.

Metabolism (Biotransformation)

Drug metabolism is facilitated by an enzyme system (cytochrome P450) in the liver, and the metabolism generally changes fat-soluble compounds of drugs to water-soluble compounds that can be excreted. Foods or dietary supplements that increase or inhibit these enzyme systems can change the rate or extent of drug metabolism.

Excretion

Renal excretion is the major route of elimination of drugs affected by renal function and urinary pH. Drugs are eliminated from the body as either an unchanged drug or its metabolite. Some drugs are eliminated through bile and other body fluids. Before being excreted, most of the drugs are absorbed in the body.

Bioavailability

Apart from ADME, "bioavailability" is another important parameter of pharmacokinetics. Bioavailability is the degree to which a drug or other substance reaches circulation and becomes available to the target organ or tissue. The percentage of the bioavailability of a drug denotes the amount of a drug available at the target site for the actual effect.

Pharmacodynamics

Pharmacodynamics is the study of biochemical and physiological effects of drugs or combination of drugs on the body or on microorganisms/parasites within or on body and the mechanisms of drug action and the relationship between drug concentration and effects. Often the drug molecule binds to a receptor, enzyme, or ion channel, producing a physiological response.

FOOD–DRUG INTERACTIONS

Food is any material that is consumed in order to provide nutritional support for the body. The food can be of either plant or animal origin; food contains essential nutrients, such as fats, proteins, vitamins, or minerals. Food can also be defined as any material that is ingested by an organism and assimilated by the organism's cells to provide energy, sustain life, and stimulate growth.

Nutrients are the components in foods that an organism utilizes for survival and growth. Macronutrients provide the bulk energy that an organism's metabolic system needs to function, while micronutrients provide the necessary cofactors for metabolism to be carried out. Both types of nutrients can be acquired from the environment.

Food interactions can affect pharmacokinetics and/or pharmacodynamics of the drug. Food can interfere with any of the pharmacokinetic stages of drug action and that too in a number of ways. The interaction may have synergistic, antagonistic, or additive effect on the drug action.

Most commonly foods interact with and affect the drug absorption. This can make a drug less effective because less of it gets into the blood and to the site of action. Second, nutrients or other chemicals in foods can affect how a drug is used in the body. Third, excretion of drugs from the body may be affected by foods, nutrients, or other substances. With some drugs, it is important to avoid taking food and medication together because the food can make the drug less effective. For other drugs, it may be good to take the drug with food to prevent stomach irritation.

DRUG–NUTRIENT INTERACTIONS

Drugs may interfere with the nutritional status of an individual as well. Some drugs may interfere with the absorption of nutrients, while others may interfere with the metabolism and/or excretion of the nutrients in the body especially vitamins and minerals. If less of a nutrient is available to the body because of these effects, it may lead to a nutrient deficiency. Sometimes, drugs affect the nutritional status by increasing or decreasing appetite, which in turn affects the amount of food (and nutrients) consumed (Bobroff et al., 2009).

THE EFFECT OF NUTRIENTS AND FOODS ON DRUGS VARIES DEPENDING ON MANY FACTORS

Interactions occur mostly on the drugs that are administered orally. Certain medications, even though not taken orally, are transported to the site of action. The effects of drugs/nutrients and food–drug interactions vary according to the type of medication administered, format of drug (capsule, tablet, liquid, etc.), dosage, route of administration (oral, intravenous, etc.), and site of absorption (mouth, stomach, intestine).

The interactions can be either positive or negative in nature. The advantages and disadvantages of drug–nutrient interactions are given in Figure 16.1.

EXAMPLES OF INTERACTIONS

Some examples of the interactions between food/nutrients and drugs are illustrated in Figure 6.1.

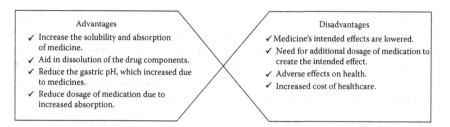

Advantages	Disadvantages
✓ Increase the solubility and absorption of medicine.	✓ Medicine's intended effects are lowered.
✓ Aid in dissolution of the drug components.	✓ Need for additional dosage of medication to create the intended effect.
✓ Reduce the gastric pH, which increased due to medicines.	✓ Adverse effects on health.
✓ Reduce dosage of medication due to increased absorption.	✓ Increased cost of healthcare.

FIGURE 16.1   Drug–nutrient interaction representative model.

Cardiovascular Drug: Warfarin

Anticoagulants such as warfarin (Coumadin®), enoxaparin (Lovenox), and heparin (Heparin), often referred to as blood thinners, help to prevent harmful blood clotting (coagulation) in blood vessels and prevent existing clots from becoming larger in size. These anticoagulants interact with nutrients such as vitamins K and E and alcohol. They also interact with foods such as garlic, ginger, ginkgo, ginseng, saw palmetto, green tea, and avocado. Vitamin K and anticoagulants have antagonistic actions, as vitamin K is responsible for the clotting of blood and the anticoagulants act as blood-thinning agents. The anticoagulants interfere with the function of vitamin K and may even reduce its levels, leading to certain complications. Similarly, vitamin E has blood-thinning properties, which are similar to the action of anticoagulants, so it may interfere with each other's actions and enhance the effect of blood thinning.

Effect of Grapefruit Juice on Drugs

Grapefruit juice contains certain compounds that increase the absorption of various drugs. This can enhance the effects of the drugs. The grapefruit juice blocks certain special enzymes present in the wall of the small intestine, and this may destroy the ingested medications and even prevent their absorption in our body. Thus, smaller amounts of the drugs get into the body than are ingested. When the action of this enzyme is blocked, more of the drugs get into the body and the blood levels of these medications increase. This can lead to toxic side effects from the medications. This compound is not found in other citrus juices. It is best to not take medications with grapefruit juice. Drink it at least 2 hours away from when you take your medication. If you often drink grapefruit juice, talk with your pharmacist or doctor before changing your routine.

Fibers

Products containing fiber when taken with any medication or vitamin supplements often slow the transport of the medication or supplement in the gut. The delay in transport may at times reduce the dissolution of the medication and the amount of medication absorbed into the blood; this would in turn reduce the effect of the product. In some cases, this delay in transport caused by fibers may increase the absorption of the medication or supplement. These interactions depend on the physiochemical properties of the medication; hence, they cannot be predicted. On a safer side, one should avoid taking medication along with a diet high in fiber.

Licorice

Natural black licorice contains glycyrrhizin. If consumed excessively (more than one ounce of natural black licorice, especially if a patient is using potassium-depleting diuretics and/or digoxin [Lanoxin®]), glycyrrhizin can induce some potent side effects. Natural licorice can be found in cough drops, candy, Chinese herbal medications, and other hidden sources (Norman Tomaka, C.R.Ph, Bulletin#44).

Coffee and Tea

Naturally brewed coffee and tea contain caffeine. Caffeine is a stimulant that, by itself, may increase the heart rate and blood pressure (temporarily). Moderate use of caffeine is not adverse in most patients (Norman Tomaka, C.R.Ph, Bulletin#44). However, patients consuming caffeine along with medication may result in a series of challenges to the medication's response. The administration of certain medications may enhance caffeine in the body or may result in the slow elimination of caffeine. Also, in some cases, other medication effects may be increased by caffeine. Tea, on the other hand, contains tannins that are responsible for taste and the "stain" associated with tea with a considerably lesser amount of caffeine than found in coffee. Tannins can result in a significant reduction of absorption of iron from nutritional supplements or foods (Norman Tomaka, C.R.Ph, Bulletin#44).

It may be best to limit caffeine consumption use with the following medications (Norman Tomaka, C.R.Ph, Bulletin#44):

- Cimetidine (Tagamet®) may increase caffeine's effect
- Quinolone antibiotics may extend caffeine's effect
- Ciprofloxacin (Cipro®)
- Norfloxacin (Noroxin®)
- Ofloxacin (Floxin®)
- Enoxacin (Penetrex®)
- Lomefloxacin (Maxaquin®)
- Theophylline products: Caffeine is chemically related to theophylline and may increase this medication's effectiveness and side effects

EFFECTS OF NUTRIENTS ON DRUGS

Dairy Products (Calcium)

Medication taken with milk or other dairy products is one of the most popular food–drug interactions. Calcium and related minerals found in food and other sources (i.e., antacids, vitamins) can sometimes chemically "hold on" to the medication and reduce absorption from the gut into the blood. This interaction can be by time spacing. It is always better to ask whether it is best to avoid taking the medication with dairy products, vitamins, or antacids (Norman Tomaka, C.R.Ph, Bulletin#44).

Some products that should not be taken with dairy products include the following:

- *Quinolone antibiotics*: When taken with dairy products, some will experience reduced absorption, especially with ciprofloxacin and noroxin.
- *Tetracycline antibiotics*: Select tetracyclines will experience minimal absorption and effectiveness when taken with milk.

- *Etidronate* (Didronel®): Taking this with dairy products may cause substantial reduction in absorption.
- *Bisacodyl* (i.e., Dulcolax®): Taking this with dairy products dissolves coating on tablet and reduces absorption while increasing stomach irritation.

ADDITIVES AND EXCIPIENTS

Vitamins may contain additives that could interfere with some medications, namely, starch, wheys, wheat, lactose (generic term), film coating (some), artificial coloring, and gluten. Additives may still be included as an excipient, even though most vitamins that are labeled, manufactured, and sold in U.S. pharmacies are now regulated by the FDA. A small amount of additives in most vitamin products may not have adverse consequences if used occasionally. However, routine daily vitamins with certain additives like lactose may pose a problem if taken with certain medications (Norman Tomaka, C.R.Ph, Bulletin#44).

VITAMIN K

Vitamin K antagonizes anticoagulant use (i.e., Coumadin). Vitamin K is easily found in green leafy vegetables like cabbage, Brussels sprouts, broccoli, cauliflower, turnip greens, and spinach. Other sources include soybeans, lentils, watercress, liver, eggs, bran, chickpeas, oats, and corn oil. It is best for patients on warfarin (Coumadin) to keep their diet routine. If the typical sources of vitamin K are used excessively or eliminated altogether, it will work against the predicted results of the blood thinner (Norman Tomaka, C.R.Ph, Bulletin#44).

VITAMIN E

Vitamin E is supplemented by many patients trying to lower their risk of cardiovascular complications due to its antioxidant properties. Aspirin, Coumadin, and other "blood thinners" may be enhanced by sudden use of vitamin E (d-alpha-tocopheryl) as it may improve blood flow. Prior checking with the physician is necessary to starting or stopping the use of this supplement (Norman Tomaka, C.R.Ph, Bulletin#44).

COENZYMEQ

Some patients with congestive heart and gum disease may benefit from CoEnzymeQ. However, "Co-Q" has shown to significantly reduce the blood-thinning effect of a certain blood thinner. It is best to ask with the physician before starting or stopping "Co-Q" use, especially while consuming blood thinners (Norman Tomaka, C.R.Ph, Bulletin#44).

BETA-CAROTENE

Beta-carotene is an excellent antioxidant with reduced toxicity often associated with other forms of vitamin A. However, the liver may be severely harmed due to the combined routine use of alcohol and beta-carotene. Thus, it is advisable for patients routinely using alcohol (not just excessive use, but routine use) to avoid supplementing any form of vitamin A, including beta-carotene. Beta-carotene, if used for long periods of time, may significantly lower blood concentrations of vitamin E. For the best benefits, patients are often advised to supplement with both of the vitamins (Norman Tomaka, C.R.Ph, Bulletin#44).

Vitamin B$_{12}$

Certain chemical factors in the stomach lining are required by B$_{12}$ (cyanocobalamin) for regular absorption from the diet. Reduced blood levels of vitamin B$_{12}$ can result from the use of certain medications for reducing stomach acid (cimetidine [Tagamet], ranitidine [Zantac®] and omeprazole [Prilosec®], and lansoprazole [Prevacid®]). B complex supplementation along with vitamin B$_{12}$ is often recommended while using these medications or in the case of stomach surgery. Potassium products, often prescribed to patients using certain diuretics, can also reduce B$_{12}$ absorption (Norman Tomaka, C.R.Ph, Bulletin#44).

B Complex

Blood levels of folic acid and other B vitamins can be lowered by many medications. Phenytoin (Dilantin®), estrogen (Premarin®), hydralazine (Apresoline®), steroids (prednisone), methotrexate (Rheumatrex®), and diuretics (Dyazide®, Maxzide®, Hctz®) all have been shown to reduce blood concentrations of folic acid and sometimes B$_6$. In most cases, simply supplementing a balanced multivitamin with B complex every day may prevent complications associated with B-vitamin depletion (Norman Tomaka, C.R.Ph, Bulletin#44).

THE BENEFITS OF MINIMIZING NEGATIVE FOOD–DRUG INTERACTIONS

It is best to avoid negative interactions having adverse effects on our body. The various benefits of avoiding or minimizing negative food interactions are that medications achieve their intended effects, that there is improved compliance with medications, that there is less need for additional medication or higher dosages, that fewer caloric or nutrient supplements are required, that adverse side effects are avoided, that optimal nutritional status is preserved, that accidents and injuries are avoided, that disease complications are minimized, and that the cost of healthcare services is reduced. By avoiding or minimizing the negative effects of food–drug interactions, one can ensure that the therapy/drug works as desired and removes any chances of adverse effects (John, 2013).

CONCLUSION

Scientists have been studying these interactions between drugs and foods/nutrients closely for several years. It is important to continue this study as more and more new drug molecules are discovered, thus making it necessary to study their interactions.

With the help of these studies, it will be easy to discover positive and useful synergistic and additive interactions that can be exploited for the benefit of the patient and for reducing the dose of therapy.

REFERENCES

Bobroff, L.B., Lentz, A., and Turner, E.R. 2009. Food/Drug and Drug/Nutrient Interactions: What You Should Know about Your Medications. University of Florida, IFAS Extension FCS8092. First Published: March 1999. Revised dates: November 2008; May 2009.

Bushra, R. 2011. Food–drug interactions. *Oman Med. J.*, 26(2): 77–83.

Chan, L.-N. 2013. Drug–nutrient interactions, *JPEN J Parenter Enteral Nutr.*, 37(4): 450–459. DOI: 10.1177/0148607113488799. Epub May 14, 2013.

Examples of Interactions. http://www.gdatf.org/about/about-graves-disease/patient-education/food-and-drug-interactions/. Accessed July 8, 2016.

John, G.K. 2013. *Presentation to Dietitians Association Australia on Drug–Food/Nutrient Interactions*, Australia, September 16, 2013.

Norman Tomaka, C.R.Ph. Graves' Disease Foundation. Food and Drug Interactions. http://www.gdatf.org/site_media/uploads/bulletins/bulletin44.pdf. Accessed July 8, 2016.

William C. Shiel Jr. Grapefruit juice—Grapefruit juice can interact with medicines! Jay W. Marks, ed., Medicinenet.com. http://www.medicinenet.com/grapefruit_juice_and_medication_interactions/views.htm. Accessed July 3, 2014.

Section VII

Future Trends

17 The Role of Food Bioactives in Disease Prevention

R. B. Smarta

CONTENTS

INTRODUCTION

As per the ancient Chinese saying, "Medicine and food have a common origin," over the years scientific advances have made the link between nutrition and health evident. The ability of foods and their components to enhance the overall quality of life has been known to mankind for ages.

"Bioactive compounds," usually referred to as "bioactives," are extranutritional constituents that typically occur in small quantities in foods. In plants the bioactive compounds are mainly secondary metabolites. Bioactive compounds in plants can have pharmacological or toxicological effects in humans and animals. Thus, one of the definitions of bioactive compounds in plants is that they are secondary plant metabolites eliciting pharmacological or toxicological effects in humans and animals.

THE PHYSIOLOGICAL ROLE OF BIOACTIVES

Bioactive compounds present in foods, plants, and animals have a physiological function in humans. These physiological functions may vary from promotion of health to modification of risk of disease or disease prevention. They may influence physiological or cellular activities, usually resulting in a beneficial health effect.

Bioactive compounds may help promote optimal health and reduce the risk of chronic diseases such as cancer, coronary heart disease, stroke, and Alzheimer's disease.

Bioactive compounds vary widely in chemical structure and function and are grouped accordingly. These compounds may act as inducers or inhibitors of enzymes, inhibitors or inducers of receptor activity, inhibitors of gene expression, and so on. These compounds can mimic an adaptive stress response in animals and humans. Bioactives have always been widely studied to evaluate their effects on health. Many bioactive compounds have been discovered so far and more and more new studies on bioactives from foods are being conducted.

BIOACTIVES VERSUS NUTRIENTS

Bioactives are not nutrients in the classical sense, as they are not essential for life, which is a fundamental criterion for a nutrient, but emerging research suggests that they are essential for good health. *Bioactives can be considered as the Mother Nature's pharmacy, making ordinary foods become natural nutraceuticals.* They are potent and have good efficacy, even in very small quantities. Bioactive compounds are much safer, because, unlike pharmaceuticals, they are developed to be used by our bodies. More precisely, in the right dosages, bioactives interact directly with the master health regulators that control our genes.

The new knowledge and deeper understanding of bioactives, together with advances in the field of gene-based nutrition, will revolutionize how we think about food and medicine. With knowledge of bioactives, we are one step closer to understanding how the foods that we eat, and those which we avoid, can help in treating and preventing many of the chronic diseases affecting humankind.

BIOACTIVE NUTRIENTS

Several epidemiological studies throughout the years have suggested that diets rich in fruits and vegetables promote health and reduce the risk of diseases.

CLASSIFICATION OF BIOACTIVES

CLASSIFICATION BASED ON THEIR SOURCE

1. Plant and food bioactives
2. Animal bioactives

The majority of the bioactive food compounds responsible for the positive effects on well-being are predominantly derived from the plant kingdom, while a few are derived from animal sources.

Within these major groups of bioactives exist a number of subclasses as well.

Plant and Food Bioactives

Plant Bioactives

Bioactive compounds in plants are the secondary metabolites produced within in addition to the primary metabolic and biosynthetic compounds produced for the plants' growth and development. Plant bioactives are by-products of the usual biochemical interactions in plants. These bioactives are usually not needed for the plant's normal growth and development, but some bioactives play an important role in the protection of the plant from predators, whereas some are harmful/poisonous to small animals and insects.

While some bioactives may be harmful to animals, many are extremely useful and beneficial to humans in disease prevention.

Some of the plant bioactive groups include:

* *Saponins*: Saponins are glycosidic, soap-forming compounds. The emulsifying property of saponins can be attributed to the presence of a hydrophilic glycone and a hydrophobic aglycone. Saponins are phytochemicals that are found in most vegetables, beans, and herbs. Commercial saponins are extracted mainly from *Yucca schidigera* and *Quillaja saponaria*. Saponins show immune-modulating and antitumor effects; they also help in reducing blood cholesterol by binding to cholesterol and bile salts, thus preventing its reabsorption.

- *Polyphenols*: Polyphenols are secondary metabolites of plants and are generally involved in defense against ultraviolet radiation or aggression by pathogens (Pandey and Rizvi, 2009). The phenolic groups in polyphenols can accept an electron to form relatively stable phenoxyl radicals, thereby disrupting chain oxidation reactions in cellular components. It is well established that polyphenol-rich foods and beverages may increase plasma antioxidant capacity. This increase in the antioxidative capacity of plasma following the consumption of polyphenol-rich food may be explained either by the presence of reducing polyphenols and their metabolites in plasma, by their effects upon concentrations of other reducing agents (sparing effects of polyphenols on other endogenous antioxidants), or by their effect on the absorption of prooxidative food components, such as iron. The consumption of antioxidants has been associated with reduced levels of oxidative damage to lymphocytic DNA. Similar observations have been made with polyphenol-rich food and beverages, indicating the protective effects of polyphenols (Vitrac et al., 2002). There is increasing evidence that as antioxidants, polyphenols may protect cell constituents against oxidative damage and, therefore, limit the risk of various degenerative diseases associated with oxidative stress such as cardiovascular diseases and cancer.
- *Tannins*: Tannins are naturally occurring plant polyphenols and are secondary metabolites produced by plants. They are of two types, namely, hydrolyzable tannins and condensed tannins. Their main characteristic is that they bind and precipitate proteins. They may have a huge impact on the nutritive value of many foods eaten by humans and feedstuff eaten by animals. Tannins are common in fruits (grapes, persimmon, blueberry, etc.), tea, chocolate, fruit dish, legume forages (clover, trefoil, alfalfa, etc.), legume trees (*Acacia* spp., *Sesbania* spp., etc.), and grasses (sorghum, corn, etc.).
- *Alkaloids*: Alkaloids are heterocyclic, nitrogen-containing compounds. They have limited distribution across the plant kingdom. They are produced by a large variety of organisms, including bacteria, fungi, plants, and animals. Some alkaloids are toxic, while many have pharmacological effects and are used as medicines, recreational drugs, and so on.

Alkaloids may be used as local anesthetic; as stimulant such as cocaine, caffeine, and nicotine; as analgesic (morphine); as antibacterial, anticancer (vincristine), and antihypertension agents (reserpine); as cholinomimetic galantamine; vasodilator agents (vincamine); as antiasthma therapeutic (ephedrine); as antimalarial drug (quinine); and others.

- *Carotenoids*: The chloroplasts and chromoplasts of plants and some photosynthetic organisms like certain bacteria and fungi contain carotenoids. Carotenoids can be produced from fats and other basic organic metabolic building blocks by all these organisms. Animals and humans cannot synthesize carotenoids, so they have to obtain these from their diet.

- *Plant sterols*: Phytosterols, which encompass plant sterols and stanols, are steroid compounds similar to cholesterol, which occur in plants and vary only in carbon side chains and/or the presence or absence of a double bond (Akhisa et al., 1991). Stanols are saturated sterols having no double bonds in the sterol ring structure. More than 200 sterols and related compounds have been identified. Free phytosterols extracted from oils are insoluble in water, relatively insoluble in oil, and soluble in alcohols (Akihisa et al., 1991).

Phytosterol-enriched foods and dietary supplements have been marketed for decades. Despite well-documented LDL cholesterol–lowering effects, no scientifically proven evidence of any beneficial effect on cardiovascular disease (CVD) or overall mortality exists (Weingartner, 2008).

- *Glucosinolates*: Glucosinolates belong to the glucosides. Glucosinolates constitute a natural class of organic compounds that contain sulfur and nitrogen and are derived from glucose and an amino acid. They are natural components occurring in several pungent plants such as mustard, cabbage, and horseradish. These natural chemicals most likely contribute to plant defense against pests and diseases, but are also enjoyed in small amounts by humans and are believed to contribute to the health-promoting properties of cruciferous vegetables.

Food Bioactives

Bioactive compounds are extranutritional constituents that typically occur in small quantities in foods. They typically occur in small amounts in foods. Bioactive compounds are present in various food-related materials such as cereals, legumes, nuts, olive oil, vegetables, fruits, tea, and red wine (Kris-Etherton et al., 2002). Food bioactives represent diet-based molecules that perform physiological roles associated with disease prevention and/or treatment. As such considerable overlap exists between food bioactives and drugs.

More scientific research needs to be conducted before we make science-based dietary recommendations. Despite this, there is sufficient evidence recommending consumption of food sources rich in bioactive compounds (Kris-Etherton et al., 2002).

Animal Bioactives

Sources of Marine Functional Food Ingredients (Bioactives)

Marine bioactives: The marine environment represents a relatively untapped source of functional ingredients that can be applied to various aspects of food processing, storage, and fortification. Numerous marine-based compounds have been identified as having diverse biological activities (Lordan et al., 2011).

Bioactive peptides isolated from fish protein hydrolysates as well as algal fucans, galactans, and alginates have been shown to possess anticoagulant, anticancer, and hypocholesterolemic activities. Additionally, fish oils and marine bacteria are excellent sources of omega-3 fatty acids, while crustaceans and seaweeds contain powerful antioxidants such as carotenoids and phenolic compounds (Lordan et al., 2011).

Macroalgae are a source of biologically active phytochemicals such as carotenoids, phycobilins, fatty acids, polysaccharides, vitamins, sterols, tocopherols, and phyco-cyanins (Lordan et al., 2011).

Microalgae are extremely diverse and represent a major untapped resource of valuable bioactive compounds and biochemicals such as pigments, antioxidants, polysaccharides, sterols, fatty acids, and vitamins (Lordan et al., 2011).

Bioactive Peptides

Certain protein hydrolysates have been shown to trigger *hormonelike* responses in humans. These may offer health benefits *in vivo* and/or *in vitro,* either in the intact form or as hydrolysates. These protein hydrolysates are also referred to as bioactive peptides. The bioactive peptides are specific protein fragments that have the ability to impart biological effect, resulting in positive impact on body functions or conditions and thus ultimately influencing health. Some positive physiological responses of bioactive peptides are antioxidative, antimicrobial, antihypertensive, cytomodu-latory, and immunomodulatory effects under *in vivo* and *in vitro* conditions. These bioactivities are observed in major body systems such as the digestive, cardiovascu-lar, nervous, musculoskeletal, and immune systems (Moller et al., 2008). The bio-active peptides can play a significant role in the pharmaceutical industry since the physiological responses they induce are the same as the targeted responses intended by small molecules and biologics (Danquah and Agyei, 2012).

Milk-derived bioactive peptides have a vast range of physiological functionality, right from antihypertensive, antithrombotic, antioxidative (effect on the cardiovascu-lar system), and opioid agonist activity and antagonist activity on the nervous system to mineral-binding, antiappetizing, and antimicrobial activities in the gastrointestinal system to immunomodulatory and cytomodulatory activity in the immune system (Korhonen and Pihlanto, 2006).

CLASSIFICATION ON THE BASIS OF SOLUBILITY (WATER AND FATS)

Bioactives derived from various sources may be hydrophilic in nature or lipophiles in nature. Long-chain polyunsaturated fatty acids derived from marine animals or plant sources and carotenoids of plant origin are examples of lipophilic bioactive nutrients (e.g., glucosinolates, which are water-soluble).

Listed here are some of the bioactive ingredients/compounds manufactured and marketed:

List of Bioactives			
Type	Bioactives	Type	Bioactives
Amino acids	Alanine	Fats, oils, and	Borage seed oil
	Alpha lipoic acid	essential fatty	Canola oil
	Arginine	acids	Cassia oil
	Asparagine		Docosahexaenoic acid (DHA)
	Aspartic acid		Eicosapentaenoic acid (EPA)
	Cysteine		Fish oil

(Continued)

	List of Bioactives		
Type	**Bioactives**	**Type**	**Bioactives**
	Glucosamine		Flax seed oil
	Glutamic acid		Gamma-linolenic acid
	Glutamine		Hemp oil
	Glycine		Omega-3
	Histidine		Omega-6
	Isoleucine		Omega-9
	Leucine		Ponticium
	Lysine		Pumpkin seed oil
	Methionine		Sinum
	Phenylalanine		Sprouted flax/chia (DHA/EPA)
	Proline		Squalene
	Serine		Sterols/sterol esters
	Threonine		Sunflower oil
	Tryptophan		Vegetable oil
	Tyrosine		
	Valine		
Antioxidants	Ascorbyl palmitate	Dietary fiber	B-glucan
	Beta-carotene/ carotenoids		Cellulose
			Chicory extract
	Flavonoids		Fenugreek fiber
	Isothiocyanates		Glucomannan
	Lutein		Guar
	Lycopene		Inulin
	Monoterpenes		Oat bran
	Organosulfur		Oligosaccharides/polysaccharides
	Resveratrol		Psyllium
	Zeaxanthin		Pulses
			Soy fiber
			Sprouted grains and seeds (soluble fiber)
			Starch-derived fiber
Botanicals	Black cohosh	Enzymes	Amylase
	Chamomile		Cellulase
	Dandelion		Chymotrypsin
	Echinacea		Lactase
	Ginkgo		Papain protease
	Ginseng		Trypsin
	Herbal tea		
	Lavender		
	Saw palmetto		
	Sea buckthorn		
	Tea		
Dairy	Casein	Prebiotics	Fructooligosacccharides (FOS)
	Conjugated linoleic acid (CLA)		Inulin
	Whey protein		

(Continued)

		List of Bioactives	
Type	**Bioactives**	**Type**	**Bioactives**
Grains	Amaranth	Minerals	Calcium
	Barley		Chromium
	Bulgar		Iodine
	Corn		Iron
	Fennel seed		Phosphorus
	Fenugreek seed		Potassium
	Flaxseed		Potassium iodide
	Kamut		Selenium
	Oats		Zinc
	Quinoa		
	Rice		
	Wheat		
Plant phenolics	Anthocyanins	Proteins	Chondroitin
	Catechins		Collagen
	Flavonoids		Dairy proteins
	Glucosinolates		Egg proteins
	Isoflavones		Ephedrine
	Lignans		Meat proteins
	Phenolic acids		Pea proteins
	Phytochemicals		Soy proteins
	Phytoestrogens		Tofu
	Phytosterol/stanol esters		
	Saponins		
	Tannins		
	Terpenoids		
Plant proteins	Anthocyanins	Probiotics	Bifidobacterium lactis
	Canola proteins		Exopolysaccharide (EPS)
	Flax proteins		Lactobacillus acidophilus
	Legume proteins		Lactobacillus reuteri
	Oat proteins		Streptococcus thermophilus
	Wheat gluten		
Soy	Flour	Supplements	Supplement
	Isoflavones		
	Protein concentrate		
	Protein isolate		
Specialty/ others	Alfalfa	Specialty/others	Dehydroepiandrosterone (DHEA)
	Apple extracts		Elk antler
	Berries		Emu oil
	Black currant		Glucosamine
	Blueberries		Glycolipids
	Blueberry powder		Gooseberry
	Broccoli extract		Grape extract
	Buckwheat		Grape seed extract
	Bulgar		Hemp

(Continued)

List of Bioactives			
Type	Bioactives	Type	Bioactives
	Carnitine		Herbs
	Chia seeds		Honey
	Chlorella		Melatonin
	pyrenoidosa		Mushroom extracts
	Chlorophyll		Mustard seed
	Chocolate		Onion extracts
	Colostrum		Phycocyanin
	Cow cockle		Pomegranate
	Cranberries		Portulaca oleracea
	Cranberry powder		Raspberry
	DNA		Strawberry powder
	RNA		Sulfolipids
	Spinach extracts		Tarragon oil
	Stevia		Wood vinegar
Seafood	Algae		
	Chitin		
	Chitosan		
	Dulse		
	Fish oil		
	Fish protein		
	hydrolysate		
	Kelp		
	Krill oil		
	Omega-3		
	Phytoplankton		
	Seaweed		
	Shark cartilage		
	Spirulina		

MECHANISMS OF ACTION OF BIOACTIVE COMPOUNDS

The bioactive compounds, when consumed in food format (along with food), elicit certain biological responses. There are several mechanisms by which they do so. Most of the bioactives have strong antioxidant potential, while others act by modifying xenobiotic metabolizing enzymes, altering lipid metabolism, or altering steroid hormones.

The interaction between diet and phytonutrients is a complex field, as thousands of dietary components are consumed each day (>25,000) through routine diets. Dietary bioactives may modify a multitude of processes in normal cells. A single, bioactive food constituent can modify multiple steps in molecular and cellular events such as nutrigenetics, nutritional epigenomics, nutritional transcriptomics, proteomics, and metabolomics (Lekshmi S.L., Dr. I. Sreelathakumari). Many of these processes can be influenced by several food components. Furthermore, the dose, timing, duration of exposure, and interactions may alter responses and, ultimately, the phenotype or manifestations.

Some specific mechanisms of actions exhibited by various bioactive components include:

- Antioxidant activity
- Modulation of activating and deactivating enzymes.
- Anti-inflammatory response and altering immunity
- Alterations of lipid and lipoprotein metabolism and platelet reactivity
- Stabilizing endothelial functions and vascularity
- Altering hormone metabolism
- Antibacterial and antiviral activity
- Cellular division, differentiation, apoptosis, and DNA stability and repair

THE ROLE OF BIOACTIVES IN DISEASE PREVENTION

The following section explores the major classes of bioactive compounds and their effect on health and their role in disease prevention. The following are some of the major bioactive compounds and their role in disease prevention.

POLYPHENOLS

Effect on CVD

Polyphenols limit the incidence of coronary heart diseases such as atherosclerosis. Polyphenols are potent inhibitors of LDL oxidation, which is considered to be a key mechanism in the development of atherosclerosis. Other mechanisms through which polyphenols may be protective against cardiovascular diseases are by improving their antioxidant, antiplatelet, and anti-inflammatory effects as well as by increasing HDL and by improving endothelial function. Polyphenols may also contribute to stabilization of the atheroma plaque. They include quercetin, green tea polyphenols (catechins), and resveratrol (Pandey and Rizvi, 2009).

Anticancer Effect

The effect of polyphenols on human cancer cell lines is most often protective and induces a reduction of the number of tumors or of their growth. Several mechanisms of action have been identified for preventive effect of polyphenols; these include estrogenic/antiestrogenic activity, antiproliferation, induction of cell cycle arrest or apoptosis, prevention of oxidation, induction of detoxification enzymes, regulation of the host immune system, anti-inflammatory activity, and changes in cellular signaling (Pandey and Rizvi, 2009). These effects have been observed at various sites, including mouth, stomach, duodenum, colon, liver, lung, mammary gland, and skin. Many polyphenols such as quercetin, catechins, isoflavones, lignans, flavanones, ellagic acid, red wine polyphenols, resveratrol, and curcumin have been tested; all of them showed protective effects in some models, although their mechanisms of action were varied (Pandey and Rizvi, 2009).

Antidiabetic Effect

Polyphenols may affect glycemia through different mechanisms such as inhibition of α-glucosidase in the gut mucosa and in turn inhibition of glucose absorption in the gut or of its uptake by peripheral tissues (Pandey and Rizvi, 2009). The hypoglycemic effects of diacetylated anthocyanins at a 10 mg/kg diet dosage have been observed with maltose as a glucose source, but not with sucrose or glucose.

Individual polyphenols, such as catechin, epicatechin, epigallocatechin, epicatechin gallate, isoflavones from soybeans, tannic acid, glycyrrhizin from licorice root, chlorogenic acid, and saponins, decrease S-Glut-1-mediated intestinal transport of glucose. Saponins additionally delay the transfer of glucose from stomach to the small intestine. Resveratrols have also been reported to act as antidiabetic agents (Pandey and Rizvi, 2009).

CAROTENOIDS

Decreased Risk of Cancer

Carotenoids have a striking effect on lung, oral, esophageal, colorectal, breast, prostate, cervical, and skin cancers. In humans, three carotenoids (beta-carotene, alpha-carotene, and beta-cryptoxanthin) are provitamin A (meaning they can be converted by the human body to vitamin A). In the eye, certain other carotenoids (lutein, astaxanthin, and zeaxanthin) apparently act directly to absorb damaging blue and near-ultraviolet light, in order to protect the macula of the retina, the part of the eye with the sharpest vision. Men and women with the highest intakes of total carotenoids, alpha-carotene, and lycopene were at significantly lower risk of developing lung cancer than those with the lowest intakes.

Effect on Cardiovascular Diseases

As carotenoids are soluble in fat and insoluble in water, they circulate in lipoproteins along with cholesterol and other fats. Evidence that low-density lipoprotein (LDL) oxidation plays a role in the development of atherosclerosis led scientists to investigate the role of antioxidant compounds like carotenoids in the prevention of cardiovascular disease (Kritchevsky 1999). A number of case-control and cross-sectional studies have found higher blood levels of carotenoids to be associated with significantly lower measures of carotid artery intima-media thickness (thickening of the carotid artery leads to atherosclerosis). Higher plasma carotenoids at baseline have been associated with significant reductions in the risk of cardiovascular disease in some prospective studies but not in others. While the results of several prospective studies indicate that people with higher intakes of carotenoid-rich fruits and vegetables are at lower risk of cardiovascular disease, it is not yet clear whether this effect is a result of carotenoids or other factors associated with diets high in carotenoid-rich fruits and vegetables (Higdon, 2004).

Effect on Age-Related Macular Degeneration

There is no cure for age-related macular degeneration (AMD), unlike cataracts wherein the diseased lens can be replaced. Therefore, efforts are aimed at disease prevention or delaying the progression of AMD (Higdon, 2004). Lutein and zeaxanthin are present in high concentrations in the macula, where they are efficient absorbers of blue light. By preventing a substantial amount of the blue light from entering the eye and reaching the underlying structures involved in vision, lutein and zeaxanthin may protect against light-induced oxidative damage, which is thought to play a role in the pathology of AMD (Krinsky et al., 2003). It is also possible, though not proven, that lutein and zeaxanthin act directly to neutralize oxidants formed in the retina. Epidemiological studies provide some evidence that higher intakes of lutein and zeaxanthin are associated with lower risk of age-related macular degeneration (Mares-Perlman et al., 2002).

BIOACTIVE PEPTIDES

Anticancer Properties

The anticancer properties of several bioactive peptides derived from various sources have been studied. These anticarcinogenic peptides have no common mechanism of action, but they eventually lead to the inhibition of mitosis and cell death. Lunasin is the most widely studied bioactive peptide for its anticancer property; it was first discovered in soy (Hernández-Ledesma et al., 2009) and later in some cereals and pseudocereals like wheat, barley, rye, rice, and amaranth. It consists of 43 amino acid residues. The antimitotic activity of lunasin is explained by eight aspartate protease residues at carboxyl end of its chain, which are able to bind to the hypoacetylated regions of chromatin (Hernández-Ledesma et al., 2009).

Lectins derived from soy are glycoproteins that can selectively bind carbohydrates (Mejia et al., 2003). Lectins play a role in agglutination of red blood cells and stimulation of pancreatic enzyme secretion, resulting in reduced intestinal absorption of nutrients. There are several reports that suggest plant lectins may have antitumor and anticarcinogenic properties. The exact mechanism of the antitumor effect of plant lectins is not yet clear, although several mechanisms have been proposed. Some of these mechanisms include the reduction of cell division, an increase in the number of macrophages, an increase in the susceptibility of tumor cells to macrophage attack, and the development of a bridge between tumor cells and macrophages (Barać et al., 2005).

Regulation of the Immune System

The effect of various bioactive peptides on immunomodulation has been vastly studied. Peptides such as lunasin, wheat gluten hydrolysates, and glutelin can enhance immune cell functions such as lymphocyte proliferation, natural killer cell activity, antibody synthesis, and cytokine regulation; reduce allergic reactions; and enhance mucosal immunity in the gastrointestinal tract (Hartmann and Meisel, 2007). Activation of NK cells is effective in patients with autoimmune disease or cancer and in elderly people, who usually have low levels of NK cell activity (Horiguchi et al., 2005).

Lunasin is usually studied among other functionalities, but Dia et al. (2009) reported its anti-inflammatory activity. It prevents inflammation by inhibiting COX-2/PGE2 and iNOS/NO pathways. Previous investigations of lunasin focused on its cancer prevention activity. However, inflammation is a critical factor in tumor progression, and cells that suffer inflammation produce various responses that can damage DNA and cause mutations that lead to tumor initiation and/or promotion. Horiguchi et al. (2005) reported that intake of wheat gluten hydrolysate can increase NK (natural killer) cell activity without severe side effects. NK cells play a major role in the rejection of tumors and cells infected by viruses. Oryzatensin, an ileum contracting bioactive peptide obtained from rice albumin, was shown to have immunostimulatory role that was mediated by histamine release. Its amino acid sequence is Gly-Tyr-Pro-Met-Tyr-Pro-Leu-Pro-Arg (Takahashi et al., 1996 in Kannan et al., 2010).

GLUCOSINOLATES

Effect on Cancer

- *Lung cancer*: Cohort studies in Europe, the Netherlands, and the United States have had varying results. Most studies have reported little association; one U.S. analysis—using data from the Nurses' Health Study and the Health Professionals' Follow-Up Study—showed that women who ate more than five servings of cruciferous vegetables per week had a lower risk of lung cancer (Feskanich et al., 2000).

- *Breast cancer*: One case-control study found that women who ate greater amounts of cruciferous vegetables had a lower risk of breast cancer (Terry et al., 2001). A meta-analysis of studies conducted in the United States, Canada, Sweden, and the Netherlands found no association between cruciferous vegetable intake and breast cancer risk (Smith-Warner et al., 2001). An additional cohort study of women in the United States similarly showed only a weak association with breast cancer risk (Zhang et al., 1999).

Bioactives and Bioavailability

Bioactive food compounds, whether derived from various plant or animal sources, need to be bioavailable in order to exert any beneficial effects. Through a better understanding of the digestive fate of bioactive food compounds, we can impact the promotion of health and improvement of performance (Rein et al., 2013). Many varying factors affect bioavailability, such as bioaccessibility, food matrix effect, transporters, molecular structures, and metabolizing enzymes. Bioefficacy may be improved through enhanced bioavailability. Bioavailability is a key step in ensuring bioefficacy of bioactive food compounds or oral drugs. Bioavailability is a complex process involving several different stages: liberation, absorption, distribution, metabolism, and elimination (LADME) phases. Therefore, several technologies have been developed to improve the bioavailability of xenobiotics, including structural modifications, nanotechnology, and colloidal systems (Rein et al., 2013).

Due to the complex nature of food bioactive compounds and also due to the different mechanisms of absorption of hydrophilic and lipophilic bioactive compounds, unraveling the bioavailability of food constituents is challenging (Rein et al., 2013). Among the food sources discussed during this review, coffee, tea, citrus fruit, and fish oil were included as sources of food bioactive compounds (e.g., polyphenols and polyunsaturated fatty acids [PUFAs]) since they are examples of important ingredients for the food industry. Although there are many studies reporting on the bioavailability and bioefficacy of these bioactive food components, understanding their interactions, metabolisms, and mechanisms of action still requires extensive work (Rein et al., 2013).

Current Activities in the Area of Bioavailability

Scientists have done a lot of research and are continuously in the process of developing knowledge and new technological solutions to incorporate bioactives into foods so that their beneficial, health-promoting properties are maximized without reducing the palatability and quality of foods.

The focus of this research is on how the inherent qualities of the food and aspects of the processing environment can affect the bioactivity and subsequent bioavailability of the bioactive components after consumption.

When it comes to incorporating bioactives in foods, challenges such as the following are faced by the researchers:

- Choosing suitable food formats
- Choosing the most appropriate processing conditions
- Protecting bioactives where necessary
- Maintaining food quality, for example, preventing adverse effects on texture and organoleptic properties, such as smell and taste

Many bioactive food components can be rendered useless by reactions with oxygen or other food components under certain processing conditions. For these *active* components to be effective for health-promoting benefits, they need delivery systems that protect them until they reach the part of the digestion process where they will be most beneficial.

INNOVATIONS IN DELIVERY SYSTEMS

All the aspects related to the delivery of bioactives in humans right from the mode of delivery to the amount delivered are very crucial. The bioactives are sensitive molecules, are prone to degradation, and may not maintain their bioavailability until they reach the target site in the body, thus rendering them less effective for the purpose of their administration.

Considering the importance of delivery of bioactives, researchers have discovered many new techniques for delivering bioactives that help in increasing their bioavailability.

MICROENCAPSULATION

One strategy being examined is to protect bioactives through microencapsulation technologies. Microencapsulation involves creating a thin film made of proteins and carbohydrates to trap bioactives inside. The resulting "capsule" is only a few microns in diameter. The film must protect the bioactives during food processing, storage, and cooking; the bioactive is then available after food consumption and digestion.

Microencapsulation has already been used to create products such as MicroMAX™, the first microencapsulated omega-3 oil food ingredient. Further research is underway to study how food matrices affect microcapsules and their contents. The knowledge will be used to develop new materials as film barriers for different bioactives in microcapsules.

The knowledge gained through this research may lead to foods that meet our active and healthy lifestyles by

- Designing foods that meet human nutritional and health needs with choice of convenience
- Promoting the health benefits of natural food components
- Providing balance choice through manufactured foods for health, well-being, and lifestyle requirements

NANOTECHNOLOGY

Many of the bioactive substances are water-insoluble and/or possess low solubility saturation in oil. The low solubility of the functional lipids impairs their bioavailability and limits their use in food formulations. On the other hand, the formulation of functional lipids into nanoparticles is expected to improve their bioavailability. The properties of functional foods depend largely on their microscale and/or nanoscale structure (Nakajima et al., 2012). The conventional preparation for functional foods is generally done by applying large-scale processes; as a consequence, the structure of the products cannot be precisely controlled. The micro-/nanotechnology has been under continuous development, as it has been applied in the formulation and characterization of functional foods.

For instance, food nanotechnology may incorporate emulsification, dispersion, and mixing (i.e., microfabrication technology, microchannel [MC] and nanochannel [NC] emulsification, membrane emulsification, micromixer, and the control of food rheology) (McClements et al., 2007).

MICROEMULSIONS

Emulsion and/or microemulsion technology is particularly suited for the design and fabrication of delivery systems for encapsulating bioactives especially lipids. Some major bioactive lipids that need to be delivered within the food industry are omega-3 fatty acids, carotenoids, phytosterols, and so on.

Microemulsion basically is a system that comprises a mixture of water–hydrocarbons and oil. The various types of emulsion techniques researched and used are conventional emulsions, multiemulsions, multilayer emulsions, solid-lipid particles, filled hydrogel particles, and so on.

COMPUTATIONAL FLUID DYNAMICS

Application of computational fluid dynamics (CFD) to food processing has also received considerable attention in recent years.

In addition to these technologies, many *in vitro* models have been applied to evaluate the digestion of lipids passing through the gastrointestinal tract.

BIOACTIVE INGREDIENTS MARKET

The bioactive ingredients market is an emerging sector. The report "Bioactive Ingredients & Product Market by Ingredient (Probiotics, Proteins, Plant Extracts, Minerals, Vitamins, Fibers, Carotenoids), by Product (Functional Foods & Beverages, Dietary Supplements, Animal Nutrition, Personal Care)—Global Trends & Forecast to 2018" has estimated the bioactive ingredient market to grow from $23.8 billion in 2013 to $33.6 billion in 2018 at a compound annual growth rate of 7.2% from 2013 to 2018.

On the whole, the market in the Asia-Pacific region dominates, with the highest growth rate and shares. The market holds power here because of the ever-growing population and urbanization in various developing nations of the region. The market here is expected to experience a growth of 7.4% from 2013 to 2018. The countries with the most potential in the bioactive industry are the BRIC countries (Brazil, Russia, India, and China).

Bioactive ingredients market has various stakeholders such as raw material suppliers, processors, product manufacturers, and end-use consumers.

An important aspect of the entire bioactives market is that it comprises two segments: bioactive products market and bioactive ingredients/components market. These two markets are interdependent on each other; shift in any one of the markets will have a direct impact on the other.

Dietary supplements form the major application of bioactive ingredients from food as earlier it served as pharmaceutical products. Hence, the majority of ingredients were served in the form of tablets, capsules, and so on. In most of the nations, people are not aware of the concept of functional food and beverages. However, the concept is gaining a degree of wider familiarity, with the growth and development of the economy. The market for dietary supplements is expected to reach $13.0 billion by 2018, whereas that for functional beverages is expected to experience the highest growth rate of 7.4% from 2013 to 2018.

CONCLUSION

While there is a growing body of research on the putative protective effects of plant bioactives on human health, the role of specific foods, and indeed specific bioactives, remains to be established. Much of the evidence for the protective effects of plant bioactives is drawn from *in vitro* or animal experiments, which are often performed with doses much higher than those to which we are normally exposed via the diet.

Before the health benefits of these substances can be established with certainty, more work is needed to establish the effect *in vivo* in humans and to demonstrate the effects of these compounds when consumed in normal amounts as part of normal diets. One major difficulty with such studies is accurately assessing actual intakes of plant bioactives, given the sheer numbers of bioactives that have been identified, the variations in concentration from plant to plant, the major differences in bioavailability of these bioactives, and the limitations of current food composition databases. In Europe, the EuroFIR project has been undertaken to provide comprehensive, high-quality information on the levels of bioactives contained in plant foods commonly consumed in Europe.

Due to the low concentration or minimal intake of certain foods, developing food products with increased levels of bioactive compounds would assist in maintaining our health and well-being through diet.

REFERENCES

Akhisa, T. and Kokke, W. 1991. Naturally occurring sterols and related compounds from plants. In Patterson, G.W., Nes, W.D., eds., *Physiology and Biochemistry of Sterols*. pp. 172–228. American Oil Chemists' Society, Champaign, IL.

Article by Linus Pauling Institute. 2009. Micronutrient research for optimum health. http://lpi.oregonstate.edu/infocenter/phytochemicals/carotenoids/. Accessed July 8, 2016.

Barać, M.B., Stanojević, S.P., and Pešić, M.B. 2005. Biologically active components of soybeans and soy protein products—A review. APTEFF, 36: 261–266.

Belović, M.M. Potential of bioactive proteins and peptides for prevention and treatment of mass non-communicable diseases. *Food Feed Res.; J. Inst. Food Technol.*, 38(2): 51–62.

BioactiveCompound/Ingredients/Products,Govt.ofCanada,Agriculture&Agri-FoodCanada. http://ffn-afn.agr.gc.ca/index-eng.cfm?page=bioactive_compounds&menupos=1.2. Accessed July 8, 2016.

Buying Bioactives, The bioactive ingredients market is estimated to grow from $23.8 billion in 2013 to $33.6 billion in 2018. April 17, 2014. http://www.preparedfoods.com/articles/113978 . Accessed July 8, 2016.

Danquah, M.K. and Agyei, D. 2012. Pharmaceutical applications of bioactive peptides. *Biotechnology*, 1(2): 5. https://www.oapublishinglondon.com/article/294.

De Mejia, E.G., Bradford, T., and Hasler, C. 2003. The anticarcinogenic potential of soybean lectin and lunasin. *Nutrition Re-views*, 61(7): 239–246.

Denny, A. and Buttriss, J. 2007. British Nutrition, Foundation, Synthesis Report No. 4: Plant foods and health: Focus on plant bioactives. http://www.ipfn.ie/download/pdf/eurofir_report_plant_bioactives.pdf. Accessed July 8, 2016.

Dia, V.P., Wang, W., Oh, V.L., De Lumen, B.O., and De Mejia, E.G. 2009. Isolation, purification and characterization of lunasin from defatted soybean flour and in vitro evaluation of its anti-inflammatory activity. *Food Chemistry*, 114: 108–115.

Feskanich, D., Ziegler, R.G., Michaud, D.S. et al. 2000. Prospective study of fruit and vegetable consumption and risk of lung cancer among men and women. *J. Natl. Cancer Inst.*, 92(22): 1812–1823.

Glucosinolate. 2016. In Wikipedia, The Free Encyclopedia. Retrieved 06:53, July 7, 2016, from https://en.wikipedia.org/w/index.php?title=Glucosinolate&oldid=722961732.

Hartmann, R. and Meisel, H. 2007. Food-derived peptides with biological activity: From research to food applications. *Curr. Opin. Biotechnol.*, 18: 163–169.

Hernández-Ledesma, B., Hsieh, C.-C., and De Lumen, B.O. 2009. Lunasin, a novel seed peptide for cancer prevention. *Peptides*, 30: 426–430.

Higdon, J. 2004. *Micronutrient Information Center*. Linus Pauling Institute, Oregon. Updated: Higdon, J. (December 2004), Drake, V.J. (June 2009). Reviewed: Johnson, E.J. (June 2009). http://lpi.oregonstate.edu/mic/dietary-factors/phytochemicals/carotenoids#reference44. Retrieved July 08, 2016.

Horiguchi, N., Horiguchi, H., and Suzuki, Y. 2005. Effect of wheat gluten hydrolysate on the immune system in healthy human subjects. *Biosci. Biotech. Biochem.*, 69(12): 2445–2449.

Kang, Y.B., Mallikarjuna, P.R., Fabian, D.A. et al. 2013. Bioactive molecules: Current trends in discovery, synthesis, delivery and testing. *IeJSME*, 7(Suppl. 1): S32–S46.

Kannan, A., Hettiarachchy, N.S., Lay, J.O., and Liyanage, R. 2010. Human cancer cell proliferation inhibition by a pentapeptide isolated and characterized from rice bran. *Peptides*, 31: 1629–1634.

Korhonen, H. and Pihlanto, A. 2006. Review: Bioactive peptides: Production and functionality. *Int. Dairy J.*, 16: 945–960.

Krinsky, N.I., Landrum, J.T., and Bone, R.A. 2003. Biologic mechanisms of the protective role of lutein and zeaxanthin in the eye. *Annu. Rev. Nutr.*, 23: 171–201.

Kritchevsky, S.B. 1999. beta-Carotene, carotenoids and the prevention of coronary heart disease. *J. Nutr.,* 129(1): 5–8.

Kris-Etherton, Penny, M. et al. 2002. Bioactive compounds in foods: Their role in the prevention of cardiovascular disease and cancer, Excerpta Medica. Inc. *Am. J. Med.,* 113(9B): 71S–88S.

Lekshmi, S.L. and Sreelathakumary, I., Department of Olericulture, College of Agriculture, Vellayani, Trivandrum, Kerala. http://ujconline.net/wp-content/uploads/2013/09/vegetables%20as%20nutraceuticals.doc.

Lordan, S., Ross, R.P., and Stanton, C. 2011. Marine bioactives as functional food ingredients: Potential to reduce the incidence of chronic diseases. *Mar. Drugs,* 9: 1056–1100.

Mares-Perlman, J.A., Millen, A.E., Ficek, T.L., and Hankinson, S.E. 2002. The body of evidence to support a protective role for lutein and zeaxanthin in delaying chronic disease. Overview. *J. Nutr.,* 132(3): 518S–524S.

McClements, D.J., Decker, E.A., and Weiss, J. 2007. Emulsion-based delivery systems for lipophilic bioactive components. *J. Food Sci.,* 72(8): R109–R124.

Möller, N.P., Scholz-Ahrens, K.E., Roos, N., and Schrezenmeir, J. 2008. Bioactive peptides and proteins from foods: Indication for health effects. *Eur. J. Nutr.,* 47(4): 171–182.

Nakajima, M., Kobayashi, I., and Neves, M.A. 2012. 16th World Congress of Food Science and Technology—IUFOST, Aug 2012. Accessed July 8, 2016.

National Cancer Institute. Cruciferous Vegetables and Cancer Prevention, Causes and Prevention of Cancer. http://www.cancer.gov/about-cancer/causes-prevention/risk/diet/cruciferous-vegetables-fact-sheet#r18. Accessed July 8, 2016.

Neves, M.A., Nakajima, M., and Kobayashi, I. 2012. Nanotechnology for bioactives delivery systems. *J. Food Drug Anal.,* 20(Suppl. 1): 184–188.

Nutraceuticals & Bioactives—Nature's Pharmacy. https://www.genesmart.com/pages/nutraceuticals___bioactives/73.php. Accessed July 8, 2016.

Pandey, K. and Rizvi, S.I. 2009. Plant polyphenols as dietary antioxidants in human health and disease. *Oxidative Med. Cell. Longev.,* 2(5): 270–278.

Prepared Foods Nutra Solutions. The bioactive ingredients market is estimated to grow from $23.8 billion in 2013 to $33.6 billion in 2018. http://www.preparedfoods.com/articles/113978-buying-bioactives.

Rein, M.J., Renouf, M., Cruz-Hernandez, C. et al. 2013. Bioavailability of bioactive food compounds: A challenging journey to bioefficacy. *Br. J. Clin. Pharmacol.,* 75(3): 588–602.

Smith-Warner, S.A., Spiegelman, D., Yaun, S.S., et al. 2001. Intake of fruits and vegetables and risk of breast cancer: A pooled analysis of cohort studies. *JAMA,* 285(6): 769–776.

Takahashi, M. et al., 1996. Studies on the ileum-contracting mechanisms and identification as a complement C3a receptor agonist of oryzatensin, a bioactive peptide derived from rice albumin. *Peptides,* 17(1): 5–12. Elsevier. doi:10.1016/0196-9781(95)02059-4.

Terry, P., Wolk, A., Persson, I., and Magnusson, C. 2001. Brassica vegetables and breast cancer risk. *JAMA,* 285(23): 2975–2977.

Vitrac, X., Moni, J.P., Vercauteren, J., Deffieux, G., and Mérillon, J.M. 2002. Direct liquid chromatography analysis of resveratrol derivatives and flavanonols in wines with absorbance and fluorescence detection. *Anal. Chim. Acta.,* 458: 103–110.

Weingartner, O., Bohm, M., and Laufs, U. 2008. Controversial role of plant sterol esters in the management of hypercholesterolaemia, *Euro. Heart J.,* 30(4): 404–409. doi:10.1093/eurheartj/ehn580. PMC 2642922. PMID 19158117.

Ying, D., Sanguansri, L., Augustin, and Maryann. 2012. Third Annual Functional Food & Beverages India, Mumbai, India, 25–27 July 2012. http://www.csiro.au/en/Outcomes/Food-and-Agriculture/Delivering-bioactives-throughfoods. aspx. p. 54.

Zhang, S., Hunter, D.J., Forman, M.R., et al. 1999. Dietary carotenoids and vitamins A, C, and E and risk of breast cancer. *J. Natl. Cancer Inst.,* 91(6): 547–556.

18 The Journey from Personalized Medicine to Personalized Nutrition

Dilip Ghosh

CONTENTS

INTRODUCTION

Today's food and dietary supplement market is considerably different than it was 10–15 years ago. Consumer demands for healthy foods have been changing considerably every year, particularly in the last decade. Consumers are more and more believing that foods with specific functionality contribute directly to their health. Foods today are not only considered as a vehicle to satisfy hunger and to provide necessary nutrients but also to prevent nutrition-related diseases and improve physical and mental well-being. In this scenario, functional food ingredients play an outstanding role. From economic perspective this increasing demand on such foods can be justified by the increasing cost of healthcare, the steady increase in life expectancy including that of infants, and the aspiration and desire of older people for improved quality of life in their later years (Roberfroid, 2007).

HOW TO DEFINE FOOD OR DIETARY SUPPLEMENTS

Dietary supplements are defined as any product that can be taken by mouth that contains a dietary ingredient intended to supplement a diet. Dietary ingredients in these products may include vitamins, minerals, herbs, or other botanicals, amino acids, and substances such as enzymes, organ tissues, glandulars, and metabolites. Another buzz word is "nutraceuticals" that are particularly of interest to the baby boomers to generation X because they have the potential to substantially reduce the expensive, high-tech, disease treatment approaches presently being employed in Western healthcare. Primarily used in functional foods and dietary supplements, nutraceutical ingredients are naturally bioactive, chemical compounds that have health-promoting, disease-preventing, or medicinal properties.

EVIDENCE-BASED FOOD AND DIETARY SUPPLEMENTS: AN EVOLVING CONCEPT

In the twenty-first century, human are facing a global pandemic of diet-related chronic disease and preventable disorders that include cardiovascular disease, obesity and diabetes, cancers, osteoporosis, and myriad inflammatory disorders, which are the leading cause of the global healthcare burden. Most of these disorders are virtually diet-related and, not surprisingly, are not responding well to pharmaceutical intervention. The heavily burdened and eroding healthcare system is in need of an etiology-based model that addresses the underlying molecular basis of a patient/consumer's dysfunction and develops therapeutic and preventive strategies that will include biochemical-molecular individuality for each person.

A genetic predisposition model of health and disease is emerging from the Human Genome Project that has opened up the etiology-based care and will be almost equivalent to the current evidence-based pharmaceutical framework (Ghosh et al. 2007).

There is convincing evidence that genes are not necessarily our destiny and that leads to the concept of genetic predisposition. This means, health and disease outcomes are not necessarily predetermined based on one's genes. These genetic outcomes, particularly with respect to diet-related disease, are typically modifiable (Ghosh et al. 2007; Ghosh and Tapsell, 2008). The current medical model of genetic determinism is now facing a challenge by the emerging concept of genetic susceptibility that is able to change one's health trajectory through the judicious use of diet and lifestyle. In this scenario, innovative, evidence-based food and dietary supplements have a significant role in changing our destiny.

WHAT PERSONALIZATION MEANS IN THE SUPPLEMENT AND INGREDIENT INDUSTRY

Personalization of nutrition advice is often proposed as one of the most promising approaches. In recent years, most of the health intervention research and methods on the effect of personalization show that advice targeted to an individual's physical parameters, lifestyle, and environmental situation is more effective in influencing their health behavior than general information. A recent and unique example is introduction of do-it-yourself cereal. A German start-up cereal company, Mymuesli, has introduced personalized muesli cereal from a blend of 80 different ingredients to meet consumers' particular tastes, dietary restrictions, and health/wellness goals. The product is also sold in personalized multiserving cartons.

It is well evident that several dietary components have been recognized to modulate gene and protein expression and thereby metabolic pathways, homeostatic regulation, and presumably health and disease. In addition, genes contribute largely to different responses to diet exposure, including interindividual variations in the occurrence of adverse reactions. Major potential areas where the development of personalized foods/nutritionals are realistically possible include type 2 diabetes and obesity, mood foods, inflammatory bowel disease (IBD), and disorders of aging where the diet–gene relationship has been extensively studied.

CURRENT SUPPLEMENT MARKET

WHAT DOES IT LOOK LIKE?

A new study has found the total economic contribution of the dietary supplement industry to the U.S. economy is more than $61 billion per year. The study also showed that the dietary supplement industry has enough activity throughout production and sales to support more than 450,000 jobs, while industry concerns paid more than $10 billion in taxes in 2006. The global supplements and remedies market including botanicals is forecast to reach $107 billion by the year 2017, spurred by growing aging population and increasing consumer awareness about general health and well-being

(Global Industry Analysts, 2012). The Economic Impact Report completed by Dobson DaVanzo, a Washington DC-based economic research firm, is the first to quantify the dietary supplement industry's overall financial impact on the U.S. economy by considering such contributing factors as supply, production, research, direct employment, manufacturing, taxes, and the extended financial effects these factors produce. The report concluded, "The dietary supplement industry is a significant economic engine that powers businesses in communities in every state across the country." According to Partnership Capital Growth, the reason for the growth is it has gone mainstream. "Ten years ago, it was just the muscleheads and the weekend warriors. Now, it's the full spectrum with men and especially women." NBJ's 2012 Global Report includes sales and growth estimates for dietary supplement industry and was very optimistic. This covers all supplement subcategories, including vitamins, herbs and botanicals, minerals, sports nutrition, meal supplements, and specialty supplements.

WHERE WE STAND NOW

Every year, several market research organizations, such as New Nutrition Business, Innova Market Insight, Institute of Food Technologists (IFT), and so forth, are publishing Top 10, Top 12 global food nutrition and health trends. These trends are mostly based on market intelligence survey without any scientific and technology input. The list of dietary active compounds (vitamins, prebiotics, probiotics, bioactive peptides, antioxidants) is endless, and formulation of final products using these functional ingredients is growing steadily. This fortification exercise was started in salt iodization in the early 1920s in both Switzerland and the United States and has since expanded progressively all over the world (Betoret et al., 2011). The fortification of cereal products with thiamine, riboflavin, and niacin has become common practice since the early 1940s. Margarine was first fortified with vitamin A in Denmark and milk with vitamin D in the United States; phytosterol enrichment came later and used by patients with high cardiovascular risk. Folic acid fortification of wheat became widespread in North America and then moved to about 20 Latin American countries. This fortification phenomenon ranges from the classical enriched milks and yogurts through infant formula enriched with prebiotics, probiotics, vitamins, and long-chain polyunsaturated fatty acids to functional beverages mainly enriched with flavonoids, vitamins, and resveratrol, snacks. Most recently, pastas rich in legumes and meats enriched with large number of bioactive compounds have been developed by fortification formulation.

During the past decade, a rapidly growing number of food supplements with a specific functionality claim have entered the marketplace. The major drivers are definitely increasing consumer demand for healthy supplements, as well as scientific and technological developments which allow for the production of new categories of food or dietary supplements with increased functionality (Schmidt et al., 2007). Moreover, new categories of functional foods are being developed that contain bioactive ingredients, generated by enzymatic conversion or produced by microbial fermentation from raw food materials. Finally, varieties of plants that are used as sources of raw food materials are carefully selected and continuously optimized with regard to the content of bioactive ingredients through selective breeding or genetic modification, while specific feeding strategies are exploited to increase the production of specific ingredients in animal-derived raw materials.

Market Economics

On the holistic basis, nutraceuticals are divided in three segments, namely, functional foods, nutritional supplements, and beverages. Functional food/medicinal food are any fresh/processed food laying claims of being health-promoting or disease-preventing product, beyond being the basic nutrient supplier. Nutritional supplements, also known as dietary supplements, are meant to supplement the food eaten and to provide the required nutrients to the body. They encompass products like vitamins, minerals, probiotics, herbs, botanicals, amino acids, sports nutritional products, and specialty nutritional products, among others.

The nutritional supplement market has shown a significant growth over the previous years, inspite of the global economic downturn that started in late 2007. NBJ 2014 report mentioned the global market for supplements hit $96 billion in 2012 and is likely reach $104 billion in 2013.

Specialty food ingredients can be defined as ingredients that have the capability to add a particular benefit to the end product. The figure earlier shows the trend of the specialty food ingredients market in terms of type. The specialty food ingredients market value is projected to reach $80,323.4 million by 2018. Functional food ingredients (nutraceuticals) are the leading specialty ingredients with the largest market share and are estimated to grow at a significant rate due to high penetration levels in end-use industries. The demand for premium products is set to propel the growth of various ingredients. Enzymes are projected to exhibit robust growth in the coming years. The demand for acidulants, flavors, colors, emulsifiers, and so on, are also steaming ahead with a remarkable compound annual growth rate (CAGR).

Vitamins and Minerals: Still a Battleground for Pharma and Consumer Product Companies

Vitamins and minerals are always on the top of the list of dietary supplements. Sales of vitamins and mineral-based supplements totaled nearly $23 billion in the United States in 2012 and are growing at a 5%–7% annual clip. This trend is justified by allocation of more shelf space by some major retailers to these supplements, giving manufacturers the room to move more brands and products. Almost all companies in this segment are showing good growth, including NBTY Inc., Jamieson Laboratories, Atrium Innovations Inc., and Thorne Research Inc., and so forth. In Americas, Venezuela shows CAGR of 14%, whereas Brazil stands second with 13% growth. In the Asia-Pacific, India is leading the market at CAGR of 10%, followed by Vietnam with 8% growth. Russia is the leader in Europe with 10% growth, whereas Turkey is very close with 9% growth. In Africa-Middle East, Nigeria shows 9% growth in vitamin and mineral segment.

The sector is shaping up to be a battleground between pharmaceutical players and consumer-products companies, many of which are trying to counter slow growth in their mainstay businesses. Active acquisitions show the critical mass and potential growth opportunity of the segment. Some significant examples of acquisitions are Schiff Nutrition by Reckit Benckiser, Wyeth (Centrum) and Alacer Corp (Emergen-C) by Pfizer, Avid Health by Church and Dwight, and so forth.

GLOBAL PROTEIN SUPPLEMENT MARKET

Protein fortification into food and beverages is increasingly becoming a solid option for meeting the global challenges of nutritional deficiencies in the developing world, while also helping to combat the rise of noncommunicable diseases, such as cardio-vascular disease (CVD), in the developed world. Specifically, a plethora of scientific research shows the use of protein supplements has a direct link in enhancing heart health, as well as helping with weight management and closing the gap of caloric and nutrient deficiency. Consequently, the protein supplement product space is highly fragmented, with many companies and protein sources, and a variety of products prepared to meet this growing and dynamic demand.

ANIMAL PROTEIN

The global animal protein market segment, with an estimated demand of 2.3 million tons in 2012, is dominated by dairy-based ingredients at nearly 50% of the global share of the animal segment. The second-largest ingredient in this market segment is egg protein, which had a 40% volume market share in 2012, due to its use in many manufactured staple foods.

Growth in the animal protein segment is primarily supported by rising demand in specific end application segments, such as the sports and fitness nutrition market, infant nutrition, and geriatric nutrition, which in turn is influenced by lifestyle and demographic shifts. In sports and fitness nutrition, whey proteins are the gold standard despite soy proteins having comparable protein digestibility-corrected amino acid score (PDCAAS). Innovation is also an important growth factor in the animal sector market. While innovation in animal protein has been going on much longer than in the plant protein segment, market participants perceive a sustained innovation stream from animal proteins in the future.

FOCUS ON PLANT PROTEINS

In 2012, the global market for plant protein ingredients used in food, beverage, and dietary supplements was estimated to be 1.7 million tons, of which soy-derived proteins were the largest segment in this market with a 56% volume share. Despite a healthy volume growth of more than 3.5%, the demand for wheat protein is expected to fall due to higher expected growth of soy proteins and newer sources such as pea protein. Specifically, pea protein is expected to grow as much as 10% over the next 5 years. Other emerging plant-based protein ingredients, such as ingredients sourced from potato, canola, rice and chia, are also expected to witness strong growth of more than 5% during the next 5 years.

BIOACTIVES AND PHYTOCHEMICALS

The market for bioactive supplements is projected to experience a growth rate of 7.2% by 2018, to touch $33.6 billion. This estimation is attributed to the widening bioactive industry, which is a result of increased consumer awareness and health concerns.

The Asia-Pacific region is the dominant market with increasing population, urbanization, and disposable income in countries such as India, China, and Thailand. In countries such as Australia, the aging population is generating market opportunities for bioactives. The improvement in the quality of ingredients with clinically proven ingredients and products entering the market is gaining the trust of consumers and is another factor driving the bioactive ingredients market (Ghosh, 2009a, b).

Based on type, phytochemicals and plant extracts prove to be the most adopted supplements with the highest projected growth rate. In regions such as North America and Europe, consumers are turning toward plant products and prefer consuming bioactive ingredients derived from plants.

In the current market scenario, fibers and specialty carbohydrates are expected to have the largest market share due to their wide application.

Functional beverages are the growing application market for bioactive ingredients, whereas dietary supplements hold the largest market share in the same market.

PREBIOTIC MARKETS

The prebiotics market by ingredients is dominated by naturally derived ingredients such as fructooligosaccharides (FOS), insulin, mannan-oligosaccharides (MOS), and others. Synthetically derived ingredients are as yet few in number and they are generally termed galactooligosaccharides (GOS). These ingredients are incorporated into food and dietary supplements that are then consumed by human beings and animals, thus helping to enhance their gut health. These markets have been segmented based on volumes and revenues and have been analyzed for market stability and growth.

WHERE TO GO FROM HERE?

Human desire for individuality is not new. It is embedded in all ancient civilizations and traditional healthcare system such as Traditional Chinese medicine and Indian Ayurvedic system. All traditional medical systems are descriptive and phenomenological—they typically diagnose patients using concepts based on the relationship between signs and symptoms. In Western-style, modern medicine model the concept of "one disease–one target–one size-fits-all" is shifting toward more personalization, including the use of multiple therapeutic agents and the consideration of nutritional, psychological, and lifestyle factors when deciding the best course of treatment. Dietary supplements have enormous potential in this personalization trend (Ghosh et al., 2013). This strategic shift in medical practice is being linked with the discipline of systems science—and systems biology in the biomedical domain. Systems science aims to understand both the connectivity and interdependency of individual components within a dynamic and nonlinear system, as well as the properties that emerge at certain organizational levels (Meyer, 2012). The concepts and practices of systems biology align very closely with those of traditional Asian medicine as well as the very idea of "health" of the current World Health Organization definition. Now we know individual dietary components can modulate and change gene function. Based on the robust evidence, healthcare professionals are now able to control gene-specific physiological expression with specific dietary intervention.

This hypothesis has just become more attainable for more people due to rising prosperity, particularly in emerging markets. Moreover the tremendous technological advancement reduces the gap between desire and reality by reaching more cost-effective personalized products and services. With rising prosperity there has also been a growth of post-materialist societies where values emphasizing self-expression and individuality have grown. The individualism mega-trend represents consumers' desires to be themselves and be recognized as having personal needs rather than being part of the mass market (Ghosh, 2008, 2010). Consumers seek products that make them stand out from the crowd and provide them with (or at least reinforce) a sense of personal and social identity.

CUSTOMIZATION: WEST VERSUS EAST

The food/dietary supplement industry is a brain child of the need for preventative personalized medicine. Born as a result of consumer demand the industry is currently developing on the back of innovation and science substantiation. Customization and personalization is the driving force for this industry, specifically in developed markets such as the United States and Europe. However, while complete personalization (based on genetic profile) is a still few years away, companies are looking at new and innovative ingredients and/or delivery mechanism to suit specific target groups. The meaning and significance of the term "customization" differ in different countries.

Cultural customization is now a real challenge to global companies. Manufacturers and marketers understand that various cultures have specific requirements for products. For example in India omega-3 a traditionally nonvegetarian product has been developed with vegetarian variants obtained from algae and flaxseed oil, in contrast to the West, particularly Europe. Both India and China are two key markets that have brought forward the importance of understanding a country's cultural psyche before launching products. For instance, the probiotic industry in India has faced challenges of a completely varied kind than seen elsewhere in the world. This is primarily because yoghurt, the primary mode of intake of probiotics, is an essential part of the indigenous diet and is normally homemade. Convincing consumers to pay premium for something so easily available has been a major hurdle for marketers.

Customization of supplemented products is based on four tenets:

1. Shift toward natural ingredients
2. Cultural customization to suit specific regions and specific target groups
3. Shift toward new delivery mechanisms
4. Disease-/condition-specific formulations

NICHE VERSUS MASS MARKET

The functional food, beverage, and supplement (FBS) market includes nutraceuticals, dietary supplements, and food supplements around the world (Table 18.1). The dietary supplement market, dominated by fiber, probiotics, protein and peptides, omega-3, phytochemicals, vitamins and minerals, and botanicals, is becoming increasingly fragmented and complex and offering opportunities for those who take

---

TABLE 18.1

Supplement Terminology

Regulatory Bodies	Related Terminology
Codex	Vitamin and mineral food supplements
United States	Dietary supplements
Europe	Food supplements
Japan	Foods (no supplement category)
Korea	Health functional foods
China	Health foods
ASEAN	Health supplements
Russia	Biologically active supplements
Canada	Natural health products
Australia	Complementary medicines
India	Dietary supplements/nutraceuticals

Source: IADSA, 2013, http://www.iadsa.org/.

---

advantage of a niche platform. Manufacturers are increasingly targeting different regions with different products. At the same time, the market is flooded with numerous generic products/ingredients without any product-specific health claims for mass market penetration. At the same time FBS market is looked upon as a market for premiumization with new value-added products promising better health through better dietary choices. For example, EGb761, a *Ginko biloba* extract produced by Schwabe Pharmaceuticals, is standardized for 24% "ginkgo flavone" glycosides and 6% terpene lactones. However, analysis of several *G. biloba* commercial products showed remarkable variations in the rutin and quercetin content as well as the terpene lactone contents, although all the products satisfied the regulatory quality control method (Sticher, 1993). Another example is St John's wort (*Hypericum perforatum* L.): Analysis of eight St. John's wort products available in the United States found that their hyperforin content varied from 0.01% to 1.89%, and only two products contained sufficient hyperforin likely to be required for antidepressant effects. Similarly, the content of the other active component hypericin varied from 0.03% to 0.29%, and for several products, the actual hypericin content did not correlate with that stated on the product label (range 57%–130% of label claim) (De los Reyes and Koda, 2002). For suppliers, functional FBS can provide growth opportunities as well as wider profit margins not available with traditional food products. Consumers are able to benefit from good health supported by product-specific efficacy support without sacrificing taste and convenience.

The movement from niche market to mass market is also a very attractive strategic option for many leading supplement companies. The sports nutrition market is changing in this direction. Its recent commercial success is also astonishing. SPINS recorded a 43% growth in fitness-inspired products in 2012, while BCC Research predicted sports nutrition products to reach $91.8 billion in 2013—logging a 24.1% compound annual growth rate (CAGR) since 2007. This segment was started with bodybuilders and their mass-building supplements but today, sports nutrition consumers range from lean, energized endurance runners to JV players looking to add mass to—gasp—regular people who do not even work out. In brief, this segment includes demographics of

- Women
- Weekend warriors
- CrossFitters
- Runners
- Mixed martial arts practitioners

Two other great examples are stevia and organic supplements. Both moved from a niche market to a mainstream platform with product innovation and positioning by intelligent marketing.

DRIVERS

The common factors driving dietary supplements/nutraceutical market are the increase in disposable income and consciousness about one's health, particularly in Asia-Pacific regions. Among all the geographies, North America has the largest consumer base for dietary supplements/nutraceutical products. Although the market is at a mature stage in this region, it witnessed a growth rate of more than 6% during 2007–2011. Developing countries like China and India possess huge potential both in terms of value and volume for dietary supplements/nutraceutical products, as the population and disposable income are on the rise in these countries.

Major factors stimulating the dietary supplements/nutraceutical market growth in the top seven countries (the United States, Japan, the United Kingdom, Spain, Italy, Germany, and France) are:

- A growing aging population
- A growing and affluent working population
- Increased awareness of evidence-based dietary supplements/nutraceuticals
- More people looking to take their health into their own hands
- Top-selling ingredients in the nutritional supplement industry
- Rising number of start-ups and supplement business owner
- Rising focus on e-commerce among consumers

The spending on purchase of healthy and organic foods is on the rise, thus giving a boost to the overall dietary supplements/nutraceutical market. One of the factors restraining the market growth is the lack of consumer trust about the health benefits claimed by supplements, including vitamins and minerals.

SEGMENT-WISE GROWTH

According to the Freedonia Group, the top-selling group of nutraceutical ingredients in the nutritional supplement industry includes proteins, fibers, and various specialized functional additives that constitute the three major groups of nutraceutical ingredients. Proteins are projected as the fastest-growing segment as manufacturers introduce innovations for protein application in foods and beverages with high-value nutrition. Herbal and botanical extracts as well as animal and marine-based derivatives are expected to have a steady, fast growth. Global demand for these products was expected to rise 8.9% annually, through 2015. Specialized functional additives such as omega-3 fatty acids, probiotics, vitamins, and minerals were predicted to grow at an annual increase of 6.7%, and was expected for the above group of dietary supplements/nutraceutical ingredients, through 2015. Innova Market Insights (2013) has identified the top five health claims for functional foods and drinks marketed to older consumers. Health optimization has become an increasing focus for an aging population, driven by rising consumer understanding of the role of a healthy diet in extending the active years. This is being reflected in promotion of the idea of healthy aging or aging well. "The most popular healthy-aging-related claims for food and drink products concern digestive/gut health, energy/alertness, heart health and immune health," and "these have general appeal among the wider population. But there are other, more specific, opportunities in age-related concerns that are currently featured much less often in product claims, including brain/cognitive health, bone health, skin health, joint health, and eye health."

Tracked product launches using eye health claims doubled in the last 5-year period, as recorded by Innova Market Insights in 2012. A range of other ingredients claimed to be beneficial in the area of cognitive health include B vitamins, CoQ10, *Ginkgo biloba*, polyphenols, acetyl L-carnitine, and green tea, but there are few specific references to aging to date, with labeling generally simply highlighting their use and relying on consumer awareness of the benefits.

Euromonitor estimated $34 billion sales segment-wise in 2012. Weight management and digestive health platforms came second and third, very strongly after general wellness domain.

HOW THE MARKET CHANGES

Regulatory Changes: Guiding Supplement Markets

The interface and steps involved in bringing product (manufacturing) and marketing (advertising) innovations that are compliant with the law are a continuous process of interaction between the innovating industry and the regulators, not necessarily in that order. It is common perception that industry initiates the need for change regulation but it is not true in all the cases. The Dietary Supplement Health and Education Act (DSHEA) is about a classic example of the regulator bringing in major change in regulations driven by consumers. Though not from the supplement industry, the following example will drive this point.

Market-Driven Regulatory Innovation: An Example

All innovatoive pharmaceutical companies had protection for their innovated new drugs by way of IP rights. The USFDA was not able to give marketing authorization for the same molecule of active drug or its formulation to any manufacturer other than innovator for a long time. The innovator not only had protection of product and market for the entire period of patent life but the brand of the drug also used to get protection as strict regulations existed before a pharmacist could switch brands. This was considered to have led to higher economics of the cost of medicines and thereby putting a higher load on expenses on drugs and healthcare management. Driven by the need to bring down the cost for healthcare management, a paradigm shift was thought and the U.S. government brought about a major change by way of Waxman–Hatch Amendment, which permitted the USFDA under specific conditions to approve generic versions of patented molecules/drugs to market after specified exclusivity period of a protected market of a first innovator. In this amendment, clear definitions of generic product and all other conditions for approval have been specified. The result was availability of generic drug formulations that are biologically and therapeutically equivalent to the innovators formulation but it also brought down cost by a high percentile lower to the innovators'/brand formulation. This amendment has been in force for more than a decade now and is a history of "Regulations opening up and driving innovations to benefit the patients that also brought benefits to generic drug industry."

Reforming Regulations

This is the toughest part and normally takes a long time, sometimes extending for too many years. Reforms call for patient and sustained efforts and personal and official interactions with not only the officials who are empowered to initiate reforms but also with political members of the legislature or senate or commissions. Often, reforms are aimed at changing the administrative and enforcing methodologies and processes, strategic changes in the way regulations look at food products and processes, and the way safety is assessed, regulated, and managed. The other aspect of reforms may extend to creating new categories shifting from restricted benefit claims to permitting bolder claims and permitting preapproved health benefit claims that border between food and drug into the food domain bringing certain categories of unrestricted food products to make them to be given under medical or nutritionist advice. A number of examples of creation of dietary supplements, nutraceuticals, food/health supplements, foods for specific health use, and functional foods fall under this bracket.

Brief Global Scenario

Different countries have taken various approaches for defining food, drug, and dietary supplements, but there are also international communication and efforts to consolidate and harmonize the activity. Markets, such as those in United States have measures to promote responsible nutrition and informed choices by a tightly controlled FDA regime when it comes to drugs. On the contrary, countries like Japan, China, and Canada have more closely knit, protective regulatory approaches with a view to protect citizens who are made of a mix of well and less literate. The governments in these countries have taken the need for performing the informed choice step and providing guidance to the consumers. Hence, in these countries, the law adopts a strategy where regulators would take a step forward by providing the informed choice and justification of functional foods claims.

Different terminologies such as "nutraceuticals," "food supplements," "dietary supplements," and "health supplements" primarily refer to processed foods containing ingredients that aid specific body functions, in addition to being nutritious.

Different countries have taken various approaches to regulate these supplementary materials. Japan has developed a concept of Food with Health Claims (FHC), under which Foods for Specified Health Use (FOSHU) are placed and a well-regulated mechanism for their categorization, approval for FOSHU seal, and claims substantiation is established and governed by Japan Ministry of Health, Labor and Family Welfare (MHLW). In the United States, the principal regulation for functional foods (Dietary Supplements) is under Dietary Supplement Health and Education Act (DSHEA), though Nutrition Labeling and Education Act (NLEA) also plays a significant role. Another well-regulated market for functional foods exists in the European Union (EU) whereby European Food Safety Authority (EFSA) has provided its scientific opinion on nutrient profiling, claims authorization, and application procedure for functional foods. Health claims on food and food ingredients are regulated in Australia and New Zealand through an integrated food regulatory system involving both governments, under the statuary agency Food Standards Australia New Zealand (FSANZ, http://www.foodstandards.gov.au/), established by the Food Standards Australia New Zealand Act 1991. A new standard to regulate nutrition content claims and health claims on food labels and in advertisements became law on January 18, 2013. India, being a new entry to regulations, is still in its infancy but with the introduction of recent new food law called Food Safety Standards Act (FSSA), a separate category for functional foods/nutraceutical has been created whereby Ayurveda or Unani medicines (AUM) and Ayurvedic Proprietary Medicine (APM) formulations are explicitly excluded from this domain. The regulatory structure for functional foods and dietary supplement regulations is not yet harmonized across the globe, and there is a need to understand the regulatory requirement of different countries. It is a fact that a single functional food may vary widely from country to country; for example, a single product may be labeled and sold as dietary supplement in the United States, and as FOSHU in Japan and as a proprietary food or an AUM or APM medicine in India.

OPPORTUNITIES AND CHALLENGES AHEAD

Hotspots

Genetics and genomics are an ideal platform for trial and experimentation of metabolism and nutrition sciences. Diet is perhaps the most important environmental factor human beings are exposed to their whole lifecycle. Nutritional factors are thought to be the cause of 30%–60% of cancers (similar in magnitude to smoking; Doll, 1992), obesity, diabetes, and cholesterol–cardiovascular diseases.

The opportunities in personalized foods and nutrition are great, but the challenges are enormous (Brown and van der Ouderaa, 2007). For many common diseases (e.g., cancer, diabetes, cardiovascular disease, rheumatoid arthritis, and dementia), there are no effective or curative treatments. Despite unprecedented investments by big pharmaceutical houses in new drug/pharmaceutical research and development, the number of new drugs approved by the regulatory agencies is extremely low. For example, only 21 drugs were approved in 2010 by the FDA, down from a yearly average approval rate of 35 drugs in the 1990s. The predominant reasons such as political, fiscal, regulatory, and scientific are very complex and shifting whole paradigm from cure to prevention. Between 2007 and 2010, 83 drug candidates that failed either in phase III clinical studies or at submission level were due (almost 90% failure rate) to either lack of efficacy (66%) or safety issues (21%). The present model of drug research and development is obviously not working, and profound changes are also needed in the way health care is organized. Personalized medicine, with its goal to predict responders and non-responders to therapy and to develop biomarkers that can be used as guides in the process of drug development, is one strategy to pursue. Personalized nutrition will piggyback on the advances made by personalized medicine. This is because of the expense and technical demands of genotyping and related disciplines. Pharmaceutical companies will be driven to genotype populations in order to minimize risk and avoid inappropriate or ineffective drug-based therapies, and medical personnel will subsequently genotype their patients in order to take advantage of knowledge of gene–drug interactions. Few will be genotyped solely to maintain or improve their health through good nutrition (Ghosh et al., 2007).

HURDLES

The first challenge for scientists entering this young discipline is to develop the fundamental knowledge base needed to start addressing this complex system. They must know the "languages" of both genetics and nutrition.

It is clearly evident that nutrients regulate the expression and function of genes. Before practical applications of nutrigenomics can arise (such as individualized nutrition recommendations or interventions designed to modify disease risks), the discipline must enhance the understanding of bidirectional nutrient–gene interactions to the point where there are overarching and integrated frameworks for thinking about how these interactions work (Zeisel, 2010).

Nutrigenomics is being applied to agriculture (enhanced plant and animal food sources) and to human health. For the purposes of this discussion, the application to individual differences in metabolism (individualized nutrition) is used to highlight how the field could proceed to address this challenge. The underlying mechanisms responsible for individual variation in metabolism and, therefore, in the responses to and requirements for nutrients, are not yet fully known. The likely involvement of genetic variation and epigenetic mechanisms makes these prime targets for study. In order to move forward and develop an overarching theory for predicting effects of genetic (epigenetic) variation on metabolism and nutrient requirements, a more detailed data set describing nutrient–gene interactions is required. Without this information any practical application to humans will be flawed.

To date, there are thousands of genes for which there is no known function. Many of these genes will likely be important for metabolism. A systematic approach is needed to discover the function of these genes. For more than 9000 genes, the United States National Institutes of Health's Knockout Mouse Phenotyping Project and the EUMODIC consortium of 18 laboratories across Europe are characterizing the functional effects of gene deletions in mice on phenotype, and hopefully they will comprehensively assess metabolic phenotypes.

The current catalog of genetic variations (single nucleotide polymorphisms [SNPs] and copy number variations [CNVs]) that cause metabolic inefficiencies is quite small, and most of the published literature considers SNPs as acting individually, rather than examining the systems effects of combinations of SNPs. There must be thousands of SNPs that alter metabolism, yet today, in the published literature there may be as many as 200 SNPs for which there are proven metabolic effects, and only a subset of these alter nutrient requirements in a significant portion of the population [e.g., the rs1801133 MTHFR SNP and folate requirement in 15%–30% of the population and the rs12325817 PEMT SNP and choline requirement in 20%–45% of the population (da Costa et al., 2006)]. Some SNPs directly alter a metabolic response to a nutrient, rather than changing the requirement for it. For example, the rs3135506 SNP in APOA5 modifies the effects of a high-fat diet on blood pressure (Mattei et al., 2009). Just as the catalogue of SNP-diet response relationships is incomplete, so too is the collection of information regarding how diet may alter epigenetic marks in DNA and histones (Lomba et al., 2010; Mehedint et al., 2010;Vucetic et al., 2010). Finally, genetic variation influences eating behaviors (Dotson et al., 2010) but these effects have not been systematically explored (this is an exciting potential collaboration between nutrigenomics and behavioral science). In part these catalogues are skimpy because nutrigenomic methods are relatively expensive when applied to large populations, and nutrition epidemiology studies often do not make genetic and metabolomic measures together.

The methods for assessing gene variation and epigenetic marks are far more mature than are the high throughput methods for studying metabolism. Traditionally, many studies of genes and metabolism used a targeted approach, measuring a small set of metabolites in pathways likely to be related to a change in a gene. Metabolomic profiling (also called metabonomic profiling) has matured sufficiently that it can be used to simultaneously measure many untargeted small molecules that are the product of many pathways in metabolism. Mass spectroscopic (Lawton et al., 2008) and nuclear magnetic resonance spectroscopic (Dumas et al., 2006) techniques are used in metabolomic profiling, each having distinct advantages and disadvantages. These methods offer an opportunity to more precisely measure the effects of genes on metabolism.

Unfortunately, measuring the effects of diet on genes faces a major challenge: the methods for measuring dietary intake are much more imprecise than are genetic or biochemical measurements. There is a dearth of novel methodology for measuring dietary exposures and there is a real need for an improved tool chest for those investigating how diet interacts with genotype to determine phenotype (Penn et al., 2010). Most nutrition scientists recognize that current diet assessment methods are not likely to provide more than an approximation (perhaps off by 30% or more) for individual dietary intake (Penn et al., 2010). Though the development of each of these methodologies is the focus of different disciplines, nutrigenomic scientists face the significant challenge of improving and adapting these methods in combination with genomic methods so that a more detailed catalogue of nutrient–gene interactions can be developed.

The grand challenge is to develop an overarching and integrated framework for thinking about how gene–nutrient interactions influence metabolism. To address this challenge, nutrigenomics has to build a cohort of multidisciplinary scientists who can talk each other's "language," develop better methods, and establish a comprehensive data set from which the great thinkers among us can develop the theory. These tasks should keep researchers busy for a decade or more (Zeisel, 2010). Another big challenge is recruitment of ethnically diverse control population. This is well recognized, and more literature has become available for certain ethnicities (e.g., Asians, African-Americans); however, there remains a wide gap in genetic knowledge pertinent to other groups such as Native Americans, Pacific Islanders, and many, many more.

The Genome-Based Health Concept

Nutritional genomics is a promising new research and development area, and as a young and blue-sky science, this is also associated with intense debate. With high hope to many researchers nutritional genomics is closely associated with "personalized nutrition," in which the diet of an individual is customized, based on his or her own genomic/genetic information, to optimize health and prevent the onset of disease. In this context "nutritional genomics is largely concerned with elucidating the interactive nature of genomic, dietary and environmental factors and how these interactions impact on health outcomes" (Brown and van der Ouderaa, 2007).

Scientists have determined that genetic expression is influenced by "endogenous and exogenous factors and therefore particularly prone to nutritional imprinting" (Ruemmele and Garnier-Lenglin, 2012). Moreover, nutrition and genes interact in two different ways. The term "nutrigenomics," is where the impact of nutritional factors on gene regulation and expression is considered. The other way, "nutrigenetics," examines the influence that genetic variations have on, or predetermine, nutritional requirements. Both interactions are important considerations in designing a personalized nutrition concept.

Traditionally (and most of the cases currently), nutrition counseling and recommendation have been offered based on population. An example of such a recommendation is the dietary reference values for calcium: Adults between 19 and 60 years of age should consume 1000 mg per day. This recommendation does not account for individual genetic variations in the ability to absorb and metabolize this mineral. Another example is that of "dietary interventions as primary prevention to reduce the risk of cardiovascular disease" (de Roos, 2013). Without a valid population-based strategy, the population-based intervention does not address the possibility of subgroups differences in response to the intervention. Personalized nutrition would address such individual variations.

One Size Does Not Fit All

Humans span a remarkable range of phenotypes. Healthy human adults largely vary in their physical appearance, physical and cognitive performance, and in their food preference and requirements. Humans are most alike at birth, but as they progress through various life stages, they diversify into numerous lifestyles.

Humans differ at the level of a wide range of basic biological variables. These variables are, in some cases, genetically determined chromosomal differences, for example, male and female, or allelic polymorphisms in structural or regulatory regions of specific genes. Differences are also due to the age and particular life stage of an individual (e.g., pregnancy, lactation, infancy, puberty, pre- and post-menopause, and elderly). Other differences are derived from environmental influences that are either exogenous and random (e.g., exposure to sunlight, toxins, and allergens), or endogenous and linked to a chosen lifestyle (e.g., excess or balanced caloric intake, meal frequency, exercise or sedentary behavior, regular sleep cycle, or frequent change between time zones or shift work). Furthermore, each of these variables may exert effects on (epi)genetic or non-genetic elements, thereby conferring persistence of a particular phenotype through some of that individual's subsequent life and altering that individual's response to dietary components (Table 18.2).

Nutrition and health research and its implementation into food products will become increasingly personalized as the ability of scientific tools to distinguish important physiological differences merges with the industrial means to deliver individual solutions. This process is not a revolution of food, but rather reflects the continued diversification of foods that has been ongoing for centuries. Practical solutions for most consumers will benefit by focusing food personalization on validated nutritional solutions to established subsets of the population. Infants, pregnant and lactating women, active or sedentary adults, athletes, frail elderly, and consumers

TABLE 18.2
Criteria Underlying Consumer Personalization

Platform	Criteria
Taste and flavor	Most immediate and easily accessed criteria.
	Genetic diversity of taste and olfactory sensation are now well established.
	Olfactory preference is most driving force
Cultural mores	Based on religious and philosophical value system.
	Halal, Kosher, vegan, religious fasting, etc.
Life stage	Specific physiological needs of the stages of life stages.
	Pregnancy, lactation, weaning, infancy, aging, recovery from illness, etc.
	Both short term and long term supplementation
Lifestyle	Products for athletes at different stages of training.
	High altitude training.
	Frequent traveler.
Lifestyle diseases	Diagnostics related to high risk disease condition as a direct result of chronic lifestyle choices.
	Excess body weight, intestinal discomfort, smoking, sedentary behavior, high-fat diet, etc.
Inherited diseases	Relevance to family history of inherited diseases.
	Food and supplement intervention is recognized an integral part of this solution such as allergies and intolerances.
	Inborn error of metabolism, phenylketonurea can well managed by metabolite-based diagnostics with low phenylalanine food and supplements.
Genetic predispositions	Personalization based on genetic variations.
	Target population-based product development.
	Strong linkage with ethical-legal-social issues.

who suffer from inherited or acquired diseases all represent large consumer groups with food requirements that both address their nutritional issues and ensure compliance by considering personal preferences in taste, texture, and appearance. Developing nutritional foods to help diseased people recover should accompany the parallel approaches in personalized medicine.

The genomics sciences have delivered proof of the principle that humans are different with respect to optimal diets. As nutrigenomics and nutrigenetics build the scientific foundation for this, and as genotyping technologies become readily accessible, consumers may gain value through information on their personal genetic code. However, only those genetic variations should be assessed that can be adequately addressed by appropriate diets.

Public dietary advice aims to encourage healthy eating, but the "one size fits all" population-based dietary guidance is no longer effective—thus opening a door to individual diets based on dietary, phenotypic, and genotypic data. Geneticists will have to examine the potential benefits of developing personalized diets to target existing nutrition growth categories such as aging, cognitive, heart and metabolic health, immunity, and weight management.

Studies have shown that people respond differently to various nutrients depending on their genes and metabolic characteristics. For example, omega 3, the healthy fat in oily fish that can help protect against heart disease, is more beneficial to people with a particular genetic makeup (Table 18.3).

SUPPLEMENTS FOR A SPECIFIC NICHE

Today's foods and dietary supplements are typically marketed to large (sub)groups of the total population. For example, phytosterol-enriched food/dietary supplements

---

TABLE 18.3
Identical Targets of Functional Foods and Drugs

Food	Target	Drugs
Enriched with phytosterol-stanol esters	Low-density lipoprotein cholesterol	Statins, ezetimibe
Containing bioactive peptides	Blood pressure	Antihypertensive drugs
Containing melatonin	Quality of sleep	Benzodiazepines
Containing omega 3 fatty acid	Depression	Antidepressants
Containing β glucan	Blood sugar values	
Low-density lipoprotein cholesterol	Insulin, oral hypoglycaemic drugs	Statins, ezetimibe
Containing prebiotics	Bowel frequency	Laxatives
Containing probiotics	Immune functioning, diarrhea (wet stools)	Loperamide
Containing extra calcium or vitamin D, or both	Bone health	Alendronate, calcitonin, oestrogens
Containing protein/bioactive peptides and alpha cyclodextrin	Obesity and type 2 diabetes	Orlistat, rimonabant

TABLE 18.4

Regulation of Genes by Nutrients

Nutrient	Gene Impact	Disease Potential
Folic acid	DNA methylation	Cancer
Fatty acid	Blind to transcription factors	Obesity
Vitamin D	mRNA stability	Kidney disease
Flavones	Increase mRNA synthesis	Cancer
Theaflavins	Decrease mRNA synthesis	Arthritis

are targeted to all adults with (moderately) elevated cholesterol levels and products with claimed pre- and probiotic activity are aimed at general healthy populations.

The recent advances in pharmaco- and nutrigenomics have formed the basis for developing the concepts of "personalized medicine" (Personalized Medicine Coalition, 2009) and "personalized nutrition" (Ghosh, 2007, 2009a, 2009b). These emerging fields rely on targeted therapies based on a person's genetic risk profile.

Pharmaceuticals (Caskey, 2010), as well as several dietary components (Afman and Müller, 2006), have been recognized to modulate gene and protein expression and thereby metabolic pathways, homeostatic regulation, and presumably health and disease (Table 18.4). In addition, genes also contribute largely to different responses to diet or drug exposure, including interindividual variations in the occurrence of adverse drug reactions (Lee et al., 2010). Major areas where the development of personalized foods/nutritionals is realistically possible include type 2 diabetes and obesity, mood foods, inflammatory bowel disease (IBD), and disorders of aging where the diet–gene relationship has been studied extensively.

PERSONALIZATION AS INDIVIDUALIZATION VERSUS CATEGORIZATION

Personalization is a major issue in contemporary nutrition science, especially in the field of nutrigenomics. From the limited interview-based survey, we see personalization as individualization and personalization as categorization, respectively; both serve their purpose in the advancement of nutrigenomic practice. With big controlled population study, Penders group (2007) also emphasized the importance of both routes of personalization. The major determinants such as what, how, when, and with whom we eat ultimately determine the large parts of our lives and eventually the trend in personalized nutrition will head toward the "creation of a new category with its own, unique, ethical agenda."

Personalization is all about differences, differences between people and differences between environments, differences between races and ultimately combined into the individual phenotype. From academic point of view, personalization is a visualized as being about each individual, but what does personalization mean from the perspective of clinical practice or from a commercial point of view? From practical point of view, "personalization" is about groups (or subpopulations) of a certain size with certain (genetic) traits, but can be discriminated between using other, relevant (genetic) traits. "Practical personalization" is conceptualized in terms of categorization as opposed to individualization. In terms of diet, categorization is the formulation of foods or development of dietary advice for the benefit of multiple individuals who share certain traits. Considering both scientific and commercial interests it is evident that these two, "personalization as individualization and personalization as categorization," will most likely continue to exist, as long as there are reasons for them to coexist. The strategic shift toward categorization should become more visible when research agendas stabilize (which is nearby) and nutrigenomics ever more evolves into common clinical practice. It is suggested, as a result of the expectation-practice interaction, the trend in personalized nutrition moves away from individuality and leads toward genetic categories of an undetermined minimum size of population. A need for changing the ethical agenda to support the changing trend in nutrition science from "individualized diet to group diet" is needed.

CONCLUSION

PERSONALIZATION IN A DIFFERENT WAY

Last year, Coca-Cola Enterprises printed over 1 billion packs of Coca-Cola, Diet Coke, and Coca-Cola Zero with 150 of the most popular names in the Unites States, ranging from Aaron to Zoe. From personalization point of view they said, "It's fantastic that we can really personalize the product for them. We're issuing the invite for people to connect and as part of that we want the public to have fun finding the names of their friends and loved ones on our products, ..." Although personalized nutrition as a proposition is exciting, and offers the opportunity for individualized interventions, "there is insufficient evidence at present; thus, dietary advice should be offered only for variables with enough evidence to support health outcomes." In addition, evidence for behavior changes consequent to a nutrition intervention is limited (Görman et al., 2013) (Figure 18.4).

TECHNOLOGY MAKES A DIFFERENCE

Understanding how food and dietary supplements modulate health is a core technology requirement for the development of future functional ingredients and supplements. So-called "the genomic toolbox" is ready to help nutritional scientists to resolve this food–gene complexity and starting to turn the wheel toward commercial success. We are not far away from reality. Coca-Cola predicts, "And soon, looking ahead, it's not going to be that far out that we will talk about personalized beverages based on people's personal genes." In 1953, Watson and Crick first described the structure of DNA. In less than 50 years, in 2001, the publication of the human genome sequence represented a revolutionary breakthrough in health and nutrition research and their market applications. Now, we are beginning to understand that DNA is not only responsible for the transfer of traits from parents to offspring, but also plays a dynamic role in how our health unfolds on a daily basis. This knowledge suggests that there are opportunities for the pharmaceutical industry to leverage

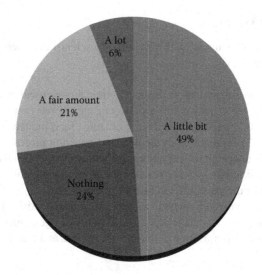

FIGURE 18.1   U.S. consumers' awareness of genomics. (From Schmidt, D. et al., *Personalized Nutrition, Principles and Applications*, CRC Press, Boca Raton, FL, 2007, pp. 205–219.)

human genome sequence data to develop new supplement based on knowledge of targets, taking into account the variations in genetic makeup between individuals (nutrigenomics/nutrigenetics).

BENEFITS TO THE INDUSTRY

What does this mean to food and dietary supplement industry? In fact, the supplement industry now has an opportunity to position nutritional bioactives to promote health and prevent disease based on knowledge of the genetic makeup of individual consumers. Few recent studies have moved a step closer to fighting certain genetic diseases with dietary interventions (Mayfield et al., 2011). Here are some opportunities for food and dietary supplement industry:

- Eighty percent of premature heart disease cases, strokes, type 2 diabetes, and 40% of cancers could be avoided with personalized nutritional supplementation.
- Personalized nutrition should target both consumers with existing ailments and younger consumers or people without existing medical conditions.
- Customization of benefits on validated nutritional solutions to established subsets of the population, such as infants, pregnant and lactating women, active or sedentary adults, athletes, and frail elderly and consumers who suffer from inherited or acquired diseases.
- The conservative forecast indicates that at least one-third of consumers will be making some changes in their nutrient intake in response to personalized nutrition by the middle of this decade.

RECOMMENDATIONS

Integrate novel business model with way forward scientific concepts for the best use of personalized nutrition.

- Introduce and implement strategically interactive research such as focus groups, interviews, and workshops to engage all relevant stakeholders in the food chain, including consumers; citizens; food industry; pharmaceutical industry; insurance; retail, health, and nutrition professional; scientific community; nonprofit organizations; public health authorities; and media.
- Consolidate findings into a coherent view about the possibilities and opportunities for future personalized nutrition approaches.
- Communicate with consumers in a simple and understandable language without using jargon of words such as "gene," "genetic," "genomics," and so forth.
- Adopt cultural customization to suit specific regions and specific target groups.

REFERENCES

Afman, L. and Müller, M. 2006. Nutrigenomics: From molecular nutrition to prevention of disease. *J. Am. Diet. Assoc.*, 106: 569–576.

Betoret, E., Betoret, N., Vidal, D. et al. 2011. Functional foods development: Trends and technologies. *Trends Food Sci. Technol.*, 22: 498–508.

Brown, L. and van der Ouderaa, F. 2007. Nutritional genomics: Food industry applications from farm to fork. *Br. J. Nutr.*, 97: 1027–1035.

Caskey, C.T. 2010. Using genetic diagnosis to determine individual therapeutic utility. *Annu. Rev. Med.*, 61: 1–15.

De los Reyes, G.C. and Koda, R.T. 2002. Determining hyperforin and hypericin content in eight brands of St. John's wort. *Am. J. Health Syst. Pharm.*, 59: 545–547.

de Roos, B. 2013. Conference on "Future food and health." Symposium II: Diet–gene interactions; Implications for future diets and health. Personalized nutrition: Ready for practice? *Proc. Nutr. Soc.*, 72: 48–52.

Doll, R. 1992. The lessons of life: Keynote address to the nutrition and aging conference. *Cancer Res.*, 52: 2024S–2029S.

Dotson, C.D., Shaw, H.L., Mitchell, B.D. et al. 2010. Variation in the gene TAS2R38 is associated with the eating behavior disinhibition in old order Amish women. *Appetite*, 54: 93–99.

Dumas, M.E., Barton, R.H., Toye, A. et al. 2006. Metabolic profiling reveals a contribution of gut microbiota to fatty liver phenotype in insulin-resistant mice. *Proc. Natl. Acad. Sci. U.S.A.*, 103: 12511–12516.

Ghosh, D. October–November 2008. Getting personal. The world food ingredients, pp. 103–105.

Ghosh, D. 2009a. Future perspectives of nutrigenomics foods: Benefits vs. risks. *Indian J. Biophys. Biochem.*, 46: 31–36.

Ghosh, D. 2009b. Personalised nutrition: The future challenges of nutrigenomics. *Food Eng. Ingredients*, 34: 30–31.

Ghosh, D. 2010. Personalised food: How personal is it? *Genes Nutr.*, 5: 51–53.

Ghosh, D. 2013. Personalised nutrition could be the way forward. *Nutraceutical Now*, Spring: 6.

Ghosh, D., Skinner, M., and Laing, W.A. 2007. Pharmacogenomics and nutrigenomics: Synergies and differences. *Eur. J. Clin. Nutr.*, 61: 567–574.

Ghosh, D. and Tapsell, L. 2008. Nutrigenomics: A genomic approach to human nutrition. In *Genomics: Principles, Applications and Regulatory Perspectives*, pp. 337–344, Chapter 14. CRC Press, Boca Raton, FL.

Global Industry Analysts. 2012. A global strategic business report. 2016, Herbal supplements and remedies. http://www.strategyr.com/Herbal_Supplements_and_Remedies_Market_Report.asp.

Görman, U., Mathers, J.C., and Grimaldi, K.A. 2013. Do we know enough? A scientific and ethical analysis of the basis for genetic-based personalized nutrition. *Genes Nutr.*, 8: 373–381.

Innova Market Insights. 2013. Global food and nutrition trends. http://www.innovadatabase.com/.

Lawton, K.A., Berger, A., Mitchell, M. et al. 2008. Analysis of the adult human plasma metabolome. *Pharmacogenomics*, 9: 383–397.

Lee, K., Ma, J., and Kuo, G. 2010. Pharmacogenomics: Bridging the gap between science and practice. *J. Am. Pharm. Assoc.*, 50: e1–e14.

Lomba, A., Martinez, J.A., García-Díaz, D.F. et al. 2010. Weight gain induced by an isocaloric pair-fed high fat diet: A nutriepigenetic study on FASN and NDUFB6 gene promoters. *Mol. Genet. Metab.*, 101: 273–278.

Mattei, J., Demissie, S., Tucker, K.L. et al. 2009. Apolipoprotein A5 polymorphisms interact with total dietary fat intake in association with markers of metabolic syndrome in Puerto Rican older adults. *J. Nutr.*, 139: 2301–2308.

Mayfield, J., Dago, D.M., Denket, D. et al. 2011. Surrogate genetics and metabolic profiling for characterization of human disease alleles. *Genetics*, 190: 1309–1323.

Mehedint, M.G., Niculescu, M.D., Craciunescu, C.N. et al. 2010. Choline deficiency alters global histone methylation and epigenetic marking at the Re1 site of the calbindin 1 gene. *FASEB J.*, 24: 184–195.

Meyer, U.A. 2012. Personalized medicine: A personal view. *Clin. Phar. Ther.*, 91: 373–375.

Penders, B., Horstman, K., and Vos, R. 2007. From individuals to groups: A review of the meaning of "personalized" in nutrigenomics. *Trends Food Sci. Technol.*, 18: 333–338.

Penn, L., Boeing, H., Boushey, C.J. et al. 2010. Assessment of dietary intake: NuGO symposium report. *Genes Nutr.*, 5: 205–213.

Personalized Medicine Coalition. 2009. The case for personalized medicine. Available from: http://www.personalizedmedicinecoalition.org/about/about-personalizedmedicine/the-casefor-personalized-medicine (accessed November 12, 2015).

Roberfroid, M.B. 2007. Concepts and strategy of functional food science: The European perspective. *Am. J. Clin. Nutr.*, 71: 1660–1664.

Ruemmele, F.M. and Garnier-Lengliné, H. 2012. Why are genetics important for nutrition? Lessons from epigenetic research. *Ann. Nutr. Metab.*, 60: 38–43.

Schmidt, D., White, C., Child, M.N. et al. 2007. U.S. consumer attitudes toward personalized nutrition. In Kok, F., Bouwman, L., Desiere, F., eds., *Personalized Nutrition, Principles and Applications*, pp. 205–219. CRC Press, Boca Raton, FL.

Sticher, O. 1993. Quality of Ginkgo preparations. *Planta Medica*, 59: 2–11.

Vucetic, Z., Kimmel, J., Reyes, T.M. et al. 2010. Maternal high-fat diet alters methylation and gene expression of dopamine and opioid-related genes. *Endocrinology*, 151: 4756–4764.

Zeisel, S.H. 2010. A grand challenge for nutrigenomics. Frontiers in genetics. *Nutrigenomics*, 1: 1–3.

19 Quality Controversies in Phytopharmaceuticals*

Dilip Ghosh

CONTENTS

INTRODUCTION

Herbal medicines are the most ancient form of health remedies known to mankind. In spite of the great advances achieved in modern medicine, plants still make an important contribution to healthcare, and several specific herbal extracts have demonstrated to be efficacious for specific conditions. Moreover, at least 120 distinct chemical substances derived from plants are considered as important drugs currently in use, and several other drugs are simple synthetic modifications of natural products (Fabricant and Farnsworth, 2001). In reality, it must also be stated that certain tightly held beliefs within traditional medicine have created an environment where strong belief "counts" more than the application of scientific principles (Cordell, 2015). Plants can be regarded as "living factories" producing a variety of chemical compounds, including primary metabolites important for the growth of the plants (amino acids, proteins, and carbohydrates) and secondary metabolites (alkaloids, terpenoids, phenylpropanoids, polyketides, flavonoids, and saccharides). All these components may work together to deliver a synergistic effect in the finished product. Certain herbal medicines, because of the complexity of their chemical content and the variety of bioactivities, can provide the polypharmacology that orthodox drugs cannot deliver. Natural products are rarely evaluated in the well-controlled clinical trials that are required to receive approval by regulatory bodies and, therefore, tend

---

* Partly adapted from Zangara and Ghosh, 2014.

to have less "scientific" evidence to support their efficacy. However, all medicinal compounds are chemicals, whether synthesized in plants, in animals, or in manufacturing laboratories; therefore, all medicinal chemical compounds should be held accountable to similar standards of quality (identity, purity, and stability), clinical effectiveness, and safety; irrespective of their source "if it is found to be reasonably safe and effective, it will be accepted" (Angell and Kassirier, 1998). Reliable and consistent quality is the basis of efficacy and safety of herbal medicinal products. Given the nature of products of plant origin, which are highly variable and complex products with numerous biologically active components, rarely completely identified, therapeutic results and safety issues vary greatly from product to product, even within a single class. Therefore, the evidence of both benefits and risks is specific to the product tested and cannot necessarily be extrapolated to other products as is the case for synthetically derived compounds. For these reasons and due to the inherent variability of the constituents of herbal products, it is difficult to establish quality control parameter, and batch-to-batch variation, in the absence of reference standard for identification, can start from the collection of raw material and increase during storage and further processing. In conclusion, to minimize variation in final botanical products, standardization of procedures should cover the entire field of study from cultivation of medicinal plant to its clinical application.

HERBAL MEDICINAL PRODUCTS

Plants have been used for medicinal purposes since time immemorial. Over the centuries diverse cultural groups have developed traditional medical systems, such as Ayurveda and traditional Chinese medicine (TCM). In the early nineteenth century, scientists began to use chemical analysis to extract and modify the active ingredients from plants. Later, chemists began making synthetic versions of plant compounds, and the use of herbal medicines was substituted by conventional drugs in most industrialized countries. In contrast, many nonindustrialized countries never abandoned medical herbalism and continued to develop their existing traditional medical systems. The World Health Organization (WHO) estimates that 80% of people worldwide rely on herbal medicines for some part of their primary healthcare (Robinson and Zhang, 2011).

The WHO recognizes herbal medicines as valuable and readily available resources and states that it is necessary to develop a systematic inventory of medicinal plants, to introduce regulatory measures, to apply good manufacturing practices, and to include herbal medicines in the conventional pharmacopoeia of each nation (WHO, 2011). In the last decades, public dissatisfaction with the cost of prescription drugs, combined with an interest in returning to natural or organic remedies, has led to a revaluation of the use of herbal preparations use in industrialized countries.

Herbal medicinal products (HMP) are any medicinal product exclusively containing as active substances one or more herbal substances or one or more herbal preparations or one or more such herbal substances in combination with one or more such herbal preparations (WHO, 1996), and with this term we comprehensively refer within this chapter to herbal drugs, herbal preparations, and finished herbal medicinal products. HMP contain complex mixtures of organic chemicals (the phytocomplex) that work together to produce an effect on the body and that are rarely completely identified. The activity of the phytocomplex is usually stronger than the sum of activities of the single active molecules, and the presence of substances apparently having no specific activity can have a very important synergistic effect (Williamson, 2001). *Ginkgo biloba*, for example, acts in several ways, including the ability to decrease oxygen radical discharge and proinflammatory functions of macrophages (antioxidant and anti-inflammatory), reduce corticosteroid production (antianxiety), increase glucose uptake and utilization and adenosine triphosphate production, improve blood flow by increasing red blood cell deformability, decrease red cell aggregation, induce nitric oxide production, and inhibit platelet-activating factor receptors (Chan et al., 2007). Another example is *Panax ginseng*; more than 200 compounds have been identified in ginseng roots, a botanical with verified capability to benefit mental and physical capacities, weakness, exhaustion, and immunity (Scaglione et al., 2005; Soldati, 2000). The pharmacological activity of ginseng is primarily due to a number of ginsenosides, but polysaccharides are also regarded as pharmacologically active in this plant (Li et al., 2009).

HMP are sold in many forms (fresh, dried, liquid/solid extracts, tablets, capsules, powders, tea bags, topicals) and, as stated by the WHO, may not contain chemically defined substances such as synthetic compounds or chemicals isolated from herbs. They normally do not possess an immediate or strong pharmacological action, but may produce more long-lasting benefits in chronic diseases like dementia (Perry and Howes, 2011). Because of the complexity and the synergy of the individual components of the phytocomplex, their combination, often resulting in complex dose- and time-dependent effects, may affect multiple neuronal, metabolic, and hormonal systems that themselves modulate behavioral processes (Zangara and Wesnes, 2012).

Although it is generally believed that most herbal preparations are safe for consumption, some herbs like most biologically active substances could be toxic with undesirable side effects that are mainly due to active ingredients, contaminants, and/or interactions with other drugs (Walker, 2004). Therefore, the use of herbal medicinal products should be carefully monitored to ensure patient safety.

PHYTOTHERAPY

Phytotherapy is commonly defined as the study of the use of extracts of natural origin as medicines or health-promoting agents. It should be perceived as an allopathic discipline, because the effects that are expected from HMP are directed against the causes and the symptoms of a disease. In Germany, for example, phytotherapy is classified as a regular discipline of natural orthodox science–oriented medicine, and HMP have to comply with similar scientific requirements as those of the chemically defined substances in terms of quality, safety, and efficacy (Keller, 1996). However, modern mass production of natural products as food supplements or herbal medicines often results in remedies that can differ greatly (dosage form, mode of administration, herbal medicinal ingredients, methods of preparation, and medical indications) from the traditions that form the basis for their perceived safety and effectiveness and from an acceptable quality standard. The potential benefit provided by the use of HMP as effective medicine is sometimes perceived to be outweighed by the clinical risks associated with the absence of standard levels of biologically active materials from natural plants (Ernst, 1998). The WHO has published monographs on the quality, safety, and efficacy of selected medicinal plants and recommendations on the cultivation of medicinal plants and on the quality control, safety, and efficacy of HMP (WHO, 1993, 2003).

QUALITY CONTROL

Quality control and standardization of HMP involve several steps that should start with the sourcing of high-quality raw material and development of criteria for precise identification of the constituents of each product, together with documentation of the role of the constituent combinations. The following step will be to optimize and control the growing conditions and each subsequent step until the finished product, in order to minimize variability and provide pharmaceutical-grade HMP. Finally, it is necessary to establish its efficacy through biological assays and determine its adverse effect profile through literature or from toxicological studies (both short-term and long-term) followed by controlled clinical trials (Bauer and Tittle, 1996). Excipients used in both pharmaceutical and nutraceuticals are no longer inert materials, but they can change the medicament characteristics, including products' quality, stability, functionality, safety, solubility, and acceptance among patients (Abdellah et al., 2015). The lack of pharmacological and clinical data on the majority of herbal medicinal products represents a major impediment to the acceptance of natural products by conventional medicine.

The quality of plant raw materials can be influenced by accidental botanical substitution (misidentification of plant species) or intentional botanical substitution (deliberate exchange with other, possibly more toxic, plant species) (Newmaster et al., 2013; Van Breemen et al., 2008). The detection of undeclared chemical or synthetic substances or other active ingredients has also been frequently reported (Blumenthal, 2002). Several studies have also highlighted different levels of active ingredients in herbal products; for example, an analysis of 25 available ginseng products found a 15- to 200-fold variation in the concentration of the active ingredients ginsenosides and eleutherosides (Harkey et al., 2001). The intentional or accidental presence in herbal medicines of toxic heavy metals in more than the permissible limit set by national regulatory authorities is another common problem (Obi et al., 2006). Toxic contaminants are reported at all steps beginning from collection of raw materials to manufacturing (Fong, 2002). The presence of pesticide residues in herbal materials has also been detected, highlighting the need for harmonization and standardization on the use of pesticides (Liva, 2009). The WHO has established maximum residue limit (MRL) for pesticides in cultivated or wild medicinal plants as well as appropriate methodologies for their detection (WHO, 2007).

HMP should be analyzed (generally through chromatographic fingerprint) for chemical consistency at various stages of development, to ensure the identity and purity of the product and correct quantification of the active ingredients or markers, and the regulators insist on the importance of the qualitative and quantitative methods for characterizing the samples, quantification of the biomarkers, and/or chemical markers and the fingerprint profiles (EMA, 2008). However, identification of all of a plant's constituents often fails because of the complexity of the plant's chemical structure, and selective analytical methods or reference compounds may not be available commercially. To overcome this problem, the German Commission E elaborated plant monographs (Blumenthal et al., 1998), and more recently, *European Pharmacopoeia* has started a program to identify and prepare the chemical reference substances for the quality control of herbal drugs and their preparations, describing the analytical methods and quality specifications for each product. The *U.S. Pharmacopoeia* is also following a similar approach, highlighting the need to lay down guidelines for a growing number of HMP (Schwarz et al., 2009).

VARIABILITY

Plants are highly variable in their content of the numerous biologically active components, and depending on their origin, the growth conditions, and the date of harvest, the content of active components in herbal drugs and herbal preparations will be influenced (Bauer, 1998; Zangara and Ghosh, 2014). Cultivated medicinal plants have specific advantages over wild harvested plants; they show smaller variation in their constituents due to greater genetic uniformity, and the main secondary metabolites can be monitored, allowing for definition of the best period for harvesting, and are therefore generally preferred. The risk of misidentification of plants is also avoided and unsustainable harvesting limited. Controlled growth systems also allow manipulation of the phenotypic variation in the concentration of medicinally important compounds present at harvest, to increase potency, reduce toxin levels, and increase uniformity and predictability of extracts (Canter et al., 2005).

However, as the majority of medicinal plants are still harvested from the wild, it is important to use standardized extracts, and to ensure that strict guidelines on good agricultural and collection practices are followed, as the ones provided by the European Medicines Agency (EMA, 2006), which cover the cultivation of medicinal plants, as well as their harvesting and postharvesting processes.

Herbal drugs are identified by macroscopic and microscopic comparison with authentic material or accurate descriptions of authentic herbs (Ding et al., 2006) and any further tests that may be required (e.g., thin-layer chromatography). It is essential that herbal ingredients are referred to by their binomial Latin names of genus and species. Other important informations are the method of extraction and the standardization procedures. These can influence how much of a particular active constituent is present in the herbal product. Some phytochemicals are more soluble in water, while others are soluble in alcohol or oil. The method varies from plant to plant, depending on the types of active constituents (Jones and Kinghorn, 2012).

Standardized extracts are processed products, where some specific and known components, recognized to contribute to therapeutic activity more than others, are adjusted to a given amount, within an acceptable tolerance. Standardization is achieved by the adjustment of the herbal substances/herbal preparations with excipients or by blending batches of herbal substances and/or herbal preparations. All the other components are still present in the extract, because the action of the plant may result from the synergistic activity of several constituents. Moreover, often all the constituents of a plant are not yet fully characterized. Different methods of standardization may yield extracts with distinct properties and make the transferability of clinical data from one extract to another almost impossible, unless bioequivalence (or phytoequivalence) and bioavailability trials are used to prove essential similarity (Barnes, 2003a,b).

Medicinal products are pharmaceutically equivalent if they contain the same amount of the same active substance(s) in the same dosage forms that meet the same or comparable standards (Birkett, 2003). These parameters of pharmaceutical similarity applied to chemically defined drugs should also be applied to HMP:

ACTIVE INGREDIENTS: SPECIFIC PARAMETERS (EXTRACTS)

- Herbal substance (quality)
- Extraction solvent (type/concentration or solvent strength)
- Production (extraction procedures)
- Drug extract ratio

FINISHED PRODUCTS: SPECIFIC PARAMETERS

- Weight of native extract per dosage form
- Weight of constituents that are solely responsible for the therapeutic effect per dosage form
- Weight of constituents possessing relevant pharmacological properties per dosage form
- Excipients per dosage form (type)
- Dosage form (type)
- Posology (single dose and daily dose)

The concept of phytoequivalence was originally developed in Germany in order to ensure consistency of HMP (Tyler, 1999). A chromatographic fingerprint for an herbal product should be identified and compared with the profile of a clinically proven reference product to determine most of the phytochemical constituents, in order to ensure the reliability and repeatability of pharmacological and clinical research. Biopharmaceutical studies researching liberation, absorption, distribution, metabolism, and excretion provide important information on the active metabolite, the effective dose, and the bioequivalence of different extracts, and are the link of *in vitro* data to clinical efficacy, as long as the therapeutically relevant compounds are known (Loew and Kaszkin, 2002).

Unfortunately, phytoequivalence is very difficult to be obtained as phytochemical profiles are so complex and closely linked to the way the "seed to patient" process has been followed. It is a common experience that batches of medicinal plants with similar specifications, as species and part of plant, may have quite different chemical compositions due to a number of factors (Canigueral et al., 2008) such as the following:

1. *Inter- or intraspecies variation*: The variation in constituents is mostly genetically controlled (Figure 19.1).
2. *Environmental factors*: The quality of an herbal ingredient can be affected by environmental factors like weather, location, and other conditions under which it was cultivated.

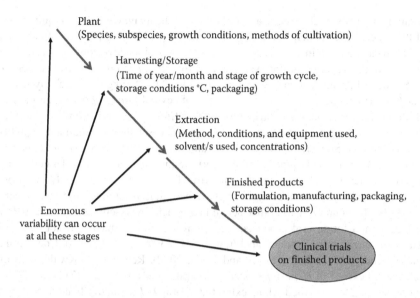

FIGURE 19.1 Stages of variability in product quality.

3. *Time of harvesting*: For some herbs the optimum time of harvesting should be specified as the concentrations of constituents in a plant can vary during the growing cycle and even during the course of a day.
4. *Part of plant used*: Different parts of the plant (e.g., roots, leaves) contain a different profile of constituents, and it is not uncommon for a herbal ingredient to be adulterated with parts of the plant not normally utilized.
5. *Postharvesting factors*: Storage conditions and processing treatments can greatly affect the quality of an herbal ingredient. Inappropriate storage after harvesting can result in microbial contamination. The most important stage of postharvest processing is drying, as dried plants can be preserved for prolonged periods of time (WHO, 1998).

CASE STUDIES

Substandard HMP containing on the label the same extract may vary in their content and concentrations of chemical constituents from batch to batch, and even the same manufacturer can market in different periods products containing different substances, although standardized to achieve a high pharmaceutical quality. This variability can result in significant differences in pharmacological activity involving both pharmacodynamic and pharmacokinetic issues. The use of a combination of herbal ingredients complicates further the issue of variability; for example, in traditional Chinese medicine (TCM), the current criteria use the concentration of several key ingredients or their total content to control the quality and ensure reproducible clinical efficacy (Li et al., 2013). Although the concentration of each bioactive component or the total concentration of all components may meet the requirements of the criteria, the concentration of each of these bioactive components often varies between batches, and in some cases one or more of the bioactive components may be absent from a preparation. For example, EGb761, a *Ginkgo biloba* extract produced by Schwabe Pharmaceuticals, is standardized for 24% "ginkgo flavone" glycosides and 6% terpene lactones. However, analysis of several *Ginkgo biloba* commercial products showed remarkable variations in the rutin and quercetin content as well as the terpene lactone content, although all the products satisfied the regulatory quality control method (Sticher, 1993). Another example is St. John's wort (*Hypericum perforatum* L.); analysis of eight St. John's wort products available in the United States found that their hyperforin content varied from 0.01% to 1.89%, and only two products contained sufficient hyperforin likely to be required for antidepressant effects. Similarly, the content of the other active component hypericin varied from 0.03% to 0.29%, and for several products, the actual hypericin content did not correlate with that stated on the product label (range 57%–130% of label claim) (Constantine and Karchesy, 1998; de los Reyes and Koda, 2002). Remotiv® (www.flordis.com. au), special extract of *Hypericum perforatum* (St. John's wort, Ze 117) herb, 1.375 g equivalent to 250 mg dried whole extract at a ratio 4–7:1, standardized to 500 mcg hypericin, negligible hyperforin <1% and flavonoids >13.5 mg, demonstrated full seed to patient control. Similarly, KeenMind® users can be assured of receiving the same benefits identified by clinical trials in which the specific KeenMind product has been used (www.keenmind.info/).

SAFETY AND EFFICACY

The efficacy and true frequency of side effects for most HMP are not known because the majority have not yet been tested in large clinical trials and because pharmacovigilance systems are much less extensive than those in place for pharmaceutical products. The development process for HMP should include traditional evidence and observational trials, but must progress to randomized, double-blind, placebo-controlled trials and pharmacovigilance protocols, and become more closely aligned with the development of new chemical entities.

Clinical trials with herbal drugs are feasible, and a significant amount of clinical data are available for some HMP such as ginseng, ginkgo, and hypericum; however, few well-controlled, double-blind, placebo-controlled trials have been carried out with herbal medicines. In a recent survey of around 1000 herbal medicines, only 156 of them had clinical trials supporting specific pharmacological activities and therapeutic applications (Cravotto et al., 2010). The major issues with clinical trials with HMP, as highlighted by a number of meta-analysis, include the lack of standardization and quality control of the products used in clinical trials, the use of different dosages of herbal medicines, inadequate study designs and statistical power, patients not properly selected, difficulties in establishing appropriate placebos, and wide variations in the duration of treatments using herbal medicines (Calixto, 2000). Clinical development of herbal medicinal products should include dose–response trials, particularly for newly developed products; however, for those products with a well-established tradition of use, they may not be required. However, any claims of efficacy for clinical indications of HMP must be evidence-based and, depending on the level of the claims, in agreement with grades of evidence recognized by the scientific community and health authorities (EMEA, 2004).

CONCLUSION

Several recent cases of adulteration and contamination of herbal medicinal products, which may have led to severe illness and possibly death in some cases, have revealed the necessity and urgency of identifying the plant material in botanicals and phytomedicines. The older system of organoleptic (or identification through microscopic observation of plant parts) is not convincing, and plants are often misidentified. Recently, DNA-based methods have been applied to these products because "DNA is not changed by growth conditions unlike the chemical constituents of many active pharmaceutical agents" (Moraes et al., 2015).

To conclude, different concentrations of the proportion of constituents in herbal medicines may lead to great variations in therapeutic results and safety issues, and consequently, the evidence of both benefits and risks is specific to the product tested and cannot necessarily be extrapolated to other products (Kronenberg and Kennelly, 2013) as is the case for synthetically derived compounds, or assume that clinical trials with one brand are relevant to any other product. Health practitioners should become more aware of these issues, in order to recommend to their patients only the exact products that have been consistently proven for safety and efficacy in clinical trials conducted according to good clinical practice (GCP) (Figure 19.2).

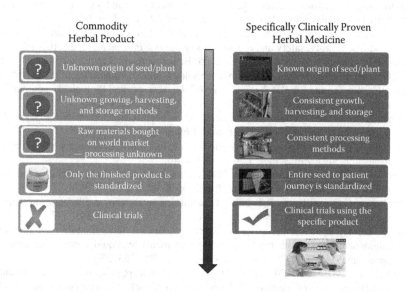

FIGURE 19.2 The "seed to patient" journey in properly standardized herbal medicine leads specifically to clinically proven medicine.

The gold standard of supportive evidence is certainly controlled, randomized, double-blind, clinical trials, but data from other type of studies such as case reports can improve and contribute to the primary evidence coming from more complex and controlled studies.

REFERENCES

Abdellah, A., Noordin, M., and Ismail, W. 2015. Importance and globalization status of good manufacturing practice (GMP) requirements for pharmaceutical excipients. *Saudi Pharm. J.*, 23: 9–13.

Angell, M. and Kassirier, J.P. 1998. Alternative medicine—The risks of untested and unregulated remedies. *N. Engl. J. Med.*, 339: 839–841.

Barnes, J. 2003a. Quality, efficacy and safety of complementary medicines: Fashions, facts and the future. Part I. Regulation and quality. *Br. J. Clin. Pharmacol.*, 55: 226–233.

Barnes, J. 2003b. Quality, efficacy and safety of complementary medicines: Fashions, facts and the future. Part II: Efficacy and safety. *Br. J. Clin. Pharmacol.*, 55: 331–340.

Bauer, R. 1998. Quality criteria and standardization of phytopharmaceuticals: Can acceptable drug standards be achieved? *Drug Inf. J.*, 32: 101–110.

Bauer, R. and Tittel, G. 1996. Quality assessment of herbal preparations as a precondition of pharmacological and clinical studies. *Phytomedicine*, 2: 193–198.

Birkett, D.J. 2003. Generics—Equal or not? *Aust. Prescr.*, 26: 85–87.

Blumenthal, M. 2002. Guest editorial: The rise and fall of PC-SPES: New generation of herbal supplement, adulterated product, or new drug? *Integr. Cancer Ther.*, 1: 266–270.

Blumenthal, M., Busse, W., and Goldberg A. et al. 1998. *The Complete German Commission E Monographs*. The American Botanical Council, Austin, TX; Integrative Medicine Communications 63, Boston, MA.

Calixto, J.B. 2000. Efficacy, safety, quality control, marketing and regulatory guidelines for herbal medicines (phytotherapeutic agents). *Braz. J. Med. Biol. Res.*, 33: 179–189.

Cañigueral, S., Tschopp, R., Ambrosetti, L. et al. 2008. The development of herbal medicinal products: Quality, safety and efficacy as key factors. *Pharm. Med.*, 22: 107–118.

Canter, P.H., Thomas, H., and Ernst, E. 2005. Bringing medicinal plants into cultivation: Opportunities and challenges for biotechnology. *Trends Biotechnol.*, 23: 180–185.

Chan, P.C., Xia, Q., and Fu, P.P. 2007. *Ginkgo biloba* leave extract: Biological, medicinal and toxicological effects. *J. Environ. Sci. Health Part C*, 25: 211–244.

Constantine, G.H. and Karchesy, J. 1998. Variations in hypericin concentrations in *Hypericum perforatum* L. and commercial products. *Pharm. Biol.*, 36: 365–367.

Cordell, G.A. 2015. Ecopharmacognosy and the responsibilities of natural product research to sustainability. *Phytochem. Lett.*, 11: 332–346.

Cravotto, G., Boffa, L., Genzini, L. et al. 2010. Phytotherapeutics: An evaluation of the potential of 1000 plants. *J. Clin. Pharm. Ther.*, 35: 11–48.

de los Reyes, G.C. and Koda, R.T. 2002. Determining hyperforin and hypericin content in eight brands of St. John's wort. *Am. J. Health Syst. Pharm.*, 59: 545–547.

Ding, S., Dudley, E., Plummer, S. et al. 2006. Quantitative determination of major active components in Ginkgo biloba dietary supplements by liquid chromatography/mass spectrometry. *Rapid. Commun. Mass Spectrom.*, 20: 2753–2760.

EMEA. 2004. EMEA/CPMP/HMPWP/1156/03. Final concept paper on the implementation of different levels of scientific evidence in core data for herbal medicinal drugs. EMEA, London, UK.

Ernst, E. 1998. Harmless herbs? A review of the recent literature. *Am. J. Med.*, 104: 170–178.

European Medicines Agency. 2006. Guideline on good agricultural and collection practice (gacp) for starting materials of herbal origin. http://www.ema.europa.eu/docs/en_GB/document_library/Scientific_guideline/2009/09/WC500003362.pdf (accessed August 2015).

European Medicines Agency. 2008. Reflection paper on markers used for quantitative and qualitative analysis of herbal medicinal products and traditional herbal medicinal products. http://www.ema.europa.eu/docs/en_GB/document_library/Scientific_guideline/2009/09/WC50000319.pdf (accessed August 2015).

Fabricant, D.S. and Farnsworth, N.R. 2001. The value of plants used in traditional medicine for drug discovery. *Environ. Health Perspect.*, 109: 69–75.

Fong, H.H. 2002. Integration of herbal medicine into modern medical practices: Issues and prospects. *Integr. Cancer Ther.*, 1: 287–293.

Harkey, M.R., Henderson, G.L., Gershwin, M.E. et al. 2001. Variability in commercial ginseng products: An analysis of 25 preparations. *Am. J. Clin. Nutr.*, 73: 1101–1106.

Jones, W.P. and Kinghorn, A.D. 2012. Extraction of plant secondary metabolites. *Methods Mol. Biol.*, 864: 341–366.

Keller, K. 1996. Herbal medicinal products in Germany and Europe: Experiences with national and European assessment. *Drug Inf. J.*, 30: 933–948.

Kronenberg, E. and Kennelly, E.J. 2013. Phytochemical identity and stability of herbal products: Challenges for clinical research. *Maturitas*, 76: 291–293.

Li, X., Chen, H., Jia, W. et al. 2013. A metabolomics-based strategy for the quality control of traditional Chinese medicine: Shengmai injection as a case study. *Evid. Based Complement. Alternat.* http://www.hindawi.com/journals/ecam/2013/836179/ (accessed August 2015).

Li, X.T., Chen, R., Jin, L.M et al. 2009. Regulation on energy metabolism and protection on mitochondria of *Panax ginseng* polysaccharide. *Am. J. Chin. Med.*, 37: 1139–1152.

Liva, R. 2009. Controlled testing. The cornerstone of all quality natural products. *Integr. Med.*, 8: 40–42.

Loew, D. and Kaszkin, M. 2002. Approaching the problem of bioequivalence of herbal randomized clinical trial. *J. Am. Geriatr. Soc.*, 288: 835–840.

Moraes, D., Still, D., Lum, M. et al. 2015. DNA-based authentication of botanicals and plant-derived dietary supplements: Where have we been and where are we going? *Planta Med.*, 81: 687–695.

Newmaster, S.G., Grguric, M., Shanmughanandhan, D. et al. 2013. DNA barcoding detects contamination and substitution in North American herbal products. *BMC Med.*, 11: 222–235.

Obi, E., Akunyili, D.N., and Ekpo, B. 2006. Heavy metal hazards of Nigerian herbal remedies. *Sci. Total Environ.*, 369: 35–41.

Perry, E. and Howes, M.J. 2011. Medicinal plants and dementia therapy: Herbal hopes for brain aging?. *CNS Neurosci. Ther.*, 17: 683–698.

Robinson, M.M. and Zhang, X. 2011. Traditional medicines: Global situation, issues and challenges. In *The World Medicines Situation*, 3rd edn. WHO, Geneva, Switzerland.

Scaglione, F., Pannacci, M., and Petrini, O. 2005. The standardised G115 *Panax ginseng* C.A. Meyer extract: A review of its properties and usage. *Evid. Based Integr. Med.*, 2: 195–206.

Schwarz, M., Klier, B., and Sievers, H. 2009. Herbal reference standards. *Planta Med.*, 75: 689–703.

Soldati, F. 2000. *Panax ginseng*: Standardization and biological activity. In Cutler, S.J., Cutler, H.G., eds., *Biologically Active Natural Products*, pp. 209–232. CRC Press, New York.

Soldati, F. and Tanaka, O. 1984. *Panax ginseng*: Relation between age of plant and content of ginsenosides. *Planta Med.*, 50: 351–352.

Sticher, O. 1993. Quality of Ginkgo preparations. *Planta Med.*, 59: 2–11.

Tyler, V.E. 1999. Phytomedicines: Back to the future. *J. Nat. Prod.*, 62: 1589–1592.

van Breemen, R.B., Fong, H.H., and Farnsworth, N.R. 2008. Ensuring the safety of botanical dietary supplements. *Am. J. Clin. Nutr.*, 87: 509S–513S.

Walker, R. 2004. Criteria for risk assessment of botanical food supplements. *Toxicol. Lett.*, 149: 87–95.

Williamson, E.M. 2001. Synergy and other interactions in phytomedicines. *Phytomedicine*, 8: 401–409.

World Health Organization. 1996. WHO Expert Committee on Specifications for Pharmaceutical Preparations, Annex 11. WHO, Geneva, Switzerland.

World Health Organization. 1998. Quality control methods for medicinal plant materials. World Health Organization, Geneva, Switzerland. http://www.gmp-compliance.org/guidemgr/files/WHO_9241545100.PDF (accessed August 2015).

World Health Organization. 2003. *WHO Guidelines on Good Agricultural and Collection Practices (GACP) for Medicinal Plants*. World Health Organization, Geneva, Switzerland.

World Health Organization. 2007. WHO *Guidelines for Assessing Quality of Herbal Medicines with Reference to Contaminants and Residues*. World Health Organization, Geneva, Switzerland.

World Health Organization. 2011. WHO Guidelines for methodologies on research and evaluation of traditional medicine. WHO, Geneva, Switzerland.

World Health Organization Research Office for the Western Pacific. 1993. *Research Guidelines for Evaluating the Safety and Efficacy of Herbal Medicines*. WHO, Manila, Philippines.

Zangara, A. and Ghosh, D. 2014. Role of seed to patient model in clinically proven natural medicines. In Ghosh, D., Bagchi, D., Konish, T., eds., *Clinical Aspects of Functional Foods and Nutraceuticals*, pp. 279–287, Chapter 19. CRC Press, Boca Raton, FL.

Zangara, A. and Wesnes, K.A. 2012. Herbal cognitive enhancers: New developments and challenges for therapeutic applications. In Thakur, M.K., Rattan, S.I.S., eds., *Brain Aging and Therapeutic Interventions*, pp. 267–289. Springer, the Netherlands.

Index

Printed in the United States
by Baker & Taylor Publisher Services